**Fracture Management for the
Small Animal Practitioner**

Fracture Management for the Small Animal Practitioner

Edited by

Anne M. Sylvestre DVM, DVSc, CCRP
Diplomate ACVS/ECVS

WILEY Blackwell

Registered Office
John Wiley & Sons, Inc., 111 River Street, Hoboken, NJ 07030, USA

Editorial Office
111 River Street, Hoboken, NJ 07030, USA

For details of our global editorial offices, customer services, and more information about Wiley products visit us at www.wiley.com.

Wiley also publishes its books in a variety of electronic formats and by print-on-demand. Some content that appears in standard print versions of this book may not be available in other formats.

Library of Congress Cataloging-in-Publication Data

Names: Sylvestre, Anne M. (Anne Madeleine), 1959– editor.
Title: Fracture management for the small animal practitioner / edited by Anne M. Sylvestre.
Description: First edition. | Hoboken, NJ : Wiley-Blackwell, 2019. | Includes bibliographical references and index. |
Identifiers: LCCN 2018056463 (print) | LCCN 2018058642 (ebook) | ISBN 9781119215943 (Adobe PDF) |
    ISBN 9781119215936 (ePub) | ISBN 9781119215813 (hardback)
Subjects: LCSH: Fractures in animals. | MESH: Fractures, Bone–veterinary | Fractures, Bone–surgery |
    Surgical Procedures, Operative–veterinary | Dogs–injuries | Cats–injuries
Classification: LCC SF914.4 (ebook) | LCC SF914.4 .F73 2019 (print) | NLM SF 914.4 | DDC 636.089/715–dc23
LC record available at https://lccn.loc.gov/2018056463

Cover Design: Wiley
Cover Images: © Cathy Popovitch, © Anne Sylvestre

Set in 10/12pt Warnock by SPi Global, Pondicherry, India
Printed and bound in Singapore by Markono Print Media Pte Ltd

10 9 8 7 6 5 4 3 2 1

To my husband for his unwavering support during the writing of this book; to the veterinarians who have encouraged me to create and finish this book; and to the veterinarians who will use the information in this book to save a limb and save a life. This book is for you.

Contents

List of Contributors

Thomas W.G. Gibson BSc, BEd, DVM, DVSc
Diplomate ACVS—Small Animal/ACVSMR—Canine
Associate Professor of Small Animal Surgery
Ontario Veterinary College
University of Guelph
Guelph, Ontario, Canada

Teresa Jacobson BSc, DVM
Sitara Animal Hospital
Lake Country, British Columbia, Canada

Catherine Popovitch DVM
Diplomate ACVS/ECVS
Resident Advisor
Veterinary Specialty and Emergency Center
Levittown, Pennsylvania, USA

Anne M. Sylvestre DVM, DVSc, CCRP
Diplomate ACVS/ECVS
President
Focus and Flourish,
Cambridge, Ontario, Canada

Kathryn Wander DVM, MS, CCRT
Diplomate ACVS
Centro Veterinario Costa Ballena
Uvita de Osa
Puntarenas
Costa Rica

Jennifer White RVT
Lead Surgery Technician
Surgery Department
VCA Canada
Mississauga Oakville Veterinary Emergency Hospital
and Referral Group
Oakville, Ontario, Canada

Harold Wotton MS BioEng
President/Chief Design Engineer
Everost, Inc.
Sturbridge, MA, USA

Preface

The contributing authors who have helped with this book were chosen because of their experience and extensive association with general practices. Often we are asked how to help an animal with a fracture when surgery is not possible at all: perhaps because the owners have very limited funds, or there is no owner, or no proximity to a veterinarian with fracture repair expertise. It is in these situations that we are called upon to stretch the boundaries of what can be done, with reasonable hope for a positive outcome and humane convalescence. Unfortunately, euthanasia is often chosen. It is a shame that an animal has to lose its life just because of a broken bone.

The goal of this textbook is to help the practitioner guide the client to make informed decisions that will best suit them and their pet.

There is often more than one way to deal with a fracture. The best repair method may not always be possible. The point is to give the client some options and to ascertain that they understand what the possible care and outcome may be. Oftentimes, in order for a pet owner to make an appropriate decision, they need to hear the conviction in their veterinarian's words and voice and they may also need to be reminded of the value and enrichment that their pet brings to the family.

The book has three distinct parts.

The first section has general information about fractures and detailed information on managing the patient.

The second part is composed of two sections that contain information on the various types of fractures and luxations sustained by dogs and cats. Details on the best method of repair, prognosis and postoperative care, potential complications, level of difficulty of the repair, and finally alternative management methods and their expected outcome are provided. The goal here is to give the general practitioner easily accessible information to help educate the client. There are three types of pet owners: those that will do everything for their pet, those that will do nothing, and all of the ones in between. It is this last category of client that will require compassionate yet strong, definitive words to help guide them to the best solution for their pet.

The last section deals with various repair techniques and how to perform them. This section contains practical tips and is intended as an adjunctive source of information for the practitioner who has had some practical continuing education in fracture repair techniques.

I thank all the contributing authors. Without you this book would not have been possible.

Anne M. Sylvestre

Section 1

General Information

1

Fracture Identification

Anne M. Sylvestre

Focus and Flourish, Cambridge, Ontario, Canada

Using proper terminology to describe a fracture is important as it allows for accurate communication among veterinarians and, to a certain extent, with clients. It only takes a little bit of practice in describing fractures to become fluent with the terminology. Fractures are described according to:

1) Number of fragments.
2) Fracture configuration.
3) Location on the bone.
4) The bone that is fractured. Descriptions of fractures involving a two-bone system (radius and ulna; tibia and fibula) are limited to the main bone involved with mention of the smaller bone if it is not fractured (e.g. two-piece transverse mid-diaphyseal fracture of the left radius and intact ulna).

1.1 Number of Fragments (Figure 1.1)

- Two-piece: Describes a bone with one fracture line and two large fragments; the simplest type of fracture to reduce. An accurately reconstructed bone will contribute to the stability and strength of the repair.
- Two-piece plus reducible wedge: Describes a fracture with two main large fragments and one smaller fragment that is large enough to be secured to the reconstructed bone with a screw or cerclage wire. This description implies that the fracture can be accurately reconstructed but with more difficulty than the two-piece fracture.
- Two-piece with small (non-reducible) fragments: Describes a fracture with two main fragments and some small fragments that are not reducible. This

configuration implies that accurate reconstruction may be difficult and that (a) bony defect(s) may be present. A repair technique of adequate strength must be chosen to overcome the forces that will not be negated due to the defect (usually bending and compressive forces).
- Multiple fragments, or, complex: Describes a fracture with more than three large fragments. Because there are numerous fracture lines, it is not possible, or necessary, to describe a predominant configuration. This descriptor implies that the fracture will be very difficult or impossible to reconstruct. A repair technique with a strong and very stable construct to bridge the unconstructed defect is necessary in order for this fracture to heal with minimal complications.

1.2 Fracture Configuration (Figure 1.2)

- Incomplete or greenstick: Describes a fracture that only involves one cortex; because the fracture is not complete there are no true pieces or fragments. Incomplete fractures occur almost exclusively in immature animals.
- Transverse: Describes a fracture line that crosses the bone approximately perpendicular (within 30°) to the long axis of the bone. This fracture configuration, once reduced, tends to counteract the compressive forces, so the repair needs only to focus on stabilizing the rotational and bending forces.
- Short oblique: Describes a fracture line that is at an angle greater than 30° to the long axis of the bone, but the length of the fracture line is less than twice the

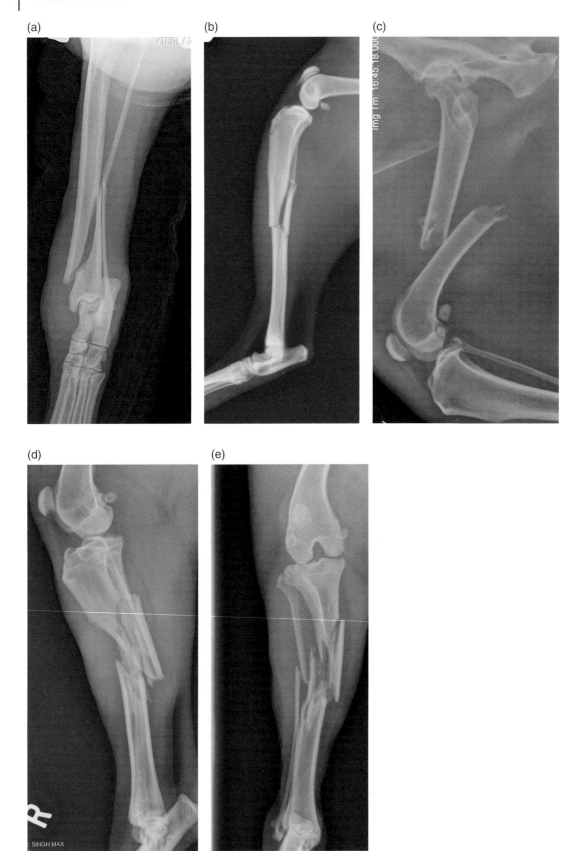

Figure 1.1 Fractures are described according to *the number of fragments* as well as fracture configuration, location on the bone and bone. (a) *Two-piece long oblique*, distal diaphyseal fracture of the (left) tibia and fibula. (b) *Two-piece with reducible wedge*, transverse fracture of the mid-diaphysis of the (right) tibia and fractured fibula. (c) *Two-piece with multiple small fragments*, short oblique, mid- to distal third diaphyseal fracture of the right femur. (d and e) *Complex, or multi-fragmented* mid- to proximal diaphyseal fracture of the right tibia and fractured fibula.

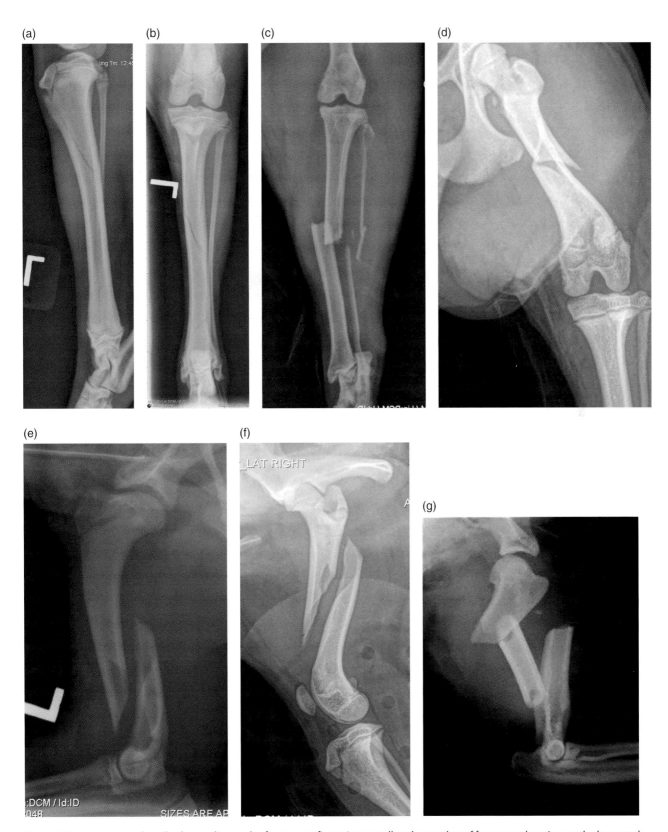

Figure 1.2 Fractures are described according to the *fracture configuration* as well as the number of fragments, location on the bone and bone. (a and b) Incomplete, or greenstick, spiral fracture of the entire diaphysis of the left tibia with intact fibula. (c) Two-piece with small fragments, transverse mid-diaphyseal fracture of the (right) tibia with fractured fibula. (d) Two-piece, short oblique, mid-diaphyseal fracture of the (right) femur. (e) Two-piece, long oblique, mid- to distal left humeral fracture. (f) Two-piece, spiral, mid-diaphyseal, right femoral fracture. An attempt was made to "stabilize" this fracture with a splint that is clearly visible on the radiographs. A femoral shaft fracture cannot be immobilized with a splint, but rather, the splint can act as a fulcrum at the fracture line and function to further cause pain and damage of the soft tissues. Splinting a femoral fracture is contraindicated. (g) Three-piece, segmental, diaphyseal, (right) humeral fracture. (h) Complex, segmental, diaphyseal, (left) tibial fracture with fractured fibula. (i) Avulsion fracture of the (right) tibial tuberosity. (j) Two-piece with small fragments short oblique mid-diaphyseal (right) tibial fracture with fissure lines (arrows). (k) Complex fracture of the distal diaphysis of the (left) femur, minimally displaced.

(h)   (i)   (j)   (k)

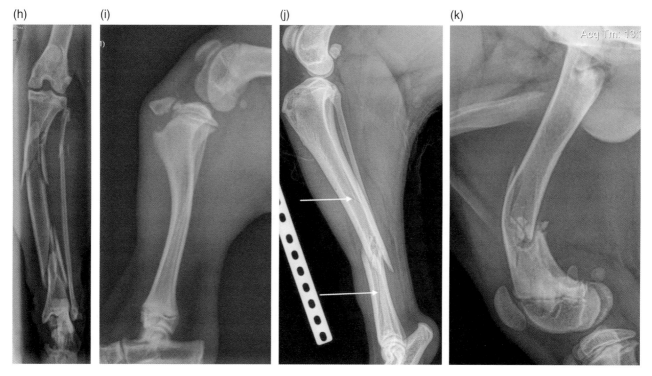

Figure 1.2 (Continued)

diameter of the bone, at the level of the fracture. This configuration is subject to the compressive forces even once reduced, and its short obliquity implies that the rotational forces will not be counteracted by cerclage wires. Therefore, an intra-medullary pin and cerclage wires are *not* an appropriate choice of repair for this configuration.

- Long oblique and spiral: Describes a fracture line that is at an angle greater than 30° to the long axis of the bone and the length of the fracture line is at least twice the diameter of the bone, at the level of the fracture. This configuration is subject to the compressive forces even once reduced, and its long obliquity implies that the rotational forces can be counteracted by cerclage wires. Therefore, an intra-medullary pin and cerclage wires *may be* (depending on the ability to reconstruct the bone) an appropriate choice of repair for this configuration. The spiral fracture is when the long oblique fracture curves around the diaphysis of the bone.
- Segmental: Describes a bone with two fracture lines that do not intersect with one another, creating at least three large fragments. The nature of this configuration implies that most of the diaphysis will be involved.

This type of fracture is the least common and tends to be challenging to repair.

- Avulsion: Although "avulsion" truly refers to the type of stress that is applied to a portion of bone to create a fracture, rather than a configuration, it is frequently used by surgeons to describe this specific fracture. Avulsion fractures occur on bony prominences where large tendons attach: acromion process, supraglenoid tuberosity, olecranon, greater trochanter, tibial tuberosity, calcaneus. Because these fractures are so specific in location and configuration, no other terms (other than location) are necessary to describe them.
- Additional terms: Fissure lines can add to the level of complexity of a fracture repair and should be mentioned in the description if they are present. The degree of displacement of the fragments can also affect decision making when it comes to fracture management. Conservative management may be adequate for a minimally displaced fracture where as a markedly displaced one may convey a sense of urgency and concern for the surrounding soft tissues. An open fracture should also be identified in the description.

1.3 Location on the Bone (Figure 1.3)

- Articular: Describes a fracture that involves the articular cartilage and by definition the epiphysis.
- Epiphysis: The epiphysis is the end of a long bone, either proximal or distal. It is usually covered in articular cartilage and is separated from the rest of the bone by the physis, or physeal scar in a mature animal.
- Physis: Describes the proximal and distal cartilaginous growth plates located between the epiphysis and metaphysis. The physes close at skeletal maturity and only a faint white line is visible on radiographs; it is termed the physeal scar. Fractures of the physes in immature animals are called Salter–Harris (SH) fractures (details below).
- Metaphysis: Describes the proximal and distal portions of the long bones between the physis and diaphysis. Bone growth occurs at the section of the metaphysis adjacent to the physis. The metaphysis is usually wider than the physis, is composed of cancellous bone and has thinner cortices than the diaphysis.
- Diaphysis, or shaft: Describes the mid-section of a long bone. It is located between the proximal and the distal metaphyses and is composed of cortical bone, which has a thicker and harder cortex than the metaphyseal bone; it often has an adipose-filled marrow cavity.
- Anatomically specific components of a bone: The location of fractures that occur at specific anatomic regions on a bone will often be described according to that anatomic part; for example, supracondylar, trochanteric, femoral neck.

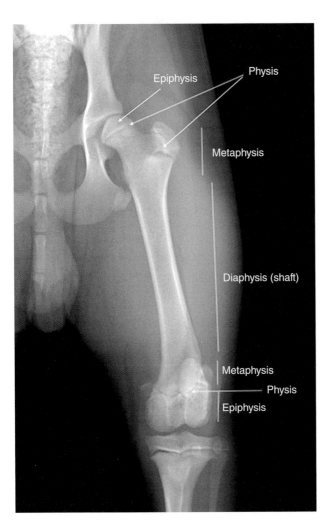

Figure 1.3 A craniodorsal radiograph of an intact femur of an immature dog is used to show the anatomic locations on the bone. The full description is found within the text.

1.4 Salter–Harris Fractures (Figure 1.4)

Salter–Harris fractures are specific to fractures involving the physes, or growth plates. There are five different types of SH fractures and they are designated by the Roman numerals I–V. In general, the prognosis declines as their numerical designation increases:

- SH I: The fracture is confined to the growth plate itself; often termed a "slipped physis."
- SH II: The fracture is along the physis and extends into the metaphysis.
- SH III: The fracture is along the physis and extends into the epiphysis, which makes this an articular fracture. SH III fractures are rare.
- SH IV: These fractures run perpendicular to the physis, extending from the articular surface through to the metaphysis. These too are articular fractures. They are most commonly seen in the elbow (lateral condylar fractures in immature animals).
- SH V: This is a compression fracture of the physis and therefore may not be evident on radiographs taken after the initial trauma. The distal ulnar physis is the one that most commonly sustains this type of SH fracture because of its conical shape. An SH V fracture is usually detected because the physis, or a portion of it, closes prematurely, resulting in an angular limb deformity.

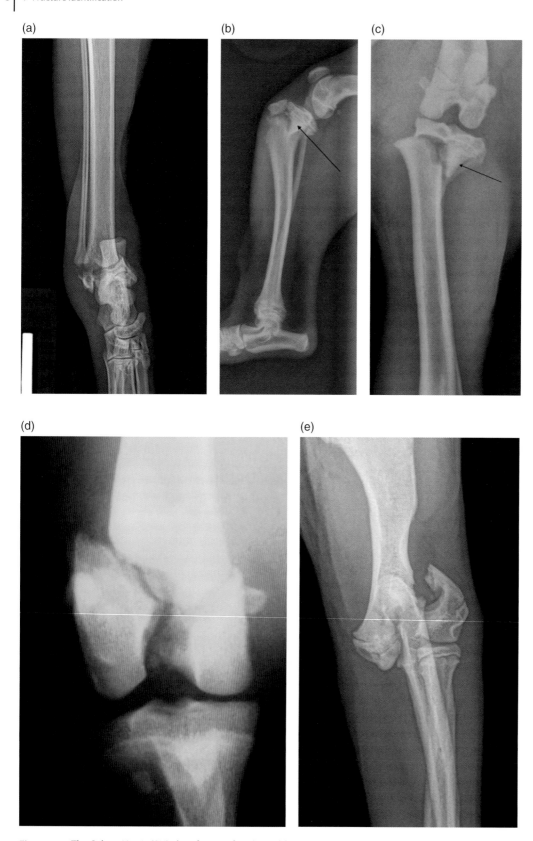

Figure 1.4 The Salter–Harris (SH) classification for physeal fractures. (a) SH I fracture of the distal (left) tibia and fibula. The fracture is located along the physis only. (b and c) SH II of the proximal (right) tibia. The fracture is located along the physis and extends into the metaphysis. The arrow points to the metaphyseal component of the fracture. (d) SH III fracture of the (left) distal femur. The fracture is along the physis and extends into the epiphysis. (e) SH IV of the (left) distal humerus. The fracture extends from the epiphysis to the metaphysis, crossing the physis.

2

Open Fractures

Anne M. Sylvestre

Focus and Flourish, Cambridge, Ontario, Canada

Open fractures are classified according to the degree of exposure of the bone to contaminants and surrounding soft tissue injury. The prognosis for first- and second-degree open fractures is similar to that of an equivalent closed fracture [1].

2.1 First Degree

This type of open fracture occurs from the inside out. At the time of the injury, the bone protrudes through the skin but the bone ends recede back under the skin as the limb settles into its postimpact position. Therefore there is usually just a small wound visible (typically no more than 1 cm) on the skin. On radiographs, pockets of gas are often visible close to the fracture (Figure 2.1). Fortunately this type of open fracture does not alter the prognosis as there are few contaminants associated with it. Once the patient has been evaluated and stabilized, the wound should be cleaned and the hair around it clipped before applying a splinted bandage to prevent further contamination until surgical stabilization is possible. The patient should be started on systemic antibiotics at the time of the initial assessment and continued for several days after repair; cephalosporin is a good choice. At surgery, the bone ends and wound are lavaged with saline.

2.2 Second Degree

This lesion occurs from the outside in and therefore allows for the introduction of contaminants and bacteria. There is a wound, of varying size but usually greater than 1 cm. The surrounding tissues will also be bruised and often there will be external debris carried into the wound at the time of impact. The bone may be protruding through the wound (Figure 2.2).

Once the patient has been evaluated and adequately stabilized, the wound should be debrided under general anesthesia. Sterile lubricating jelly can be used to cover the wound before shaving and scrubbing the surrounding area. The loose hair will get trapped in the jelly and can then be washed away. Sterile technique should be used to debride the wound. The wound should be swabbed for a culture and then the patient can be started on systemic antibiotics. Foreign debris can be removed with the aid of copious lavaging and *gentle* rubbing with finger tips or gauze square. It is best to repair the fracture immediately after debriding the wound because the stabilized bone will help prevent further trauma to the soft tissues therefore preserving the existing blood supply to the area. If for some reason the fracture cannot be repaired immediately, then a splinted bandage can be applied to the limb to prevent further contamination. Systemic antibiotics are continued for several days after repair; cephalosporin is a good choice.

2.3 Third Degree

These are usually a result of a high-velocity trauma and have extensive soft tissue damage and bony fragmentation. Severe shearing injuries and bullet wounds are examples of third-degree open fractures (Figure 2.3). This type of open fracture carries a less favorable prognosis because the management of such a case is usually more extensive and expensive. Once the patient is stable enough for general anesthesia, the wound should be addressed as detailed in Section 2.2. Serial debridements are often necessary with these wounds. Tissue that is obviously necrotic should be excised; if there is any doubt as to the viability of a tissue, it is best to leave it and re-assess over the next 24–72 hours. Caution should be exercised when debriding not to further compromise blood flow to the tissues. Stabilization of the fracture should be performed after the first surgical debridement as the stabilized bone will help prevent further damage and therefore preserve existing blood flow to the area. These cases are best left in the hands of a trained surgeon. Amputation of the limb may be the best alternative for the patient with a third-degree open fracture if a veterinarian with the necessary skills is not available to the client.

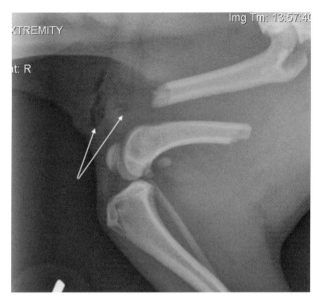

Figure 2.1 A radiographic example of a first-degree open fracture. Pockets of air are visible within the soft tissues (arrows).

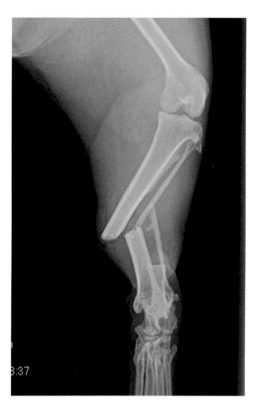

Figure 2.2 A radiographic example of a second-degree open fracture. The bone is visibly protruding through the skin.

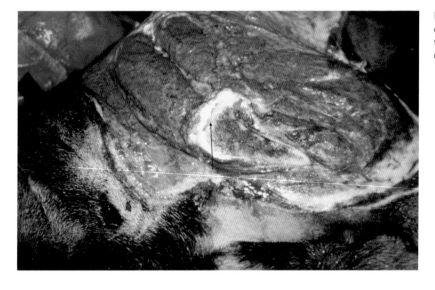

Figure 2.3 An example of a third-degree open fracture. This dog was dragged along the pavement. The shoulder joint is exposed (arrow).

Reference

1 DeCamp, C.E., Johnston, S.A., Déjardin, L.M., and Schaefer, S.L. (2016). Fractures: classification, diagnosis and treatment. In: *Brinker, Piermattei and Flo's Handbook of Small Animal Orthopaedics and Fracture Repair*, 5e, 139–144. St Louis, MO: Elsevier.

3

Patient Management

Anne M. Sylvestre

Focus and Flourish, Cambridge, Ontario, Canada

The focus of this chapter is to discuss managing a fracture. However, a full and thorough examination of the entire patient is necessary to rule out any and/or all co-morbidities. If the fracture occurred due to a low-velocity trauma, such as jumping off furniture, then co-morbidities are less common but should still be considered possible. A patient that suffered a more substantial trauma, such as a vehicular accident, should have thoracic radiographs and basic blood work done as a minimum data base. The more life-threatening issues (cardiovascular shock, hemorrhage, respiratory compromise, head trauma, etc.) must be addressed first. Consideration is given to management of the fracture once the patient is adequately stabilized systemically.

3.1 The Patient

3.1.1 Upon Admission

The most important factors to address for the fracture are (1) stabilizing the fracture to control pain and prevent further soft tissue damage; (2) offering proper pain management with opiates and anti-inflammatory drugs, if appropriate; (3) controlling swelling wherever possible; (4) assisting the patient with ambulation.

Immobilizing a fracture is possible for all long bones by applying a Robert Jones or splinted bandage (Chapter 4), *except for the femur* (Figure 3.1). A patient with a femoral fracture should be confined to a small area and provided with pain relief. The large muscle mass of the thigh and the concurrent swelling of the tissues around the fracture will help to hinder some of the motion between the fragments. There are *no conditions* under which a femoral fracture can be splinted or bandaged. A bandage (splinted or Robert Jones) can usually be applied once the patient has been given opiates.

The systemically stable patient should be scheduled for a definitive repair of the fracture at the earliest convenience, preferably within 24–72 hours of the trauma. A patient who is stable, with the limb comfortably immobilized and the pain managed, can be discharged to the client to return on the day of surgery.

3.1.2 Immediate Postoperative Care

Pain management with narcotics and non-steroidal anti-inflammatory drugs (NSAIDs) is important. The degree of pain will vary depending on the severity of the trauma, soft tissue damage and duration of the surgery, as well as the patient's tolerance for pain. The severe pain experienced with a fracture tends to subside quickly (24–48 hours) once the fracture is stabilized with implants or external coaptation.

Support with an abdominal sling or chest harness should be offered when taken outside especially if the patient is still unsteady because of the drugs, and if there are slippery surfaces to contend with.

If a bandage is not required postsurgically then the pain and swelling can be helped with icing of the fracture site as well as gentle passive range of motion (PROM) of the joints adjacent to the fracture.

If the limb is bandaged then appropriate monitoring of the bandage is indicated (Chapter 4).

3.1.3 Upon Discharge From Hospital

A good pain management regime is important. A narcotic for the first 7–14 days is indicated; an NSAID is also beneficial providing it is not contraindicated for that patient.

The patient's limb may or may not be bandaged or splinted postoperatively. If there is a lot of soft tissue swelling, then the surgeon may opt to place a bandage on the limb for 3–7 days to help decrease swelling.

(a)

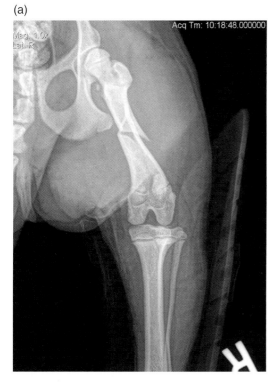

(b)

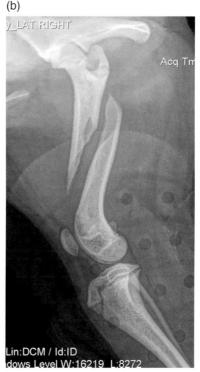

Figure 3.1 Mediolateral (a) and craniocaudal (b) radiographs of a femoral fracture that was "stabilized" with a lateral splint. Clearly the splint is not advantageous to this fracture and is likely deleterious as the top of the splint is level with the fracture line and can act as a fulcrum. Femoral fractures should not be splinted.

The surgeon would opt to add a splint based on several criteria: (1) the complexity of the fracture; (2) the degree of stability offered by the repair; (3) the location of the fracture; and (4) the patient's personality. The duration for which the splint would be applied will vary based on the same criteria. Two to four weeks is a common average. As a general rule-of-thumb, one never goes from the rigid support of a splint to no support, so a soft padded bandage would be applied once the splint is removed for 1–2 weeks. Bandaging may also be necessary in order to manage a wound. The duration of the bandaging in this case will be dependent on the extent of the wound.

Home care instructions must be made clear to the owner (see below) and should be made available to them *before* the pet is discharged into their care so that they can be prepared.

The patient may be discharged with a harness to assist with ambulation if there are multiple fractures or other concurrent orthopedic issues (Figure 3.2).

Bandage/splint care discharge instructions must also be made clear and reviewed with the client (Chapter 4). These same instructions, along with a schedule of bandage change appointments, should be written and handed to the client at the time of the discharge.

A recheck appointment should be scheduled at the time of discharge. The patient will need to be seen for suture removal at 10–14 days and perhaps sooner, based on the extent of the trauma.

A follow-up phone call the following day will help the client navigate through their pet's home management: caring for a pet with a fracture can be overwhelming for some clients. The patient should be re-evaluated on a regular basis (monthly) until the fracture has healed.

3.1.4 Outside and Walks

Taking a pet outside, if simply to get some fresh air, is good. However, they must *always* be on a leash, even if in a fenced-in backyard. Activity should be restricted to going out on a leash for urination and bowel movements only for the first 4 weeks. Once splints and/or bandages have been removed and as the patient's healing progresses, short controlled slow walks on a leash may be allowed and may be better for the patient than uncontrolled bursts of activity in the house. Exercise is restricted to short, slow, controlled leash walks until the injury has fully healed. An appropriate walk for the convalescing pet is on a 4-ft leash and done at a slow pace. The goal of leash walking as an exercise is to increase mobility, increase blood flow to the injured area, increase strength and promote cardiovascular endurance as well as the patient's confidence in using

(a)

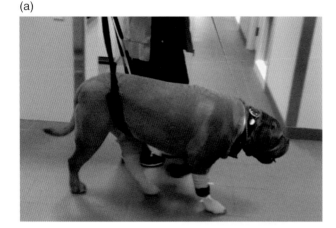

(b)

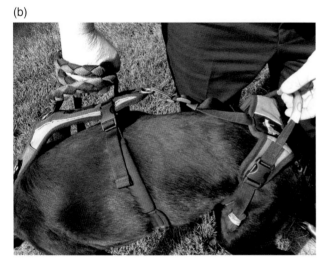

Figure 3.2 The dog in figure (a) is being supported with an abdominal sling. A large towel can also be used as an abdominal sling. The dog in figure (b) is being supported with a pelvic sling as well as a chest harness. Pelvic slings are commercially available and can be more comfortable to the patient as they do not bunch up in the inguinal area or place pressure on the bladder. The pelvic sling may be preferred for long-term use.

the limb. Walking on easy surfaces (such as a sidewalk) is best until the fracture has healed. Walks should be not too long—short more frequent walks are better for the recuperating dog. A 5–10-minute walk is ample to start with. The dog should always end the walk as he/she started it: no increase in lameness, no slowing down toward the end of the walk, no lameness or stiffness later in the day. If such effects are noted, then the walk was too long and the duration should be reconsidered for the next day. If the dog is doing well, then the walks can be gradually lengthened to a maximum of 20 minutes. Once the follow-up radiographs show that the fracture has healed, then a gradual return to regular

activity over a 4-week period is advised. The owners should start by lengthening the duration of the walks and adding difficulties (uneven terrain, hills, stairs); then gradually and slowly re-introducing the pet's usual activities.

3.1.5 Follow-up Radiographs and Healing Times

Ideally, follow-up radiographs are taken every 4 weeks until there is radiographic evidence of a bridging callus. Most fractures in healthy adult patients will heal within 6–10 weeks. In the immature patient, the healing time is much faster, therefore follow-up radiographs may be taken sooner; at 2 weeks in the pediatric patient.

It is important to always take two views of the fractured bone so that the radiographs can be properly assessed.

- Bony union is evaluated by looking for evidence of callus formation. The fracture is considered healed once the callus bridges across the fracture line in at least one view (Figure 3.3).
- The integrity of the implants is assessed by looking for evidence that a pin or screw is backing out or has broken (Figure 3.4). Such an occurrence indicates that the fracture site is not stable. Increasing the stability by placing the limb in a splint may be adequate, but a revision surgery may be necessary.
- Evidence of infection, osteomyelitis, which can appear as radiolucency around an implant (Figure 3.5).

3.1.6 Implant Removal

Most implants are *not* routinely removed once a fracture has healed; however, their extraction should be considered if they are bothersome to the patient. It is considered safe to remove implants once there is radiographic evidence that the fracture has healed.

Intra-medullary pins and K-wires can irritate the surrounding soft tissues, resulting in a seroma formation or soft tissue swelling over the end of the pin/wire; the patient may show a lameness and indicate pain when the area where the pin protrudes is palpated. Removal of a pin or K-wire is a minor procedure when the end of the pin/wire is palpable; at times pins can be removed under heavy sedation.

Plates are removed if they are irritating to periarticular tissues or if there is a persistent draining tract, indicating that there is an infection. Some surgeons will routinely plan on removing a plate from the radius of toy breed dogs because of possible stress protection. Removal of a plate, although not usually a complicated procedure, does requires general anesthesia and is done under full aseptic technique in the operating room.

(a)

(b)

(c)

(d)

(e)

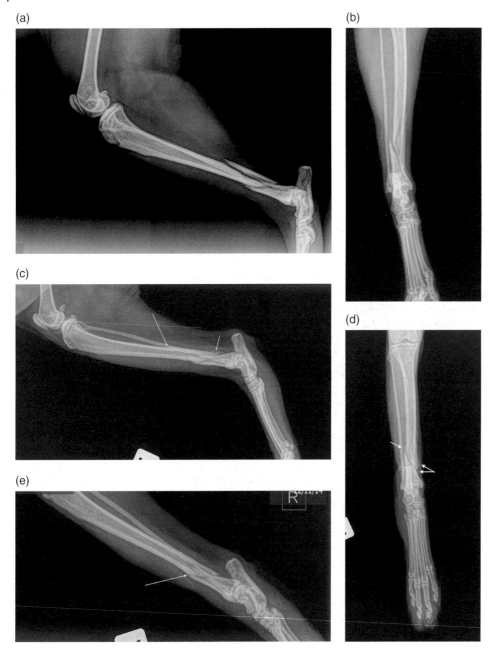

Figure 3.3 Mediolateral (a) and caudocranial (b) views of a two-piece and a wedge distal tibial fracture with intact fibula taken at the time of presentation. The fracture was treated with a splint. Follow-up radiographs taken at 4 weeks (c and d) show no significant displacement of the fragments and early callus formation across the main fracture line (short arrow). There is already a bridging callus at the proximal aspect of the wedge (long arrow). Radiographs taken at 8 weeks (e and f) show a bridging callus across the main fracture line (arrow) and the proximal wedge fracture line is barely visible. Radiographs taken at 12 weeks (g and h) show that the fractures have all healed. *Source:* Photos courtesy of the Animal Hospital of Cambridge.

3.2 The Owner

Written and verbal instructions should be given to pet owners at the time of discharge. Whenever possible, owners should be given home preparation instructions in advance of bringing their pet home so that they can properly prepare the home environment.

3.2.1 Slippery Floors

Dogs should have non-slippery surfaces to walk on in the home. Inexpensive runners can be purchased and placed in the areas where the pet most frequently travels within the house. As the fracture heals, the runners are gradually removed.

(f)   (g)   (h)

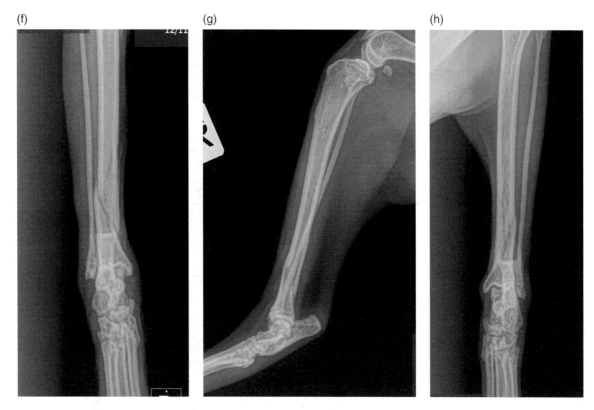

Figure 3.3 (Continued)

3.2.2 Stairs

Preventing the pet from going up or down stairs freely is important. Baby gates are the simplest solution for blocking stairs. If stairs are unavoidable, the owners can be instructed to assist their dog by going up the stairs with them in a slow, controlled manner, ensuring that the dog walks, rather than hops, the steps. Owners may need to place their dog on a leash or hold their collar to accomplish this. If the stairs have a slippery surface, the owner can give further assistance by using a chest harness (for a forelimb fracture) or an abdominal or pelvic sling (Figure 3.2) for a hindlimb fracture. Small dogs should be carried up and down stairs.

3.2.3 No Jumping

Preventing jumping onto furniture can be a challenge. Placing obstacles such as large pillows or removing the cushions from the pet's favorite chair or couch may be sufficient. An alternative and easily accessible place for the pet to lie should be made available. Jumping can be one of the more detrimental "activities" that the recuperating pet may attempt.

3.2.4 Common Stressors

Having the owners identify the conditions/situations that tend to trigger their dog to have episodes of uncontrolled activity will be helpful. The doorbell ringing or people walking by "the large bay window" are common examples. Eliminating the stressors as much as possible will help control the bursts of activity level within the home. Simple solutions such as placing a note on the doorbell or closing the curtains are usually available.

3.2.5 Crates

If the dog is crate trained, the owners can make use of the crate to help confine their pet to a safe and comfortable environment, especially when the pet is unattended in the house. If a pet is not accustomed to a crate, then it may be perceived as a negative place, a punishment of sorts, and therefore may not be appropriate for the postoperative or posttrauma patient. Some dogs may be more amenable to being confined in a large ex-pen that is placed in a "central" location in the house so they do not feel isolated or removed from the family.

3.2.6 Icing

For the patient without a bandage, the owner can assist their pet's recovery from surgery by icing the area for 10–15 minutes two to four times daily. Putting ice cubes in a freezer bag and then wrapping it with a thin cloth

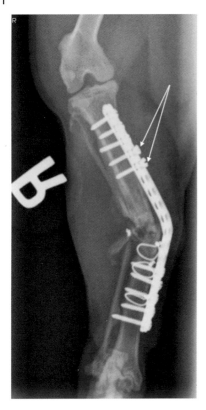

Figure 3.4 Craniocaudal projection of a cat tibia with a problematic fracture repaired with stacked cuttable plates that failed. Besides the obvious bend in the plate at the fracture line there are two screws backing out (arrows).

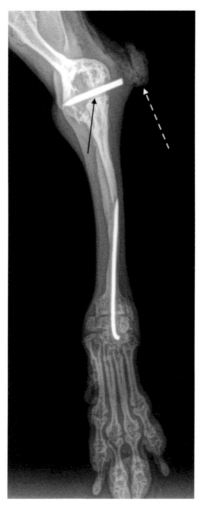

Figure 3.5 A toy breed dog presented non-weight bearing on its left forelimb and a draining tract on the lateral aspect of the elbow. He had had a lateral condylar fracture repaired with a pin that became infected. The lucency around the pin is visible (black arrow) as is the draining tract (dotted arrow) on the radiograph. Unfortunately this dog also had a fracture of the radius repaired with a pin. All implants were removed but the patient never did use the limb well.

(pillow case or thin towel) before placing it on the surgical site is a simple and readily accessible technique. Icing can be used to help reduce the swelling until the sutures are removed.

3.2.7 Gentle Passive Range of Motion (PROM)

These exercises are encouraged to help decrease pain, swelling, and to restore proper motion to the joint. Even if the fracture is not articular, the joints on either side of the fracture as well as those that were immobilized by a splint will benefit from PROMs. Videos on how to execute PROM exercises are available on YouTube or through iBooks [1].

3.2.8 Urination and Bowel Movements

It is important that the pet re-establishes an appropriate and regular pattern for urination and bowel movements. Pets healing from a fracture can be predisposed to constipation because of the narcotics used to control pain and a reluctance to position themselves for defecation; also fluid therapy while in the hospital can result in a

more frequent need to urinate. Careful consideration on the owner's part regarding access to water and timing of access to the yard for urination may be necessary to ensure that all parties have an uninterrupted night of sleep. Patients healing from a pelvic or hindlimb fracture are especially at risk for constipation. Stool softeners (canned pumpkin, psyllium or even lactulose) for the first week or two may be helpful in preventing issues with bowel movements.

3.2.9 Food and Water

Fresh water should be readily accessible. If the pet has difficulty ambulating, then having more than one water bowl may be necessary. Raising the food and water bowls may be helpful for the patient with a forelimb issue. Caloric intake should be adjusted to ensure proper amounts are being fed for a healing, non-exercising pet.

3.2.10 Cats

An easy way to restrict the activity of cats is to confine them to a large crate or pen. The pen must have a "roof" to prevent jumping or climbing out. An upside down child's playpen or large dog crate works well for this purpose. The area must be large enough for the cat to have a small bed, litter box, food and water dishes as well as sufficient space to move around. Many cats like to have a "place to hide," such as a box within the crate as well. Placing the crate in an area of the house where there is some activity will help to keep the cat somewhat mentally stimulated and not feel too isolated. The cat can be allowed to have supervised exercise periods outside of the crate as the fracture is healing. Jumping and vigorous activity should be avoided until the healing is complete.

3.3 Managing Osteoarthritis (OA)

Managing OA is a topic on its own and the reader is encouraged to seek more information on this subject [2]. Weight control and appropriate activity are two very important building blocks of a good OA management program.

The patient should have a body condition score (BCS) of 3/5 or 5/9. Dogs that are overweight will place excessive stress on their joints and cardiovascular system, making exercise uncomfortable and unpleasant. Since joint motion is essential for chondrocyte metabolism, exercise becomes the hallmark of a healthy joint.

Motion will also maintain joint capsule flexibility, especially if some degree of joint pathology and therefore fibrosis, is present; as well as keep the supporting muscles and tendons functioning properly. A good exercise program is instrumental in keeping the OA joint comfortable. The level of activity must be tailored for each individual. The morning stiffness that many OA suffers experience is an example of how a lack of motion can affect the joint.

Nutritional supplements such as omega-3-fatty-acids, glucosamine sulfate, chondroitin sulfate and manganese can also have a positive effect on joints and should be given consideration. The patient's lifestyle may need to be altered somewhat to keep the OA pet pain-free and drug-free. Most pets will still be able to maintain an active lifestyle, but the duration and intensity of the activities may need to be modulated.

The use of NSAIDs may be helpful when a patient is experiencing an acute or sub-acute flare-up of the OA. Many pets that are following a good OA regime will be able to have a pain-free and fulfilling lifestyle without the use of daily medications.

Alternative modalities such as massages, acupuncture, LASER, and chiropractics can be helpful to keep the arthritic patient more mobile and using fewer drugs.

References

1 Pyke, J. and Sylvestre, A.M. (2013) iRehab my dog. https://itunes.apple.com/ca/book/i-rehab-my-dog/id1070374203?mt=11.

2 Johnston, S.A., McLaughlin, R.M., and Budsberg, S.C. (2008). Nonsurgical management of osteoarthritis in dogs. *Vet. Clin. North Am. Small Anim. Pract.* 38 (6): 1449–1470.

4

Bandages and Splints

Jennifer White[1] and Anne M. Sylvestre[2]

[1] Surgery Department, VCA Canada Mississauga Oakville Veterinary Emergency Hospital and Referral Group, Oakville, Ontario, Canada
[2] Focus and Flourish, Cambridge, Ontario, Canada

4.1 The Bandage

A bandage, or splinted bandage is applied to fulfill a specific purpose; for example, providing stability, decreasing swelling or protecting a wound. The construct of the bandage will vary according to its function. Bandages are not benign: they can create superficial and deep wounds, articulation issues and can be a source of pain, frustration, and expense. The key to minimizing complications associated with a bandage is to create one that is properly constructed; fits the patient well; has adequate, even tension throughout; the bony prominences are protected; and is diligently monitored and changed frequently.

This chapter will focus on bandages and splints applied for orthopedic purposes only. The reader is encouraged to seek out other resources for information on bandages applied specifically for managing wounds [1].

4.1.1 Layers of a Bandage

A bandage consists of several layers. To be effective and comfortable, it is important that the layers be applied in the correct sequence (Figure 4.1).

4.1.1.1 Contact Layer

Also known as the primary layer. This layer is placed directly over a wound or incision. The type of material used as a contact layer will vary according to the stage of healing that the wound is in. The reader is encouraged to seek out other resources for information on various types of primary contact materials for managing wounds [1]. A simple non-adherent product (e.g. Telfa™ pad) is typically used for surgical incisions.

4.1.1.2 Padding Layer

Often referred to as the secondary, or intermediate, layer, the padding layer functions to help reduce swelling and hinder motion. The thickness of this layer will dictate the degree of immobilization offered by the bandage. Cast padding is the most commonly used material for this layer. It conforms well to the limb, comes in a variety of sizes, and is easy to use. A bulk roll of cotton can also be used but it does not conform well to the limb and is difficult to apply evenly. The bulk cotton roll is used almost exclusively for a Robert Jones bandage. This layer cannot be applied too tightly as the materials used will readily tear under tension.

4.1.1.3 Compressive Layer

This is a component of the tertiary or outer layer. A conforming gauze roll (e.g. Kling™) is used to compress the padding layer into place, giving shape to the bandage. An appropriate amount of even tension is required for the bandage to remain securely positioned on the body part without constricting it. Getting the tension just right comes with a bit of practice and experience.

4.1.1.4 Protective Layer

Another component of the tertiary or outer layer. This layer gives a bit of stiffness to the bandage, helping to hold its shape and to repel dirt and moisture. A cohesive bandage material such as Vet Wrap or Coflex™ is used for this final layer of the bandage.

4.1.2 Creating the Bandage

It is best to leave the two middle digits exposed when applying a bandage in order to better assess the bandage for tension and the development of potential complications as well as minimizing the creation of an interdigital dermatitis. Leaving more than just the two middle digits exposed will increase the risk of venous return obstruction and therefore swelling of the digits.

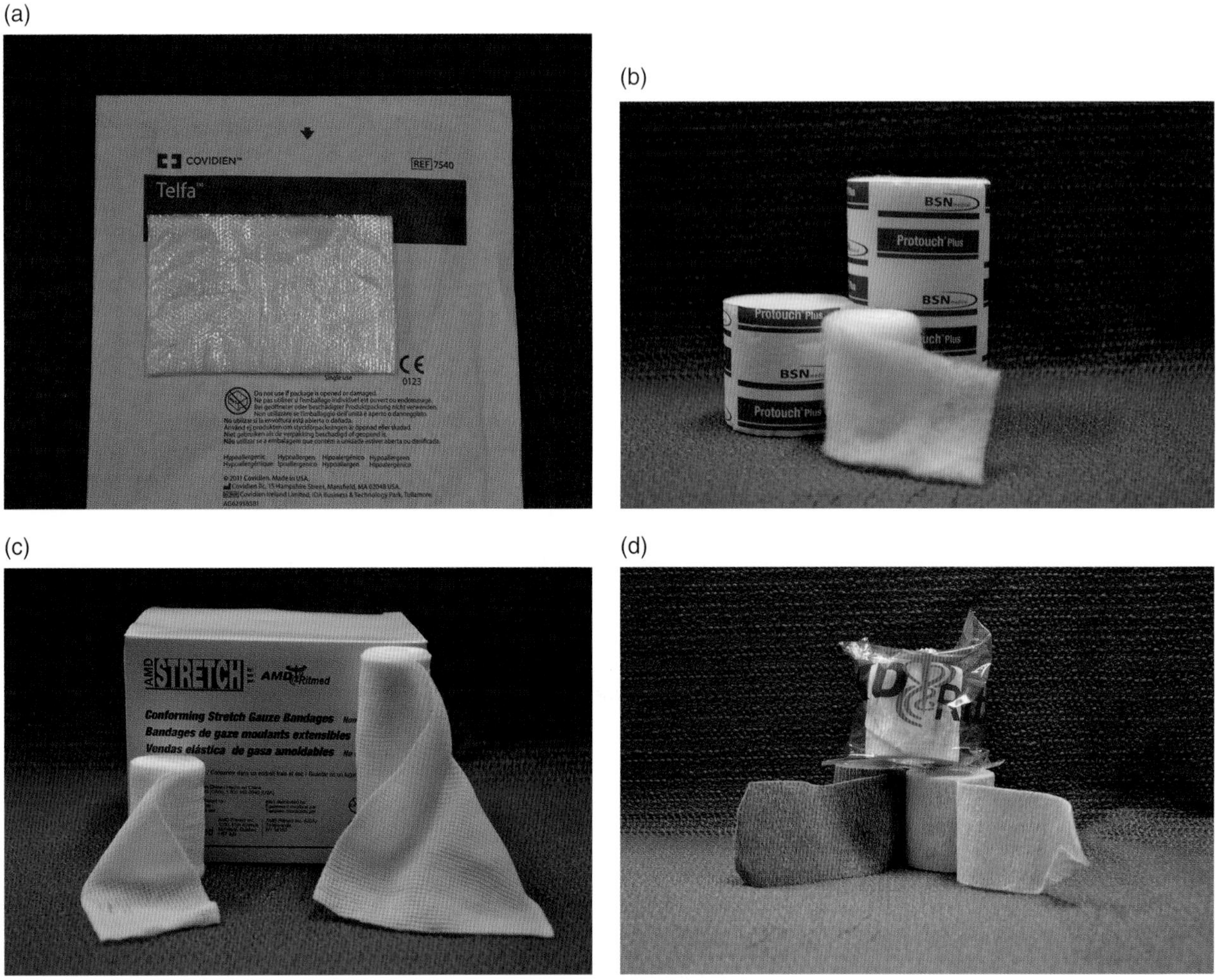

(a)

(b)

(c)

(d)

Figure 4.1 The layers of a bandage. (a) Telfa™ pad is an example of a contact layer; (b) cast padding is applied over the contact layer and/or directly against the skin; (c) a conforming gauze roll such as Kling™ is used to compress the padding; and (d) a water-resistant cohesive layer, such as Vet Wrap or Coflex™ is then applied to protect the bandage.

4.1.2.1 Managing the Digits

(Figure 4.2) Moisture between the digits and around the pads can promote interdigital yeast dermatitis. This problem can be controlled with frequent and regular bandage changes, washing the paw with a chlorhexidine soap at the time of bandage change, then rinsing and drying the area before reapplying a new bandage. Some dogs are more prone to interdigital dermatitis from moisture and debris build-up and can benefit from having a small amount of cotton placed between each digit to help keep the area dry. Trimming the hair between the digits and around the pads can also help prevent interdigital debris build-up.

4.1.2.2 Donuts

Donuts are used to protect the skin over protuberant areas of the limb from being damaged by the bandage. Accessory pads, olecranon, calcaneus, medial, or lateral metacarpo/metatarso-phalangeal joints are areas that commonly require donuts. Adequate tension on the compressive layer will also help to decrease the formation of skin wounds by limiting the amount of motion between the skin and the bandage. Donuts can be created in advance. The key is to ensure that the protuberance does not extrude beyond the "donut hole." A donut can be created in a number of ways:

- A hole of appropriate size is cut into layered cast padding or gauze squares, of appropriate thickness (Figure 4.3).
- Gauze roll or cast padding is used to create the donuts. The material is wrapped several times around two, or more, fingers to create a ring of the approximate size necessary. A sufficient length of the roll of gauze or cast padding is left intact and used to bind the donut by weaving it in and out of the ring until the entire ring/donut is bound (Figure 4.4).

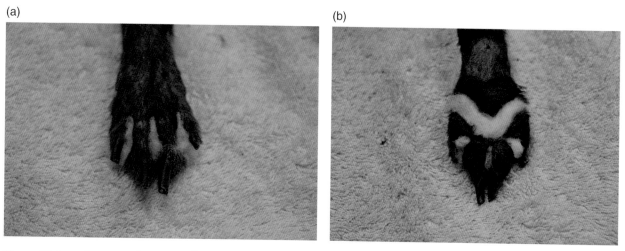

Figure 4.2 A small amount of cotton can be placed between the digits (a) and, if necessary, along the metacarpal or metatarsal pad (b).

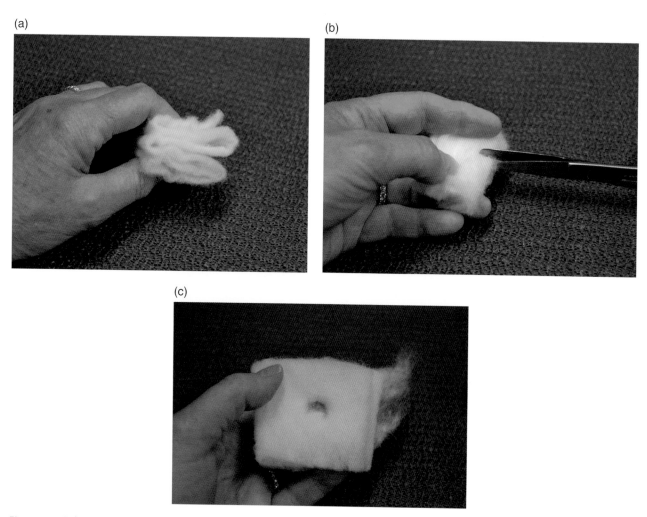

Figure 4.3 A donut can be created by folding cast padding on itself several times (a). The pad cushion is folded in two and a slit or wedge is cut into the fold (b). The slit is then stretched to the desired size (c).

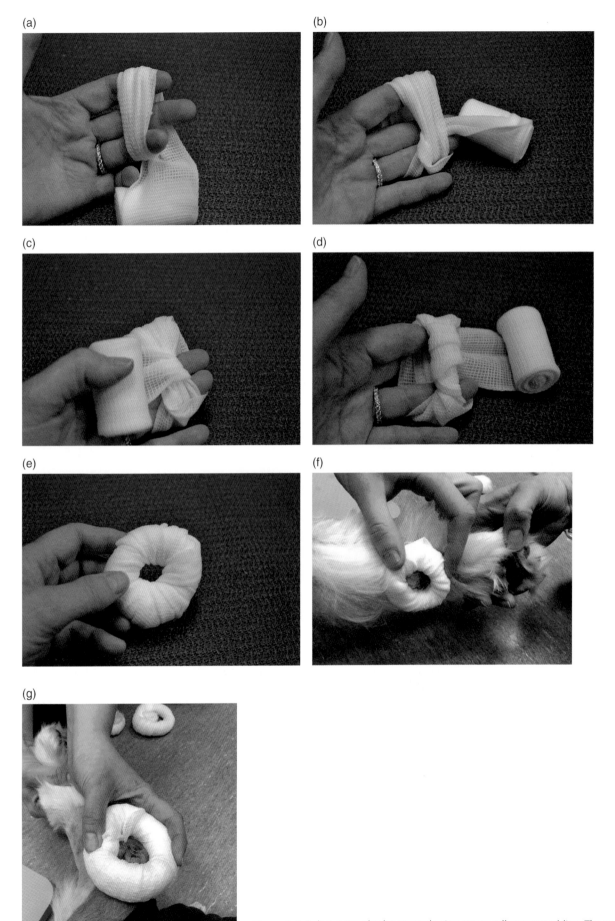

(a)

(b)

(c)

(d)

(e)

(f)

(g)

Figure 4.4 A donut can also be created using gauze roll or cast padding. The material is wrapped several times around two, or more, fingers to approximate the size of the desired hole (a). The material is then woven around the formed ring by moving it in and out of the circle until the entire ring/donut is bound (b–e). The protuberance should not extrude beyond the donut (f and g).

(a)

(c)

(b)

(d)

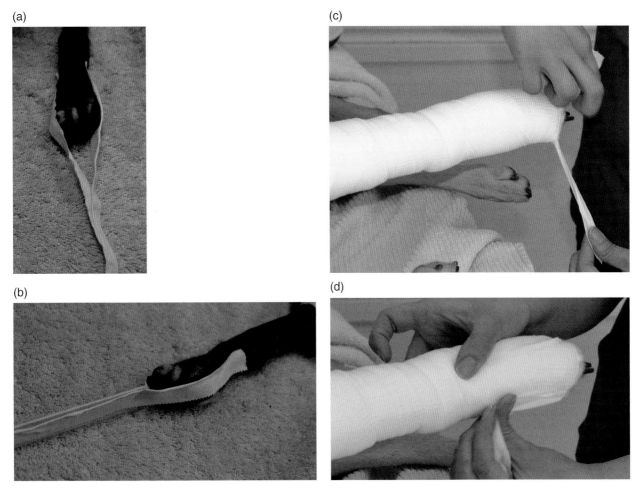

Figure 4.5 A stirrup is applied to the paw with two strips of 0.5″ or 1″ white porous tape that extend several centimeters beyond the paw. The ends are lightly taped to one another (a), or taped to a tongue depressor (b). Once the compressive gauze layer has been applied, the strips are separated and then twisted to adhere to the gauze (c and d).

4.1.2.3 Stirrups

Orthopedic bandages can be bulky and stirrups will help to keep the two middle digits exposed and the distally located bandage materials from shifting. If the stirrups are used to "hold the bandage up," then the bandage is not likely fulfilling its purpose. Appropriate tension is applied to the compressive layer to prevent a bandage from slipping down. If a stirrup is desired, it can be applied to the medial and/or lateral aspect(s) of the paw (from just below the carpus/tarsus). A single strip can also be applied to the dorsum of the paw. It is best to avoid placing a strip onto the digital pads as the adhesive can cause damage when removing the tape. A strip is created using white porous tape of appropriate width, and it should be long enough to surpass the end of the paw by several centimeters. The strip ends can be lightly taped to one another, or to a tongue depressor placed in between the two, to prevent them from becoming

bunched up. The strips of tape will be twisted and made to adhere to the compressive gauze layer once it has been applied (Figure 4.5).

4.1.2.4 Contact Layer

If there is a wound or incision, an appropriate contact layer is selected to cover it. Resources are available for the appropriate selection of a contact layer [1]. Bandages used for orthopedic conditions often do not require a contact layer.

4.1.2.5 Padding Layer

The bandage is started at the digits and the material unraveled in a proximal direction with each turn overlapping the previous one by approximately 50%. The cast padding material is applied evenly, removing any wrinkles or bunching that may occur. If an additional roll of material is needed, it is best to have the new roll overlap the end of the previous one by at least 10–15 cm. This will allow for better continuity, preventing breaks in the bandage, and ensuring that it works as one unit.

To prevent the leading edge of the bandage from protruding distally and to allow for easier viewing of the two central digits, the author (JW) starts the bandage in a fashion that creates an upside down "V" over the dorsum of digits 3 and 4, leaving them a bit more exposed while still cradling the palmar/plantar surface of the paw. Figure 4.6 has a full description.

4.1.2.6 Compressive Layer

The compressive layer is applied over and started in the same manner as the cast padding layer. Because this layer will compress the bandage, it is important to start distally and move proximally. If using JW's upside down "V" technique, it is important not to apply tension to the gauze roll (Kling) until the distal-most point has been reached. The tension should be evenly applied throughout the bandage. One successful technique used by the author (JW) is to apply compression, using the heel of the hand, as the gauze roll is being pulled toward the back of the limb and then relaxing the compression as it is brought forward. The bandage is created in this steady and rhythmic fashion ensuring an even and not excessive application of compression (Figure 4.7).

The stirrups are taped to the compressive gauze layer.

4.1.2.7 Protective Layer

The final layer is applied/started in the same fashion as the previous two. The working tension was applied with the conforming gauze layer so the protective (Vet Wrap) layer is applied with just enough tension for it to fit smoothly and evenly over the bandage (Figure 4.8).

4.1.2.8 Adding a Splint

If extra stability is required, then a splint is placed between the compressive (conforming gauze roll) and the protective (cohesive bandage material) layers. The splint is secured in place with white porous tape and another layer of the gauze roll to prevent the splint from shifting within the bandage. Wrapping the gauze around the most distal and proximal components of the splint will help prevent it from moving proximally or distally during weight bearing.

A) *Commercially available splints*: These come in a variety of shapes and sizes to fit specific body parts and patient types. The commonly used ones are: forelimb splints, hind limb splints and palmar/plantar splints (Figure 4.9). A tongue depressor can also be used as a splint with the small patients.

B) *Creating a splint from fiberglass tape* (Figure 4.10): A splint can readily be custom-made using fiberglass material (e.g. DeltaLite™). There are many ways of creating a custom splint. It is important to wear gloves and have access to water when creating a fiberglass splint. A large dog may require the use of two packages for the splint to be strong enough. The splint can be applied directly on the conforming gauze (Kling) or a stockinette can be placed over the Kling. The fiberglass material will adhere to the material that it is in contact with; at the next bandage change, that material will be cut out and will become part of the splint. The padding and compressive layers of the bandage should be in place before opening the fiberglass package. The roll of fiberglass can be placed in the water for several seconds (as per the manufacturer's directions) and then applied to the bandage. The author's (JW) preferred technique is to unroll the fiberglass material into position over the limb, creating the desired basic splint shape and length. The layers are then carefully lifted up and placed in the water for a few seconds. The excess water is removed and the wet splint is placed back onto the bandage and molded into its final shape. Even pressure with open, flat palms is used to mold the material to the limb. It is important not to create "indentations" in the fiberglass material while it is hardening. The splint is then wrapped in place with conforming gauze roll, with gentle even compression to help maintain the splint's shape as it hardens. The final protective layer is then applied. The fiberglass material needs to cure for a full 15–20 minutes before the patient can walk on it.

C) *Creating a bivalve cast* (Figure 4.11): Typically, the patient will be under general anesthesia for this procedure. A bivalve cast offers more support and immobilization than a splint but is easier to manage than a full cast; the amount of stability offered by the cast can be lessened by applying only one half of it (simply using it as a splint) and the patient will not need to be re-anesthetized to have the cast removed. Before creating the bivalve cast, the padding and compressive layers are applied. It is important not to overly pad the bandage as the cast will loosen once the cast padding layer becomes compressed over time. To create the cast, the appropriate size roll of fiberglass is removed from the package and placed in water for several seconds, allowing the water to reach the core of the roll. The fiberglass material is then applied as another bandage layer, over the pre-placed padding and conforming gauze layers, starting at the digits and wrapping around the limb while moving in a proximal direction and overlapping each layer by 50%. Even pressure should be applied to help mold the cast to the limb and care is taken

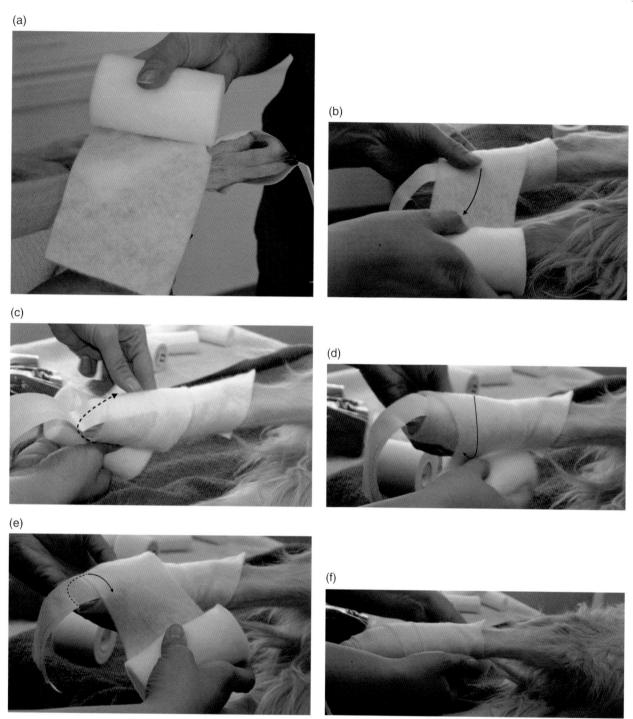

Figure 4.6 A preferred bandage starting technique (JW) is shown here. The leading edge of the bandage material is placed on an angle and started slightly proximal to the digits (a). The cast padding is unraveled in a distal direction for one or two turns maintaining that same starting angle aiming for the medial (or lateral) digital pads (b). The angle of the material will cause it to catch the paw on an edge and then it is continued on an upward angle (c); crossed over the dorsum, which allows for the angle to be adjusted back downwards (d) to catch the other side of the paw (e). The bandage material is then continued up the limb overlapping the previous layer by 50% (f). This starting technique tends to better cradle the palmar/plantar aspect of the paw and leaves the two center digits a bit more exposed dorsally for easier monitoring; it also prevents the leading corner of the material from protruding beyond the bandage. Note: the other two layers are placed in the same manner but when applying the compressive (Kling) layer it is important to simply position the gauze roll at the start and to start applying the pressure only once it has reached its distal-most point as seen in c. A video of this technique is available at www.focusandflourish.com.

(a)

(b)

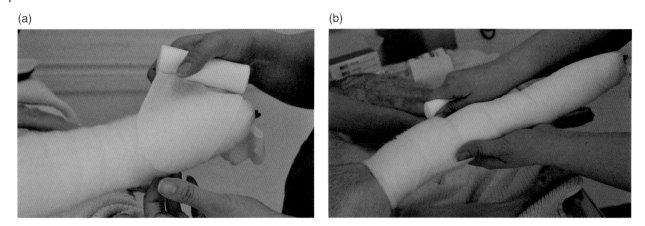

Figure 4.7 The compressive layer using conforming gauze roll is applied in the same manner as the cast padding (a). Even compression is applied with this layer. JW applies compression, using the heel of the hand, as the gauze roll is being pulled toward the back of the limb (b) and then relaxing the compression as it is brought forward. The steady rhythm of compression ensures that she applies it evenly over the padding layer.

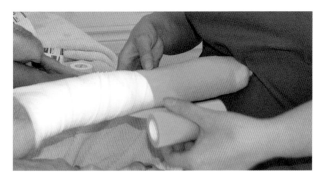

Figure 4.8 The final protective layer is applied using a cohesive bandage material that is water-resistant. The layer is applied in the same manner as the two previous ones with just enough even tension for the material to lie smoothly.

not to create indentations or creases in the fiberglass material along the way. The fiberglass material is allowed to fully harden (approximately 15–20 minutes) and then it is cut along the medial and lateral or cranial and caudal surfaces using a cast saw. The two halves of the cast are separated, to ensure that the cuts are complete. The two half cast forms are securely tapped back together, recreating a full cast, and then the final, protective, bandage layer is applied. As the fracture heals, the amount of support can be decreased by simply removing one half of the cast. The bivalve cast is managed with the same home care instructions and regular changes as for any bandage.

(a)

(b)

(c)

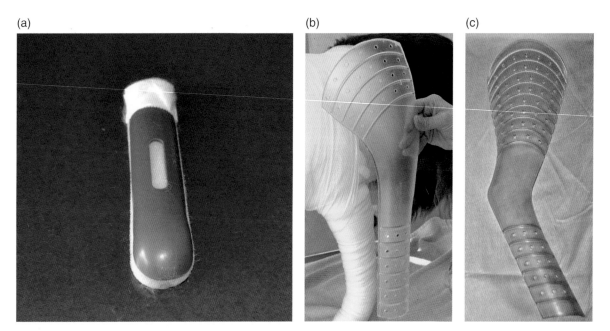

Figure 4.9 Common commercially available splints that can be cut to the appropriate length to fit the patient. Spoon or metasplint (a), a left forelimb splint (b), and right hind limb splint (c).

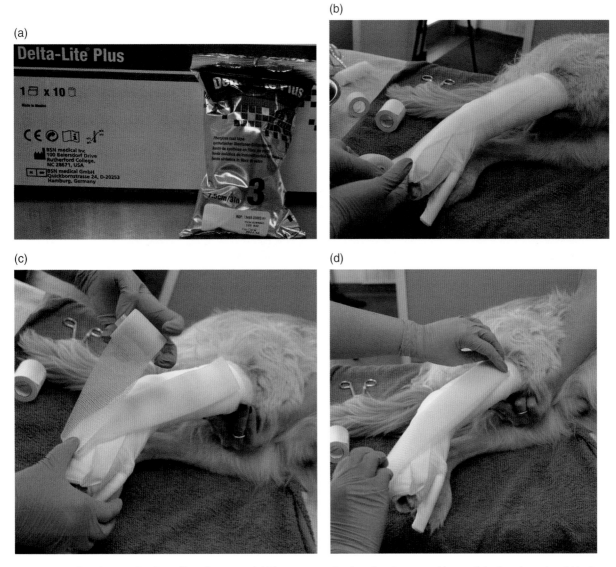

Figure 4.10 Creating a splint from fiberglass material. The compressive (conforming gauze) layer of the bandage should be in place before opening the package containing the fiberglass casting material (a). Gloves must be worn. The fiberglass material is unrolled into position over the limb, creating an approximate desired splint shape and length (b–d). The layers are then carefully lifted up and placed in water for a few seconds (e). The excess water is removed (f) and the wet splint is placed back onto the bandage and molded into its final shape by applying even pressure with open, flat palms (g). It is important not to create "indentations" in the fiberglass material while it is hardening. The splint is then wrapped in place with a layer of conforming gauze, using gentle, even compression to help maintain the shape as it hardens (h). The fiberglass needs to cure for a full 15–20 minutes before the patient can walk on it.

4.1.2.9 Finishing Touches

An adhesive protective material can be used to cover the ends of the bandage, preventing the patient from picking at any cotton padding that may be protruding at the edge of the bandage. The adhesive material is loosely wrapped around the end of the bandage, partly on the bandage and partly on the adjacent skin/hair. Applying the adhesive bandage material around the tip of the paw will help give more durability to a walking style bandage. This element is optional but does help to keep the bandage neat and tidy (Figure 4.12).

4.2 Forelimb

4.2.1 Velpeau Sling

The Velpeau sling is a non-weight bearing bandage that places the elbow and carpus in flexion and slightly lateralizes the humerus. This sling is ideal for medial shoulder luxations and for scapula and shoulder conditions that would require the patient not to bear weight on the limb. The Velpeau sling is contraindicated for lateral shoulder luxations and most humeral fractures, and,

(e)

(f)

(g)

(h)

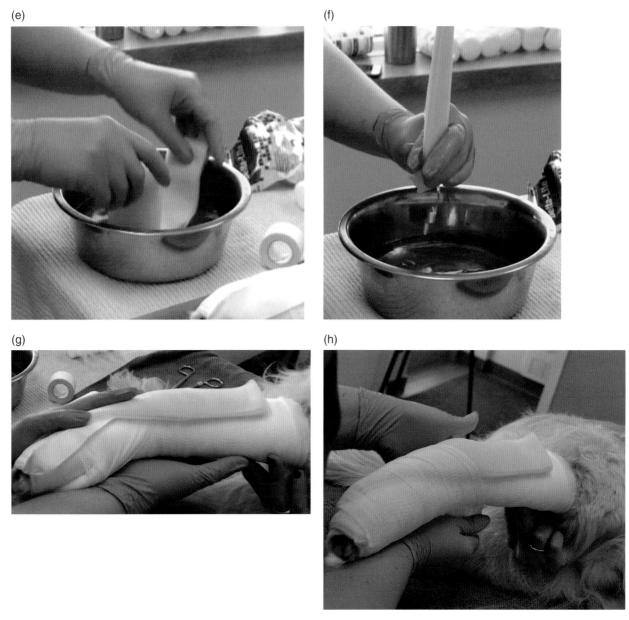

Figure 4.10 (Continued)

because the carpus and elbow are held in flexion, it is best to avoid in patients with osteoarthritis in these joints. A spica bandage would be a better choice for these patients.

The patient will commonly be under general anesthesia when this bandage is applied. This makes it difficult to create a smooth, well-fitting, and secure bandage. It is therefore important to monitor the patient/bandage carefully over the following 48 hours for signs of respiratory distress, discomfort from the bandage and the flexed joint position, and to ensure that there is no slippage of the bandage or the limb from the bandage.

The Velpeau sling should be left on for a maximum of 10 days. Once the sling is removed, gentle passive range of motion exercises of the carpus and elbow joints are indicated as well as activity restriction to short controlled on leash walks to allow the tissues to re-adapt to weight bearing.

Cats can wiggle out of this bandage just as easily as they can wiggle out of the Ehmer sling. It may be better to consider a spica bandage/splint or, perhaps, confinement to a small area like a crate.

(a)   (b)   (c)

(d)   (e)   (f)

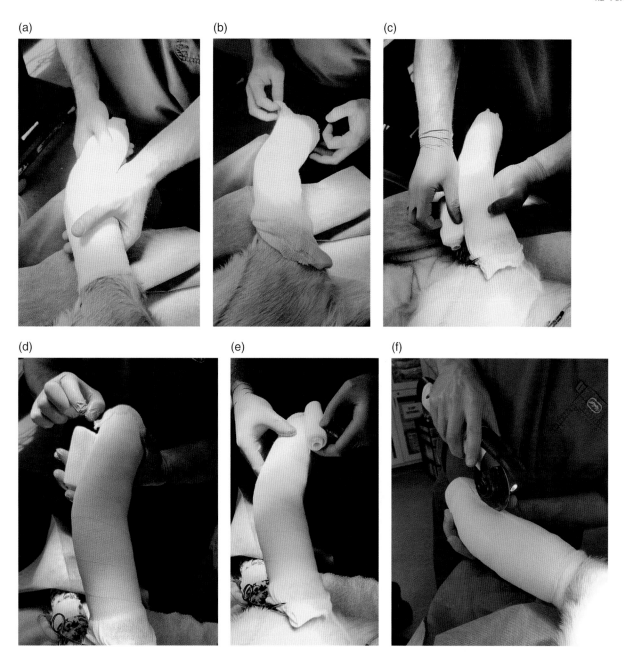

Figure 4.11 Creating a bivalve cast. The antebrachium has been wrapped with cast padding and compressed with the conforming gauze layer (a). A stockinette has been placed over the conforming gauze layer (b). It is important to wear gloves when handling the fiberglass material. The roll of fiberglass material has been dipped in water (as per the manufacturer's instructions) and is being applied to the limb in the same manner as the previous bandage layers, starting distally and moving proximally, with even overlap (c). The stockinette ends are folded back to be incorporated into the cast itself (d and e). Once the fiberglass material has hardened, it is cut using a cast saw (f and g). In this example only a palmar splint will eventually be needed so the cast is cut on the medial and lateral sides. If a lateral splint is desired, then the cast would be cut on the cranial and caudal surfaces. Two half casts are created (h). The two halves are securely taped back into place and the protective cohesive wrap is applied over the fiberglass cast (i and j). When less support is appropriate, only the palmar portion of the bivalve cast will be used. *Source:* Photos courtesy of the VCA Canada Mississauga Oakville veterinary emergency Hospital and referral group.

(g)　　　　　　　　　　　　　　(h)

(i)　　　　　　　　　　　　　　(j)

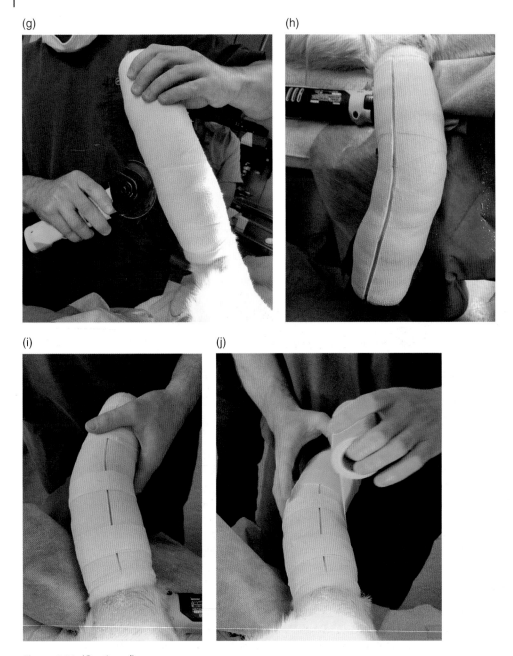

Figure 4.11 (Continued)

Figure 4.13 has details on how to apply the Velpeau sling. There are different ways that this sling can be applied: the "cross your heart" style or the simply "wrapped around the chest" style. The key points are that the carpus and elbow are maintained in flexion close to the body and that the bandage adequately supports these joints so that the patient cannot wiggle the limb out of the bandage.

4.2.2 Spica Bandage

The spica bandage is ideal for immobilizing the upper portion of the forelimb by stabilizing it to the thorax. It is useful for conditions of the elbow and above (humerus, shoulder, and scapula) that require immobilization or support but where weight bearing is acceptable or indicated. This bandage requires a lot of materials to apply

(a)

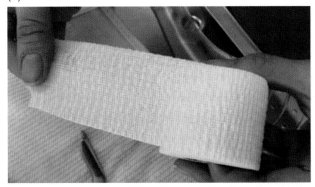

(b)

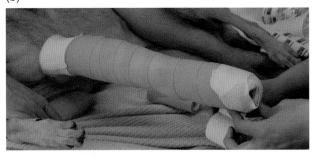

Figure 4.12 Ultralight elastic adhesive material (a) is used to protect the distal and proximal ends of the bandage (b).

small patient so that it does not become too bulky, too heavy, and too restrictive.

Commercially available forelimb splints work well for adding extra immobilization within a spica bandage for issues of the proximal radius/ulna to mid-humerus. A custom-made splint using fiberglass material (as described above) may offer more immobilization to the proximal humerus and shoulder areas. It is important that the splint is strong yet not too heavy. For larger dogs, two rolls may be necessary. The custom-made splint is applied laterally, it should begin in the mid-metacarpal region; extend straight up the limb and curve over the back, beyond the midline, taking on the shape of a "candy cane" when done. The splint can readily be made to gently curve in a palmar direction distally. Placing another layer of conforming bandage material with mild, even compression will help to nicely mold the splint to the bandage. The fiberglass material should be allowed to harden for at least 15–20 minutes before moving the patient. If the patient is in lateral recumbency the antebrachium is placed and supported in a natural standing position with pressure applied to the paw to simulate weight bearing; this will help maintain a natural degree of flexion in the elbow and shoulder. Once the fiberglass material is sufficiently stiff (5 minutes), the limb can simply be supported on a towel for the reminder of the curing process.

4.2.3 Antebrachial Bandages

This is a versatile and commonly used bandage. It is easily adapted to being a splinted bandage as well. The bandage can be created to include or exclude the elbow. However, the bandage is best tolerated by the patient, with significantly decreased morbidity, if it does not include the elbow. Therefore, careful consideration should be given to the purpose of the bandage/splint before deciding how to apply.

4.2.3.1 Antebrachial Bandage *Including* the Elbow (Figure 4.15)
This bandage or splint is indicated when the support is necessary for a mid- to proximal radius and/or ulna fracture in any patient; a more distally located fracture on the radius and ulna in a larger breed of dog. This type of bandage should be monitored carefully for morbidity issues. This "high" antebrachial bandage often slips down to the level of the elbow, causing it not to function as well to immobilize the proximal radius; it tends to irritate the skin on the cranial aspect of the elbow area and in the axilla; and it can readily produce a decubital ulcer over the olecranon. If long-term bandaging/splinting is anticipated, it may be better to apply the spica bandage/splint for the early treatment period and then finish the

properly but it functions very well and tends to be well tolerated by many patients and their owners.

There are various ways of applying this bandage. It can be anchored to the body by simply wrapping around the chest or around the chest and contralateral shoulder ("cross your heart" style of body bandage). For the bandage to be comfortable it must be appropriately padded and secure in position so that it does not slip. The "cross your heart" style where both shoulders are incorporated into the bandage is preferred by the authors (JW, AMS). Although this version of the bandage requires more materials than the single shoulder type, it tends to slip less, therefore maintaining better immobilization of the bandaged limb and being more comfortable to the patient. When a bandage moves, the conforming gauze layer can slip over the cast padding and lie in direct contact with the skin. The delicate skin located close to the axilla is easily cut by the conforming gauze material.

Figure 4.14 has detailed information on how to apply a spica bandage. It is easiest to place this bandage with the patient standing.

The quantity of material used for a 26 kg dog: six rolls of 4″ cast padding, five rolls of 4″ conforming bandage and three rolls of 4″ cohesive bandage material. Caution should be exercised when applying this bandage to a

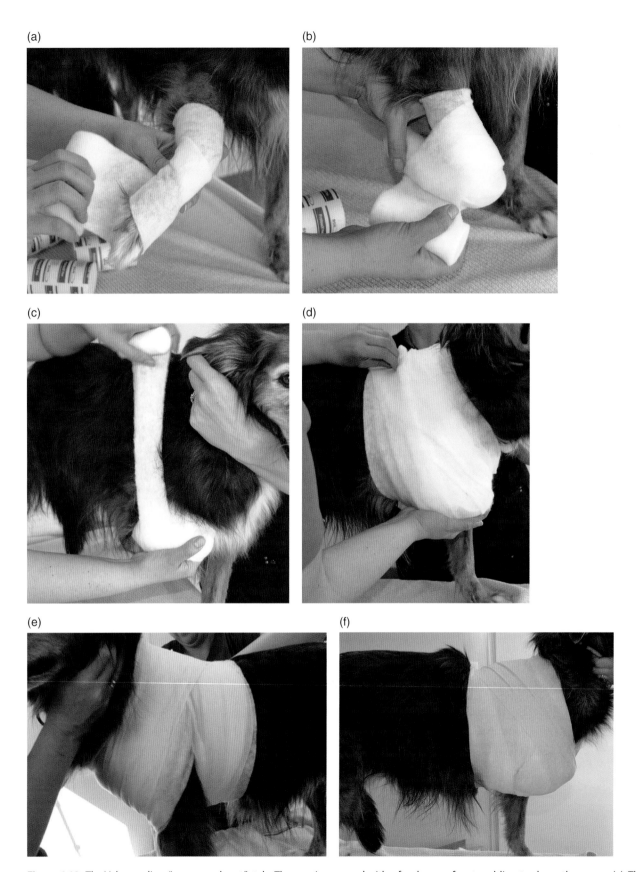

Figure 4.13 The Velpeau sling, "cross your heart" style. The paw is wrapped with a few layers of cast padding to above the carpus (a). The carpus is then flexed and the cast padding is then wrapped around the flexed carpus (b). The elbow is then placed in flexion and cast padding is continued around the thorax (c), behind the far shoulder, then back around again, incorporating the flexed carpus and elbow; this time the bandage material will be placed in front of the far shoulder. The bandage material is wrapped around the thorax several more times until the affected forelimb is securely held to the chest (d); with each wrap the material is made to alternate between passing behind and in front of the far shoulder (e), creating the "cross your heart" style of bandage. The same pattern is repeated with the conforming gauze and protective (cohesive bandage) layers (f).

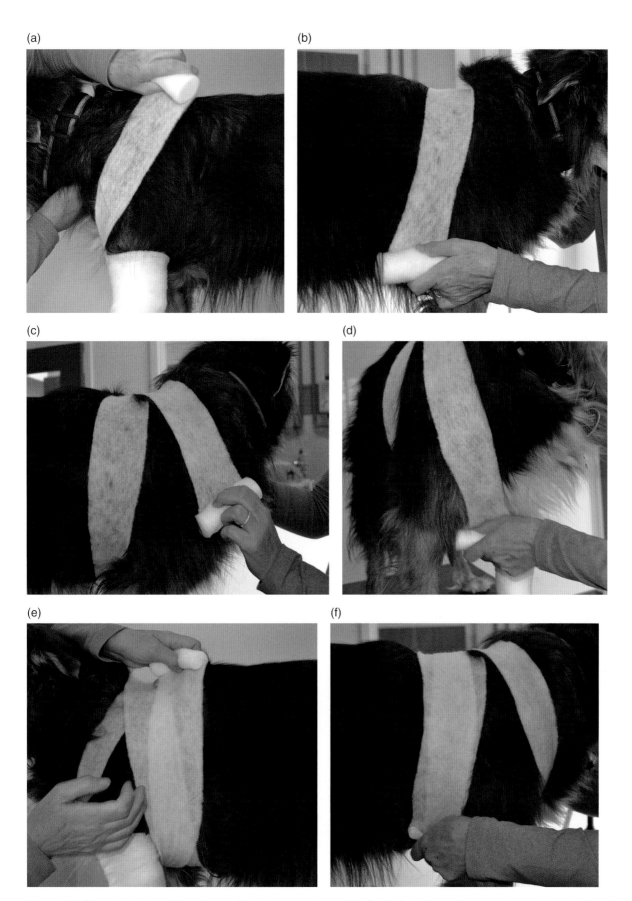

Figure 4.14 The spica bandage. The cotton padding is wrapped around the forelimb, starting at the paw and moved proximally as described for the antebrachial bandage including the elbow (Figure 4.15). To move the bandage up the chest, the cast padding is brought from within the axilla forward and upward over the point of the shoulder (a), around the thorax by passing behind the far shoulder (b), to return over the back and this time passing in front of the far shoulder (c), between the front limbs (d) and then behind the near (affected) shoulder (e), over the back once again and behind the far shoulder (f), and forward between the front limbs (g), and over the point of the affected shoulder (h).

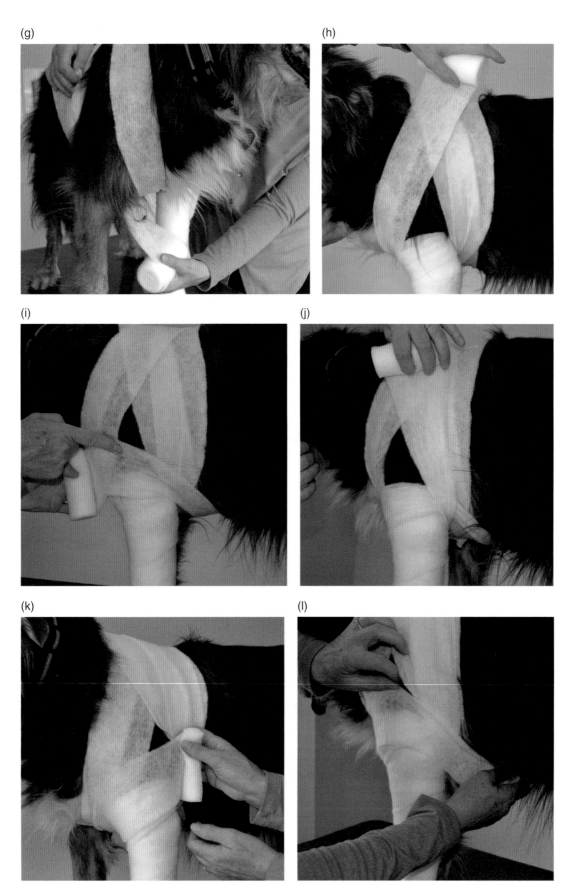

Figure 4.14 (Cont'd) This basic pattern creates the "cross your heart" portion of the bandage. It is repeated with the addition of an extra wrap around the affected shoulder to bind the limb to the body portion of the bandage. To achieve the shoulder wrap, the bandage material is continued as follows: from over the point of the shoulder (h), around the thorax, behind the far shoulder; placed around the near shoulder (i) and then continued over the back in front of the far shoulder (j), between the forelimbs, around the thorax by going behind the far shoulder and then forward between the forelimbs (as in d–g); the bandage material is placed around the affected shoulder (k–m).

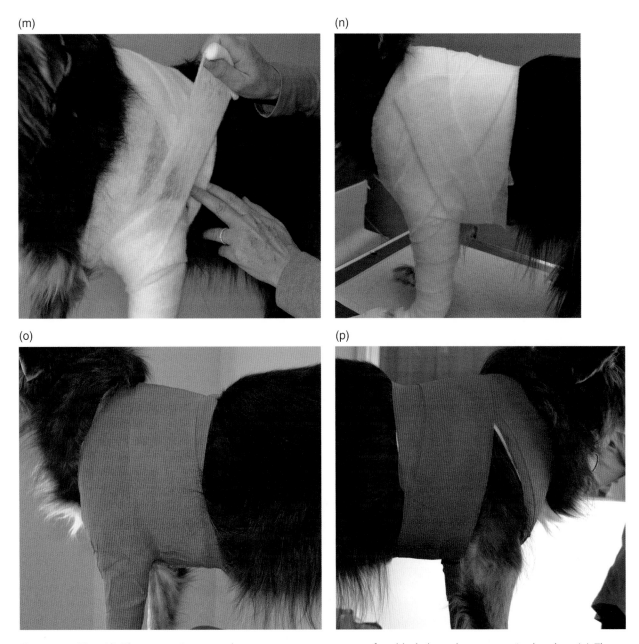

Figure 4.14 (Cont'd) The pattern is repeated as necessary to create a comfortable, balanced yet supportive bandage (n). The compressive and then protective layers are applied in the same manner (o–q). Should a splint be necessary, it is applied after the compressive layer and before the protective layer. (r and s) A commercially available splint. (t and u) A custom-made fiberglass splint being applied. It begins in the mid-metacarpal region, extends straight up the limb, and is curved over beyond the dorsal midline, taking on the shape of a "candy cane" (v). The distal portion of the splint can be molded in a palmar direction for a more comfortable fit. The antebrachium is elevated and supported in a natural standing position (w). A video of this bandage being applied is available at www. focusandflourish.com.

(q)

(r)

(s)

(t)

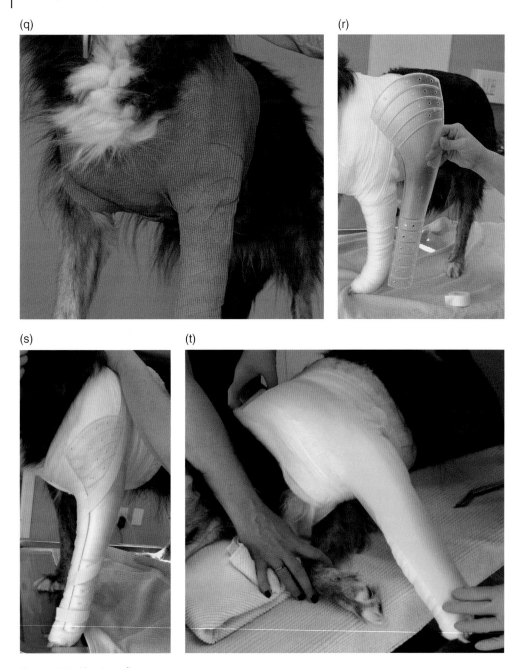

Figure 4.14 (Continued)

treatment with this "high" antebrachial bandage. The spica uses more bandage materials but tends to have lower morbidity and it better immobilizes the proximal radius/ulna/elbow area than the antebrachial bandage. As an example, a fracture of the proximal radius/ulna that is being treated conservatively might be placed in a spica splint for 4 weeks and then the distal antebrachial bandage including the elbow for 4 weeks could suffice.

A commercial metasplint or custom created fiberglass splint can be added to the bandage if increased support is necessary. The splint should extend to the point of the elbow and distally should include the paw. The metasplint is adjusted by cutting through the ridges using a heavy pair of scissors or a saw. The paw should be nicely cradled within the curve of the splint, extending just past the digital pads.

4.2.3.2 Antebrachial Bandage *Excluding* the Elbow (Figure 4.16)

This bandage or splint is indicated when the support is necessary for the distal radius/ulna in a midsize, or smaller, patient; an isolated mid- to distal ulnar fracture

(u)

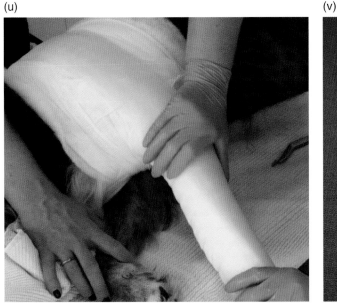

(v)

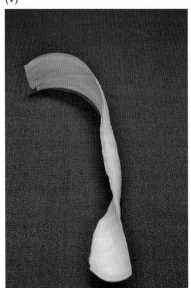

(w)

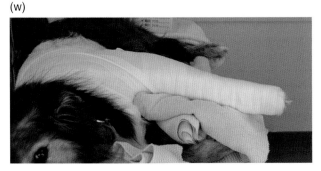

Figure 4.14 (Continued)

in a larger dog; or a carpal injury. The properly applied bandage/splint can offer adequate stability for these cases while significantly decreasing bandage morbidity.

This type of splinted bandage is frequently used in smaller patients. A tongue depressor can be used as a splint in the toy breed dogs, as it offers adequate stability but is lightweight. The splint should be cut down to the appropriate length, to just below the elbow joint. Distally, the splint may incorporate the paw or extend just below the carpus to allow the patient to walk on the paw, depending on the level of stability necessary.

4.2.4 Bandages for a Manus

A bandage that is applied to the paw to deal with a meta-carpal issue must include the carpus. When bandaging for a phalangeal issue, however, the carpus *can* be excluded; some clinicians feel that the bandage is more secure when the carpus is included. A bandage applied for a phalangeal

issue will need to cover the digits completely in order to be effective, making it impossible to visually monitor the toes. Owners will need to be instructed to use other indicators such as comfort, behavior, and smell.

Figure 4.17 has detailed information on how to apply a bandage to the manus for managing issues of the meta-carpal bones.

Figure 4.18 has detailed information on how to apply a bandage to the manus for phalangeal issues.

4.2.5 Carpal Flexion Sling

The purpose of the carpal flexion sling is to prevent the patient from weight bearing on the limb. It may be used in a variety of circumstances where weight bearing is undesirable but the limb does not require immobilization. For example, a reconstructed shoulder may need to be protected simply by preventing weight bearing. With the carpal flexion sling, passive range of motion exercises can also be performed on the joints of the limb if desired.

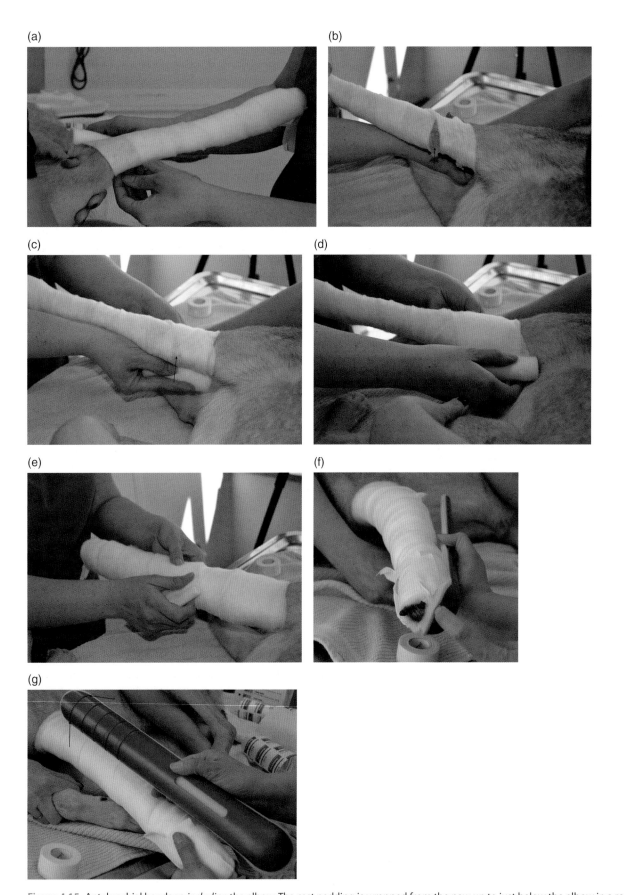

Figure 4.15 Antebrachial bandage *including* the elbow. The cast padding is wrapped from the paw up to just below the elbow in a routine manner (a); it is then pulled above the point of the elbow (arrow) and wrapped around the distal humeral area, as high into the axilla as possible (b). The material is then brought back down over the elbow to join the existing cast padding below the joint ((c) arrow indicates location of the point of the elbow). Several layers are applied around the elbow and just below it to help prevent slippage and to offer more support and padding at the elbow. The bandage material should be placed as high as possible into the axilla (d). Cast padding is added to the entire antebrachium to create a bandage of the desired and even thickness (e). The compressive (conforming gauze) and protective (cohesive bandage) layers are applied in the same manner. A splint can be added to the bandage. The paw should be cradled within the curve of the splint, extending just past the digital pads (f). The splint should extend to the proximal level of the olecranon; it is fitted by cutting through the ridges (appropriate cutting level for this patient indicated by arrows) using a heavy pair of scissors or a saw (g).

This type of sling maintains the carpus in flexion and therefore should not be used for more than 10–14 days.

Figure 4.19 has detailed information on how to apply a carpal flexion sling.

4.3 Hind Limb

4.3.1 Ehmer Sling

The Ehmer is a non-weight bearing sling that is ideal for maintaining a luxated coxofemoral joint in place after it has been reduced. The sling is applied in a manner such that the stifle is turned inward and the tarsus turned outward in order to help hold the femoral head within the acetabulum. The patient will likely already be under general anesthesia for a hip reduction procedure. If not, general anesthesia or heavy sedation is necessary to properly apply this sling. An Ehmer sling should not be left on the patient for more than 10–14 days.

Cats do not tolerate this sling very well at all; they tend to successfully maneuver themselves out of this sling. It may be better simply to place the cat in a crate to restrict its ability to move around and try to jump, for 2 weeks.

Figure 4.20 has detailed information on how to apply an Ehmer sling. It is best to use only white porous tape to apply this bandage. The cotton padding and Kling are omitted, and it is imperative not to use materials that are stretchy. Complications will occur with Ehmer slings that have been made with an elastic material such as a conforming material (Kling), or a cohesive material (Vet Wrap or Elastoplast™).

Owners should be forewarned that sedation may be needed to remove the bandage, although products available that dissolve the glue of the white porous tape make removal easier.

4.3.2 Robert Jones Bandage

This bandage used to be very popular. It is used for temporary immobilization of a fractured limb (tibia or radius) and to help decrease swelling. The bandage can be cumbersome and difficult to apply. It is used less frequently today as a splinted soft padded bandage will often serve the same function and is easier to apply and less bulky for the patient.

Figure 4.21 has detailed information on how to apply a Robert Jones bandage. Cotton rolls are used to create this bandage, as cast padding rolls cannot adequately provide the necessary amount of stiffness. Stirrups must be used with this bandage in order to keep the digits visible. The cotton padding is applied to the limb starting at the digits and moved proximally. The cotton sheets can be split in thickness and in width and rolled into strips to help ease the application. Once the cotton has been placed, the compressive layer (Kling) is applied with *a lot* of tension. Finally the protective (Vet Wrap) layer is applied. When done the bandage is quite large, firm and should emit a hollow sound (like a ripe watermelon) when pinged.

4.3.3 Crural and Tarsal Bandages

This is a versatile and commonly used hind limb bandage. It is easily adapted to being a splinted bandage. The hind limb bandage can be difficult to apply to because of its shape, especially in the small, chondrodystrophic dogs. This bandage or splint can be used for some stifle issues, and problems along the tibia or in the hock joint.

The bandage can be created to include or exclude the stifle joint. However, the bandage is better tolerated by the patient and has less morbidity if it does not include the stifle. Therefore, careful considerations should be given as to the purpose of the bandage/splint before deciding how to apply.

4.3.3.1 Bandage to *Include* the Stifle (Figure 4.22)
If the support is necessary for a mid- to proximal tibial fracture in any patient, and a more distally located fracture of the tibia in a larger breed dog (such as a Labrador), then a full bandage, including the stifle, should be applied. The bandage often slips down to the level of the stifle, causing it not to function as well; it can cause skin lesions along the caudal surface of the stifle area and on the patella. Good bandage monitoring practice is essential to ensure that the bandage fulfills its function and does not injure the patient.

A commercially available hind limb splint can be used. These are applied to the lateral aspect of the limb and placed between the compressive and protective layers of the bandage. Alternatively, a custom-made lateral fiberglass splint can be used. The fiberglass splints can be heavy especially for the smaller patients.

4.3.3.2 Bandage to *Exclude* the Stifle (Figure 4.23)
If the support is necessary for a distal tibia fracture in a midsize to small patient, or for a tarsal injury, then the stifle can be excluded. The properly applied bandage/splint can offer adequate stability for these cases while significantly decreasing bandage morbidity.

A commercially available hind limb splint can be used. These are applied to the lateral aspect of the limb and placed between the compressive and protective layers of the bandage. It must be cut down to size and the sharp edges filed down and covered with tape so as not to injure the patient. Alternatively, a custom-made lateral fiberglass can be used. The fiberglass splints can be heavy, especially for the

(a)

(b)

(c)

(d)

(e)

(f)

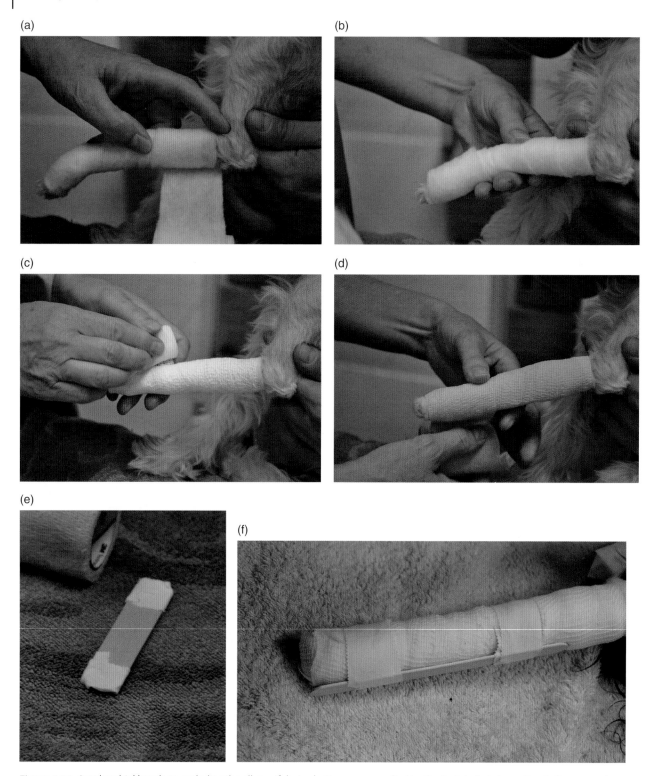

Figure 4.16 Antebrachial bandage *excluding* the elbow. If desired, stirrups are applied to the limb to help keep the digits exposed. The cast padding is wrapped from the paw up to just below the elbow and back down. (a and b) Cast padding is added to the desired thickness. The compressive (conforming gauze) and then protective (cohesive bandage) layers are applied in the same manner (c and d). A tongue depressor can be used as a splint in the small patients; it should be cut to the appropriate length and the ends covered to prevent injury to the patient (e). Distally, the splint may incorporate the paw (f) or extend just below the carpus to allow the patient to walk on the paw (g), depending on the amount of stability necessary. The splint is taped onto the compressive (conforming gauze) layer and then the final, protective layer is applied to the bandage (h).

(g)　　　　　　　　　　　　　　　(h)

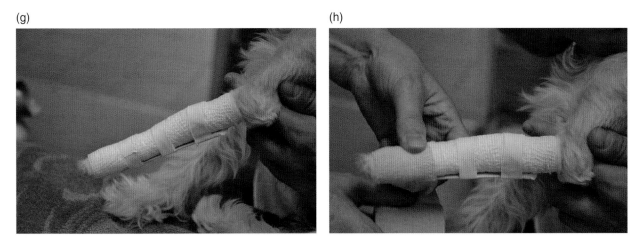

Figure 4.16 (Continued)

(a)　　　　　　　　　　　　　　　(b)

(c)　　　　　　　　　　　　　　　(d)

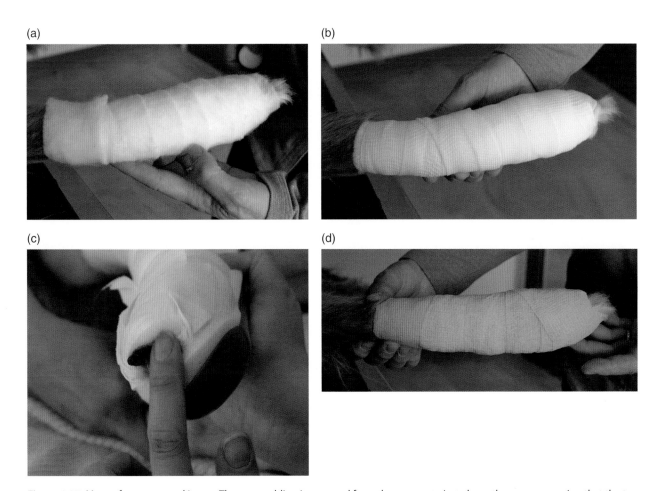

Figure 4.17 Manus for metacarpal issues. The cast padding is wrapped from the paw up to just above the carpus ensuring that the two central digits are exposed (a). The compressive layer (conforming gauze) is applied (b). If a splint is necessary, it is applied here and should cradle the digits (c). The protective (cohesive bandage) layer is then applied (d).

(a)

(b)

(c)

(d)

(e)

(f)

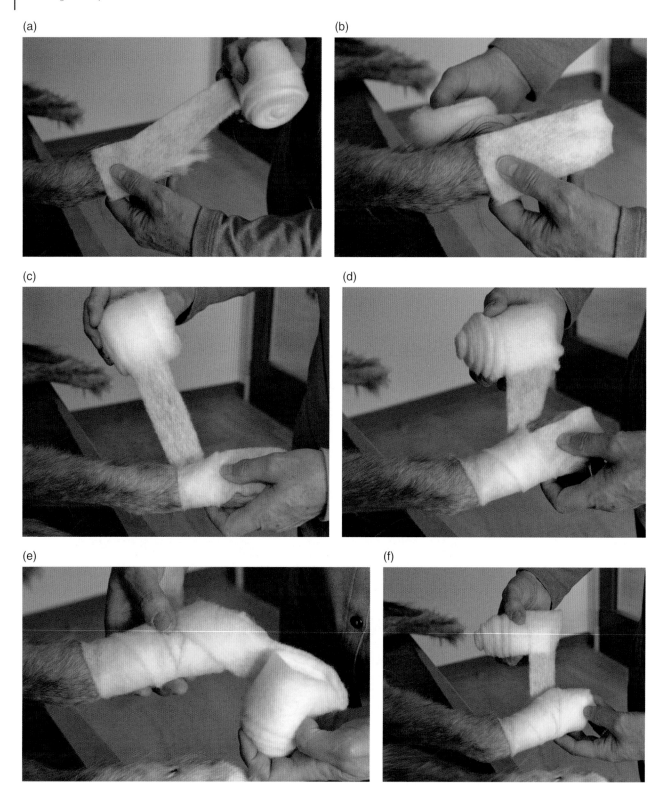

Figure 4.18 Manus for phalangeal issues. The leading edge of the cast padding is placed over the dorsum of the paw, starting distal to the carpus (a). The cast padding is then brought distally to cover the digits and back up along the palmar surface (b). It is then wrapped around the paw, at its proximal-most edge and the wraps are continued distally (c and d). To adequately cover the digits, the bandage material is made to criss-cross over the medial, lateral, and central aspects of the paw (e–i), and then back up to the proximal edge of the bandage (j). The compressive layer is applied in the same fashion (k–m) followed by the protective layer (n and o).

(g)

(h)

(i)

(j)

(k)

(l)

(m)

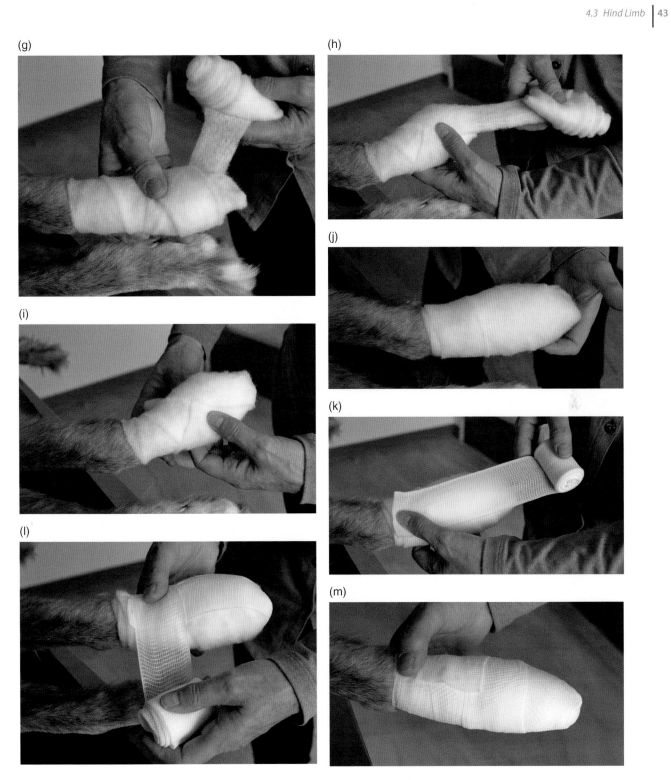

Figure 4.18 (Continued)

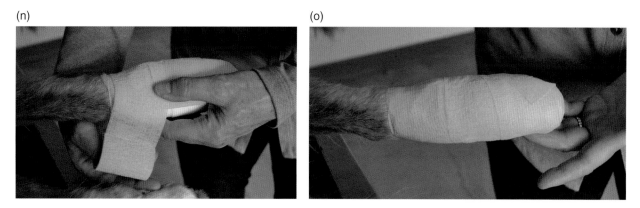

Figure 4.18 (Continued)

(a)

(b)

(c)

(d)

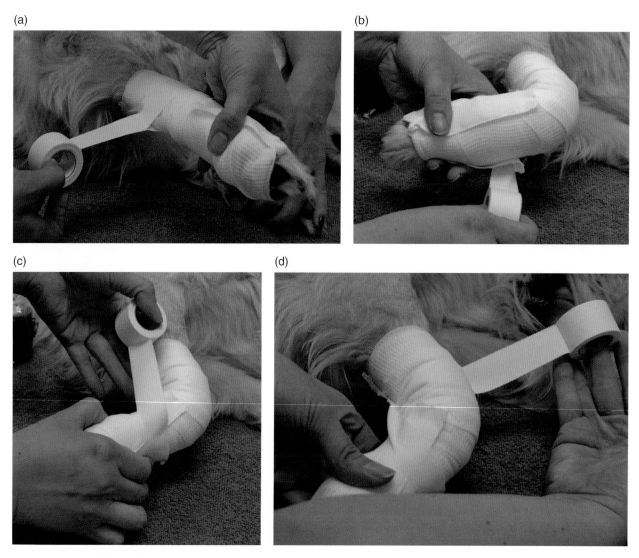

Figure 4.19 Carpal flexion sling. The tape can be applied directly on the skin or a light covering of cast padding and conforming gauze, or a stockinette, can be applied to the limb to protect the skin first. A loop of tape is placed around the distal third of the antebrachium (a). The carpus is then placed in flexion; the tape is turned to loop across the mid-metacarpal area (b and c); twisted again and brought back around the antebrachium, above or on the initial loop (d). Again the tape is twisted and brought distally around the metacarpal area, on or close to the previous loop (e). The tape is applied in this figure-8 fashion between the metacarpal and antebrachial areas, preferably moving further proximally and distally with every loop created, causing the tension to be distributed over a greater area (f and g). For added security, the tape is made to encircle the paw (h and i). A protective layer can be added to help keep the bandage clean and dry (j). No tension is created when applying the protective layer.

(e)

(f)

(g)

(h)

(i)

(j)

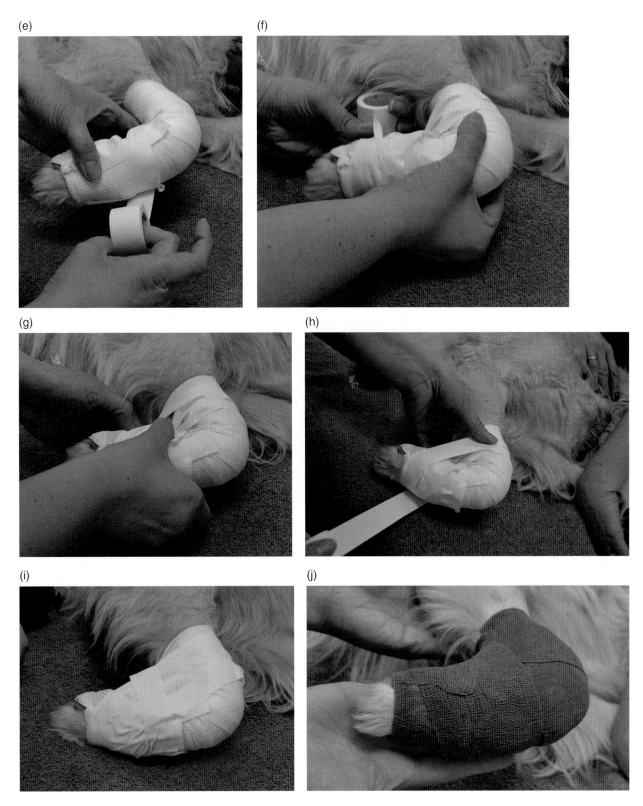

Figure 4.19 (Continued)

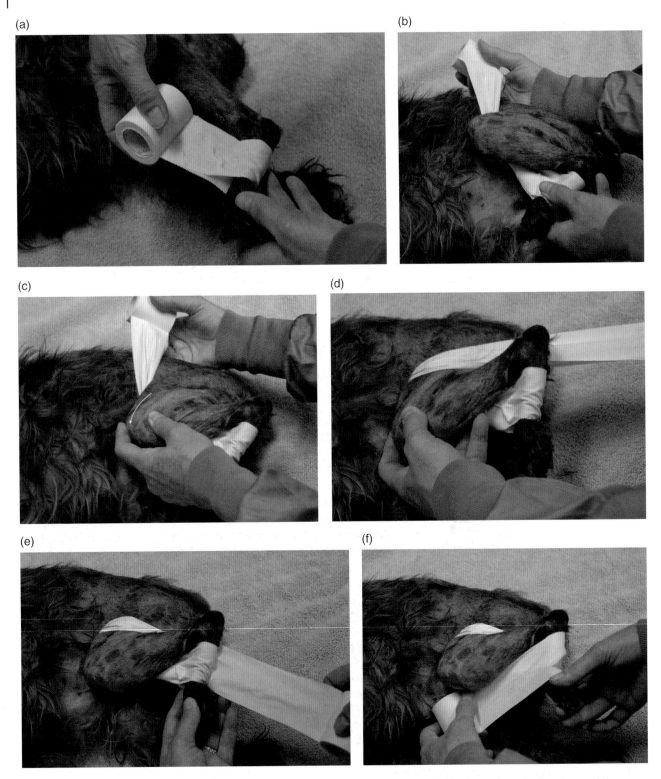

Figure 4.20 The Ehmer sling: Wide white porous tape is used for this bandage. A non-constrictive loop of tape is placed around the metatarsals (a). The hock and stifle are placed into flexion and the tape is pulled along the medial aspect of the thigh, high up into the groin (b). The skin is "pulled distally" toward the stifle (c) before the tape is brought back down onto the lateral aspect of the thigh (d); a slight twist is then placed in the tape in order to keep the adhesive side against the patient's limb while bringing it down medial to the hock (e), covering the initial loop that was placed on the metatarsals (f). Another twist is placed in the tape to extend it back up the medial aspect of the thigh (g). This loop of taping is repeated one to two more times (h). It is important to ensure that strands of hair or folds of skin from the abdomen or groin area are not tethered to the tape. To see a video on how to apply an Ehmer sling go to www.focusandflourish.com.

(g)

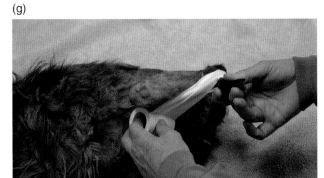

(h)

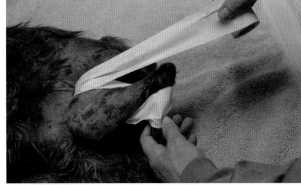

Figure 4.20 (Continued)

smaller patients, so careful consideration is important when choosing.

4.3.4 Bandages for a Pes

For an injury to the hind paw at the level of the metatarsals, the bandage or splinted bandage should extend to the level of the proximal calcaneus. A bandage applied for a phalangeal issue will cover the toes completely in order to be effective, and need only extend to the area just distal to the hock joint. Owners will be unable to visually monitor the toes and will need to use other indicators such as comfort, behavior, and smell. If increased stability is needed, a metasplint can be added within the bandage along the plantar aspect of the paw to the proximal calcaneus; a tongue depressor may be sufficient in the toy breeds.

Figure 4.24 has detailed information on how to apply a bandage to the pes for managing issues of the metatarsal bones.

Figure 4.25 has detailed information on how to apply a bandage to the pes for phalangeal issues.

4.3.5 Robinson and 90-90 Slings

These slings are used to prevent a patient from weight bearing on a hind limb. There are not many indications for these types of slings but perhaps a dog with a complex femoral fracture and a difficult repair might benefit from this sling. It is a personal preference whether to apply a Robinson or 90-90 sling to prevent a patient from weight bearing. Like the Ehmer sling, the 90-90 tends not to work well on cats as it falls off the stifle too easily. It is likely best to simply confine a cat to a large crate in order to restrict its usage of the limb.

Figure 4.26 has detailed information on how to apply a 90-90 sling.

Figure 4.27 has detailed information on how to apply a Robinson sling.

4.4 Bandage Care

4.4.1 Home Care Instructions

The bandage should be monitored carefully. The owners should be asked to examine (look, touch, and smell) the bandage at least twice per day. Should any of the following concerns be detected, then the patient should be brought back for bandage evaluation and probable change:

- Slipping of the bandage/splint.
- Wetness of the bandage.
- Swelling at the exposed digits. The owners should be instructed to look for increased separation of the digits and moisture between the toes (Figure 4.28).
- Malodorous smell (including urine).
- Evidence of chewing (Figure 4.29).
- Evidence of discomfort (pet stops using the limb, chews excessively, is depressed).

(a)

(b)

(c)

(d)

(e)

(f)

(g)

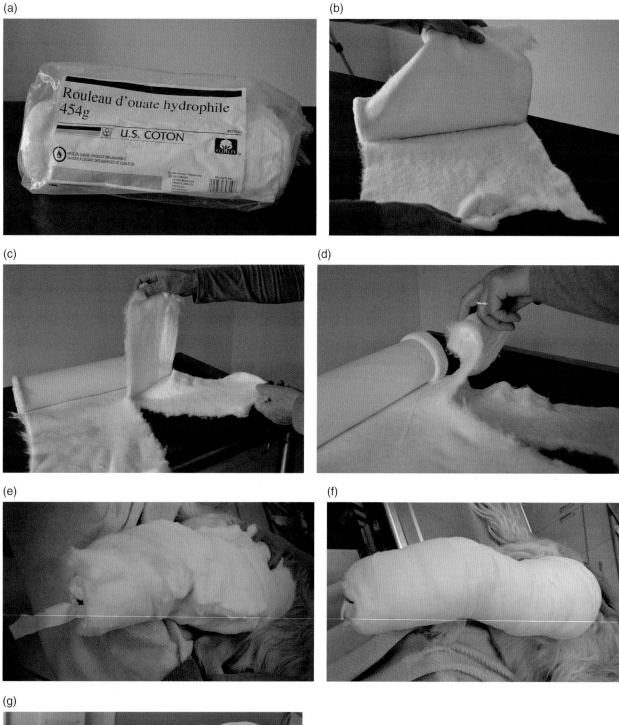

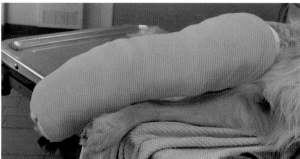

Figure 4.21 The Robert Jones bandage. A roll of cotton (a) is used to create this bandage as cast padding rolls cannot adequately provide the same amount of stiffness. To make the cotton easier to handle, it can be split in thickness by simply "peeling" half of it up (b); if desired it can also be torn into more manageable strips that are then rolled up for easy application (c and d). Stirrups must be used with this bandage in order to keep the digits visible. The cotton padding is applied to the limb starting at the digits and moved proximally (e). The compressive layer is then applied with a lot of tension (f). Finally, the protective layer is applied (g).

(a)

(b)

(c)

(d)

(e)

(f)

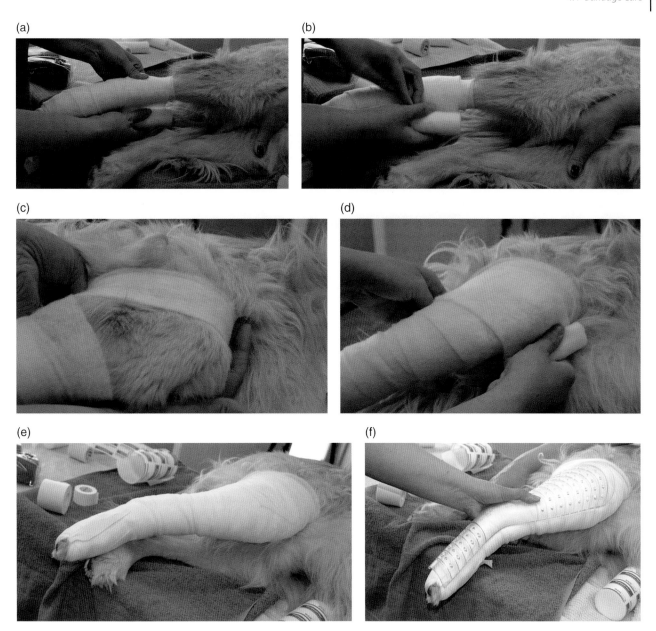

Figure 4.22 Hind limb bandage *including* the stifle. If desired, stirrups can be applied to the medial and lateral surfaces of the paw. The cast padding material is started at the paw and moved in a proximal direction (a). It can be helpful to add extra padding over the "skinnier" mid- to distal tibial area, helping to even out the circumference of the shank; the extra padding can help to prevent the bandage from slipping down below the stifle (b). Once the bandage material reaches the level of the tibial crest it is brought above the stifle joint (c), as high into the groin as possible, for a few wraps, and the material is brought back down over the stifle with the usual 50% overlap of the bandaging material (d). Cast padding is added until the bandage is of the desired and of even thickness. The compressive layer is then applied in the same manner (e). If desired, a commercially available hind limb splint is applied to the lateral aspect of the limb. (f) The splint is secured into place with adhesive tape and conforming gauze (g). The bandage is then finished with the addition of the protective layer (h).

(g)

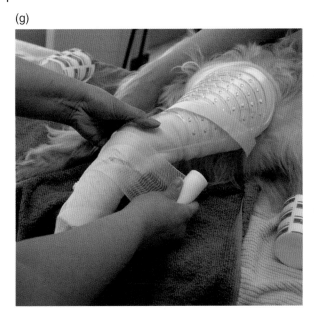

(h)

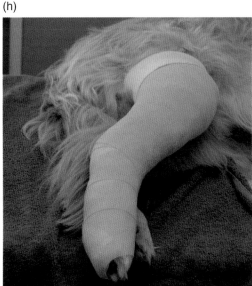

Figure 4.22 (Continued)

When the pet goes outside, the bandage should be protected from the wet environment with a plastic bag (an IV bag works well for this) and, preferably, a commercially available bandage protector (Figure 4.30).

Bandages/splints should be changed weekly; sooner if there is a problem. It is advisable to book the bandage appointments before the pet leaves the hospital. Any missed appointments and reminder phone calls should be noted in the patient's record. Owners must be made to understand that the regular and frequent bandage changes are important to help prevent the formation of serious complications. Once a problem occurs (decubital ulcers, severe dermatitis, necrosis of the digits or paw; malunion), it can be expensive and time-consuming to manage the issue.

4.4.2 Bandage Changes

- The bandage/splint should be changed weekly. If splinting for a fracture, some patients may need to be sedated for the first one or two bandage changes but are usually amenable to a bandage change without sedation subsequent to that.
- While removing the bandage, abnormalities such as urine stain or donut slippage should be noted and corrected.
- The limb should be thoroughly examined for signs of skin lesions and interdigital dermatitis. If these are noted, then measures can be taken to prevent them from becoming a problem. Donuts are applied where

necessary. The paws are washed with a chlorhexidine solution and the paw is allowed to dry before reapplying the bandage. A blow dryer can be used for this. Talcum powder can be sprinkled onto the paw and between the toes to help keep the areas dry. A little bit of cotton padding can also be inserted between the digits to help absorb moisture.
- The bandage/splint is reapplied.

4.4.3 Bandage/Splint Complications

Significant problems can be seen with poor bandage application and care. Below are some of the more common problems noted:

- Bandage is too loose and falls off.
- Bandage is too tight and digits swell; necrosis of the digits or paw occurs (Figure 4.31).
- More than two digits exposed allowing for poor venous return and the paw swelling (Figure 4.32).
- Inappropriate layering, typically conform is applied before cast padding, resulting in an ineffective and poorly fitting/compressed bandage. The Kling against the skin will also bunch up and be uncomfortable, leaving visible indentations in the skin (Figure 4.33).
- Urine-soaked bandages causing skin irritation (Figure 4.34).
- Conforming gauze applied beyond the level of the cast padding allowing inappropriate tension and potential lacerations in the skin to occur caused by the Kling

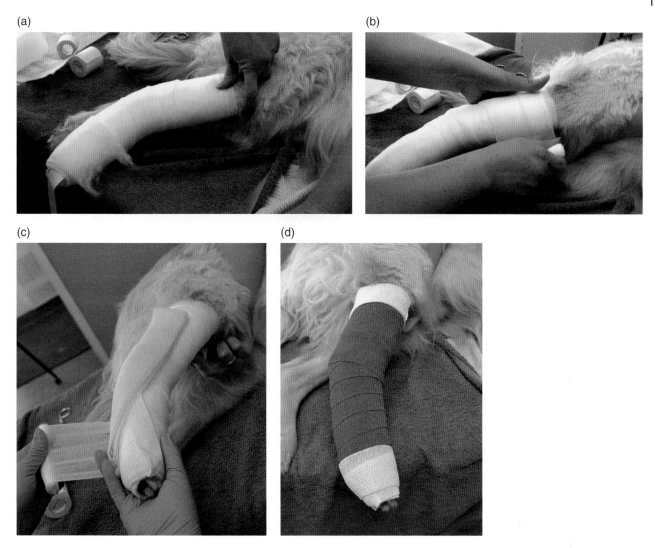

Figure 4.23 Hind limb bandage *excluding* the stifle. If desired, stirrups can be applied to the medial and lateral surfaces of the paw. The cast padding material is started at the paw and moved in a proximal direction to just below the tibial crest ((a) index finger indicates position of tibial crest). Cast padding is added until the bandage is of the desired and of even thickness. The compressive layer is then applied in same manner (b). A custom-made lateral fiberglass splint is applied (c) followed by the protective layer (d).

(especially seen when the bandage wraps around the thorax or abdomen).

- Splint placed within the incorrect layer, causing discomfort, uneven tension and often skin lesions (Figure 4.35).

- Decubital sores. These can be very difficult to treat (Figure 4.36).
- Tarsal bandage with a straight metasplint (Figure 4.37).
- Bandaging/splinting of a femoral fracture (Figure 3.1).

(a)

(b)

(c)

(d)

(e)

(f)

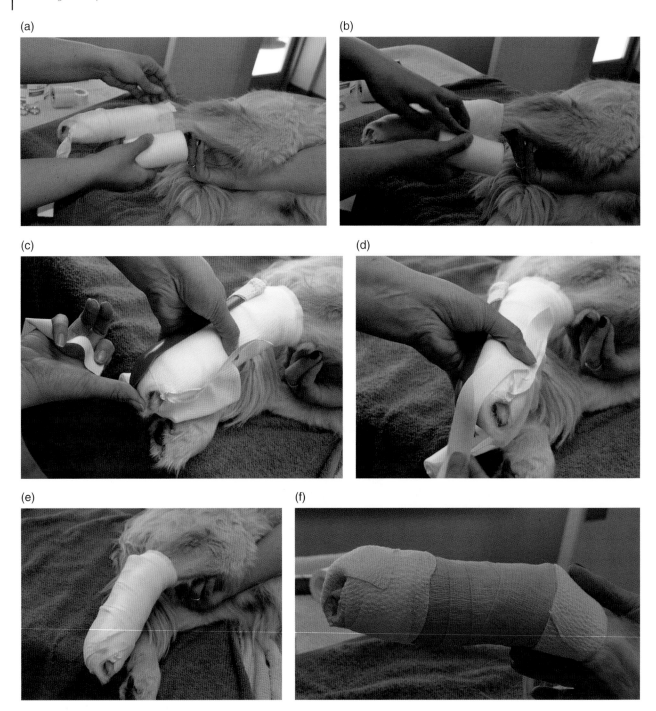

Figure 4.24 Pes for metatarsal concerns. The bandage should extend to the proximal calcaneus area with some padding extending just proximal to that level to ensure that the skin is protected from the splint (a and b). The compressive layer is applied. Should a splint be necessary, it is fitted to the plantar aspect of the paw, ensuring that the digital pads are comfortably cradled within the metasplint (c). The splint is secured in place using adhesive tape (d) and then conforming gauze (e). The final protective layer is then applied (f).

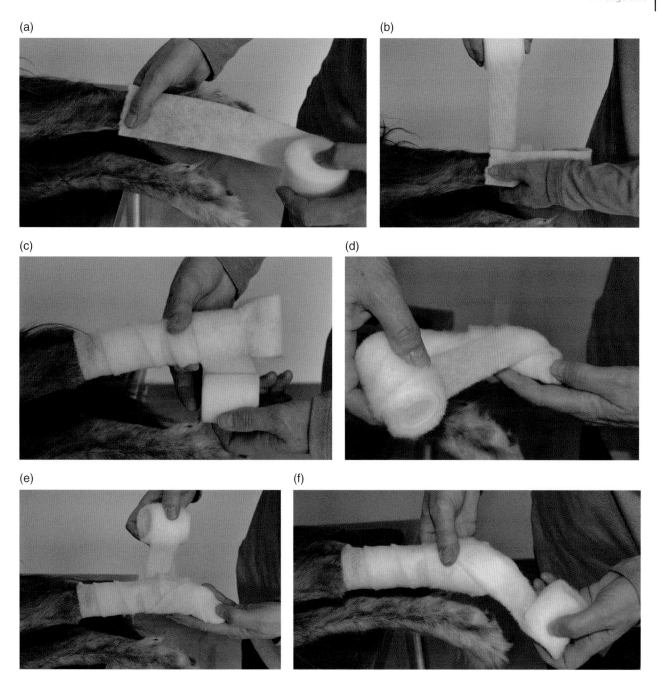

Figure 4.25 Pes for phalangeal issues. The leading edge of the cast padding is placed over the dorsum of the paw, starting distal to the tarsus (a); the cast padding is then brought distally to cover the digits and back up along the plantar surface and is then wrapped around the paw, at its proximal-most edge (b) and the wraps are continued distally (c). To adequately cover the digits, the bandage material is made to criss-cross over the medial, lateral, and central aspects of the paw (d–h) and then back up to the proximal edge of the bandage (i). The compressive layer is applied in the same fashion (j) followed by the protective layer (k and l).

(g)   (h)

(i)   (j)

(k)   (l)

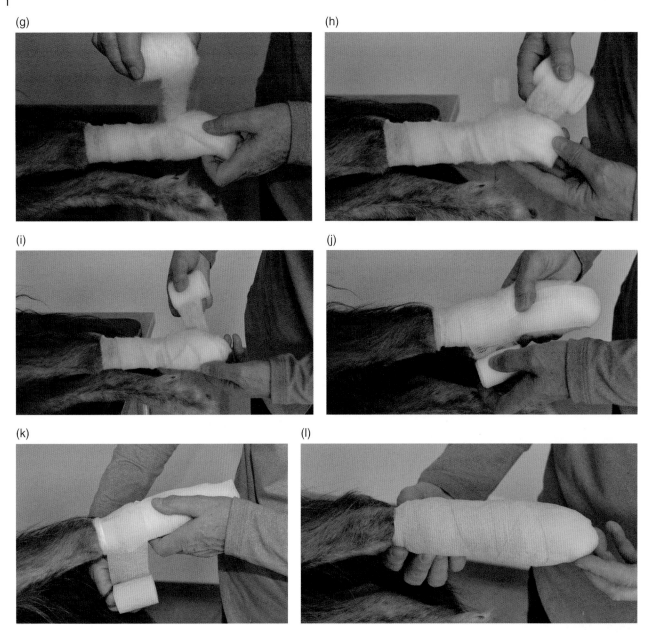

Figure 4.25 (Continued)

(a)

(b)

(c)

(d)

(e)

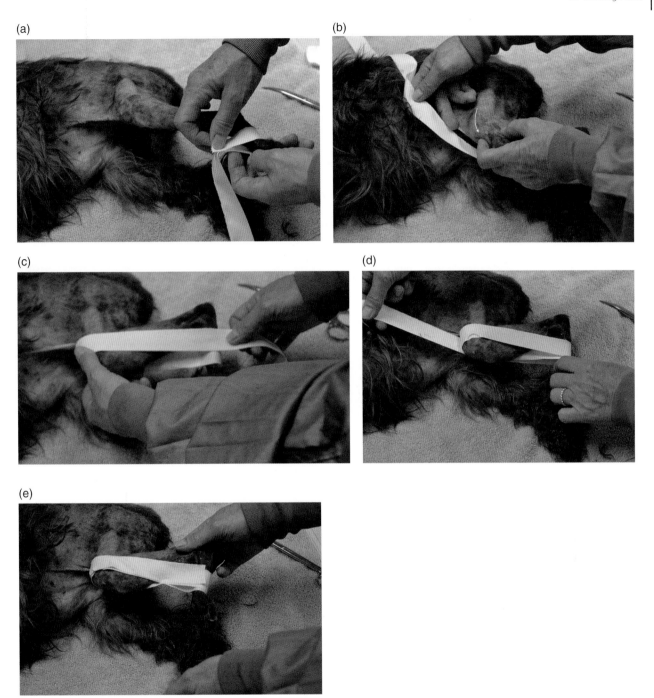

Figure 4.26 The 90-90 sling. It is best to use adhesive porous tape and to avoid any type of stretchy bandaging material. A loop of tape is placed around the metatarsals, and the tape is "stuck to itself" creating a non-compressive loop or sling for the paw (a). This loop is placed so that the tape is poised to be pulled up the medial aspect of the limb. The hock and stifle are each positioned at 90° of flexion. The tape is then brought up the medial aspect of the limb and up around the mid-femur area, while pulling the skin of the thigh toward the stifle to help prevent the tape from sliding off the stifle (b). The tape is brought back down the lateral side back to the metatarsals (c). This loop (metatarsals around the mid-femur and back down to metatarsals) is repeated (d and e). The sling should be "tested" by trying to slide it off the stifle before recovering the patient from anesthesia.

(a)

(b)

(c)

(d)

(e)

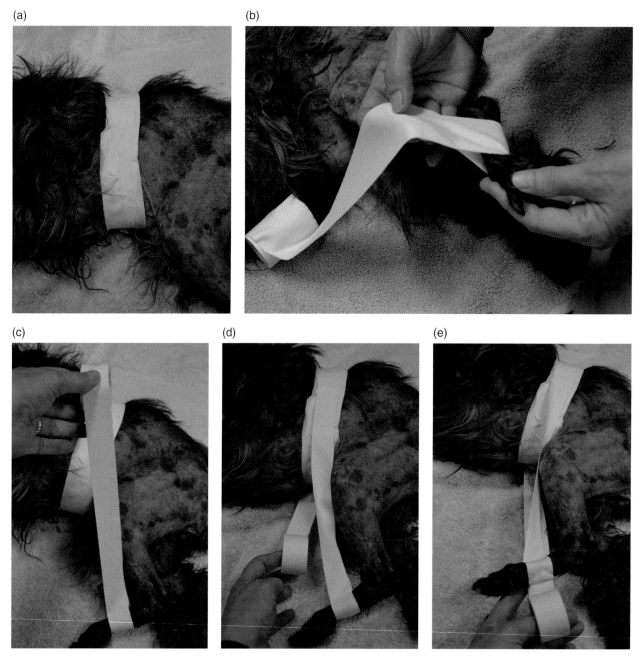

Figure 4.27 The Robinson sling. Two to three loops of tape are placed around the abdomen (a). A non-compressive loop or sling is placed around the metatarsal area (b). This loop is placed so that the tape is poised to be pulled up the lateral aspect of the limb. The tape is then brought up toward the tape on the abdomen, while the paw is held at the desired height off the ground (c). The tape is continued over the dorsum and around the far side of the abdomen, over the existing tape, and back down to the metatarsals (d and e). The loop is repeated at least one more time to add strength to the sling. An extra strip of tape is used to bind the two long straps together (f–h).

(f)

(g)

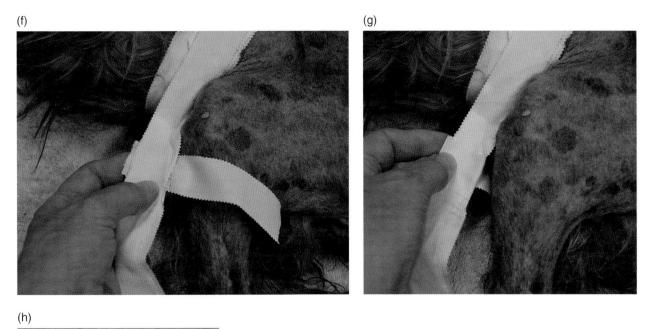

(h)

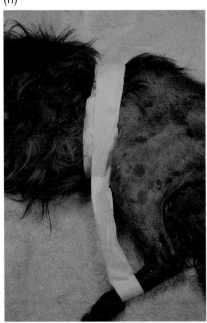

Figure 4.27 (Continued)

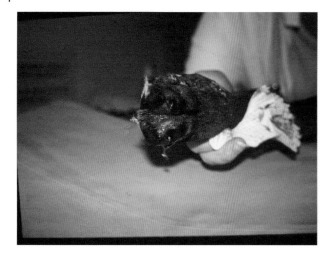

Figure 4.28 The bandage was appropriately positioned but applied too tightly causing swelling of the two central digits. The separation of digits and interdigital moistness are evident. The swelling regressed completely within an hour of removing the bandage.

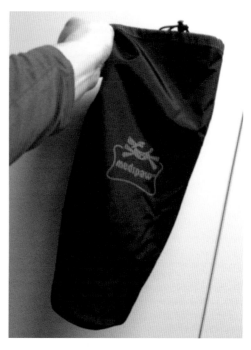

Figure 4.30 An example of a commercially available bandage protector.

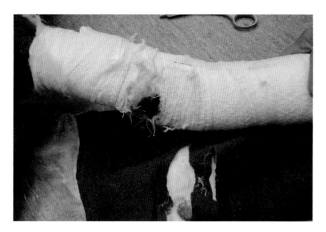

Figure 4.29 The patient had been chewing at the bandage for 2 days. The bandage had just been reapplied 5 days prior. The patient had not chewed the previous bandages. He was clearly uncomfortable with this one.

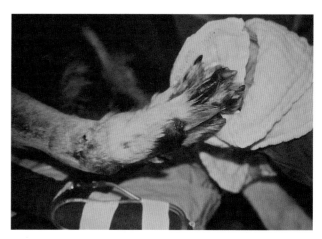

Figure 4.31 This limb was amputated because of poor bandage management. The bandage was too tight and the owners failed to return for bandage changes despite multiple phone calls. The limb would likely not have been so necrotic if a timely bandage change had occurred.

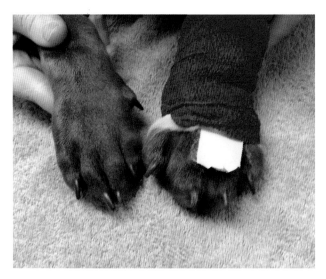

Figure 4.32 This patient has more than the two central digits protruding from the bandage, which resulted in swelling.

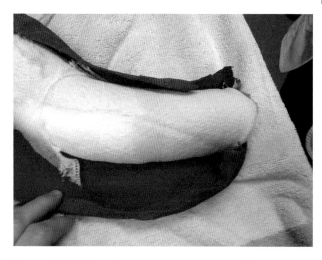

Figure 4.34 This bandage was not wet to the touch but was clearly urine-soaked. This is not uncommon in male dogs.

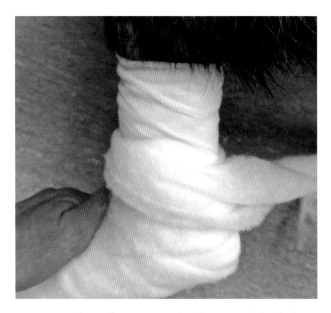

Figure 4.33 The conforming gauze bandage was applied before the cast padding, resulting in an ineffective, uncomfortable bandage.

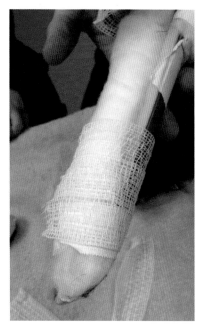

Figure 4.35 The splint was placed between the cast padding and conforming gauze bandage layers. The cast padding became unevenly and inappropriately compressed and the splint has markedly slipped.

(b)

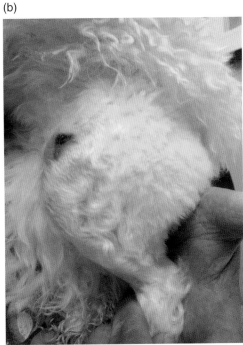

(a)

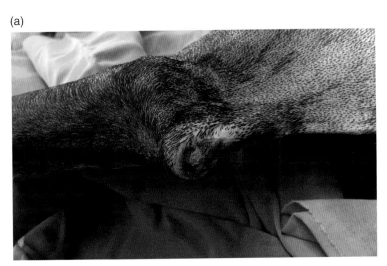

Figure 4.36 A decubital ulcer has developed on the olecranon (a). This patient had an antebrachial bandage that included the elbow. A decubital sore was noted on this patient's stifle after removal of a crural bandage that included the stifle (b).

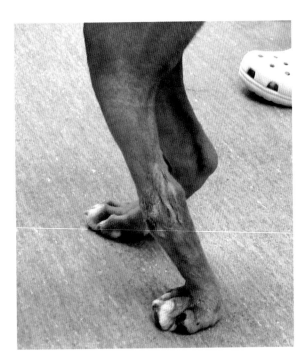

Figure 4.37 This young dog was placed in a straight splint for 1 week, for a tarsal injury. Fortunately he returned to normal after a few weeks of rehabilitation.

Reference

1 Swaim, S.T., Renberg, W.C., and Shike, K.M. (2011). *Small Animal Bandaging, Casting and Splinting Techniques.* Oxford: Wiley-Blackwell.

Section 2

The Forequarter

5

Mandible and Maxilla
Teresa Jacobson

Sitara Animal Hospital, Lake Country, British Columbia, Canada

An anatomical review of the mandible and maxilla is available in Chapter 24, Figures 24.1, 24.2, and 24.3.

5.1 Mandibular Fractures

Mandibular fractures require repair if they are causing a malocclusion or if they are unstable [1]. From the symphysis to the canine teeth of the mandible is the most common area to be affected in the cat. Fractures of the mandibular body from the canine to the angle of the mandible are the most common oral fractures in the dog [2].

When there is a fracture of the mandible there is often a deviation of the mandible to the side of the fracture due to the abnormal alignment of the dental arcade. Deviation of the mandible or a "dropped jaw" appearance is also seen in rostrodorsal luxation of the temporomandibular joint (TMJ). A thorough oral examination of the patient under general anesthesia should be performed as a foreign body may also result in an inability to close the mouth.

5.1.1 Mandibular Symphyseal Separation

This is most often a ligamentous injury in cats (Figure 5.1) and the displacement is often minimal if it is the only injury. Patients present with an occlusal abnormality that is most noticeable with the mandibular canine teeth. The symphysis may be separated with no apparent break in the soft tissues. It can also be separated with obvious laceration to the soft tissues or with tissue trauma and communication with bone [2]. Fractured teeth are not an uncommon presentation with symphyseal separation [2].

Treatment of choice: This separation is best repaired with mandibular symphyseal wiring (Figure 5.2). This technique can be performed by a general practitioner and does not require specialized equipment or advanced training. Chapter 24 has further details.

Postoperative management: After surgery, most cats do not require a feeding tube if this is their only lesion and will usually eat immediately after surgery. The wire may be removed in 3 weeks as this is essentially a sprain. Stabilization for longer (i.e. 6 weeks) is necessary for a fracture repair.

Prognosis: Complications can occur if the wire is too tight: there will be excessive swelling of the soft tissues around the wire. This is a ligamentous injury and requires support not rigid stabilization. Also if the jaw has not been carefully aligned, it will heal abnormally causing a malocclusion. The prognosis for these patients is very good to excellent.

5.1.2 Rostral Mandibular Fractures

Rostral mandibular fractures often occur near or through the alveolus of a mandibular canine (Figure 5.3).

Treatment of choice: The mandibular canine tooth in a rostral mandibular fracture should not be removed unless it is periodontally affected. The mandibular canine tooth is a strategic anchor for the fracture repair (Figure 5.4). These can be repaired with interdental wiring using the Ivy loop or Stout loop techniques reinforced with an acrylic splint (Figures 5.5 and 5.6). Some patients with severe bone loss secondary to periodontal disease may not heal well. Sometimes a fibrous union in a small dog or cat is sufficient to provide stability for comfort and function. Teeth that are periodontally affected must be removed before the fracture repair is attempted. The teeth need to be monitored and endodontically treated if so indicated.

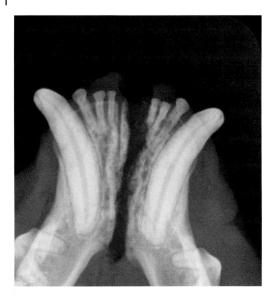

Figure 5.1 Symphyseal separation with rostral mandibular fracture between 301 and the symphysis.

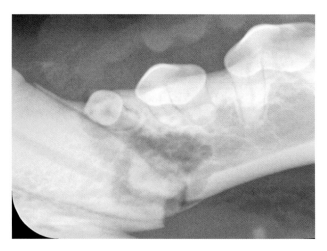

Figure 5.3 A minimally displaced rostral mandibular fracture involving teeth 304 and 305.

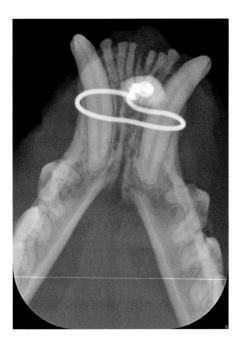

Figure 5.2 Mandibular symphyseal wiring to realign the mandible into normal occlusion.

Postoperative management: The patient should be fed a gruel or soft food, if an esophageal feeding tube has not been placed, until the fracture has healed. Chew toys should also be avoided. The patient's mouth should be rinsed with saline twice daily to keep the repair site clean. The implants can be removed once the fracture has healed (approximately 8 weeks).

Prognosis: The prognosis for the repair of an acute traumatic fracture is very good; however, patients with pathological fractures secondary to periodontal disease may not do as well due to the extensive bone loss.

5.1.3 Fracture at the Level of the Mandibular First Molar

Fractures at or just mesial or distal to the first molar are often due to trauma or periodontal disease (Figure 5.7). These fractures are especially challenging when they are pathological due to the severe lack of bone remaining in the mandible associated with periodontal disease.

Treatment of choice: These fractures are best left to a trained dental surgeon. When referral is not an option an inter-fragmentary wire can be used to stabilize the alveolar border (the tension side) of the mandibular fracture. Addition of interdental wiring using the Stout technique reinforced with acrylic can also be used to stabilize these fractures. The wire and acrylic reinforcement must extend across the arcade to the canine tooth on the opposite side of the fracture site in order to provide adequate fracture stability. Pathological fractures benefit from the placement of bone grafts and are best left in the hands of a dental specialist.

Postoperative management: Postoperatively the patient has restricted use of the jaw by eliminating any objects other than soft food.

Prognosis: The prognosis depends on the stability of the fracture repair and the amount of bone remaining in the mandible. Pathological fractures secondary to periodontal disease do not do as well due to the extensive bone loss and often benefit from bone grafts.

(a)

(b)

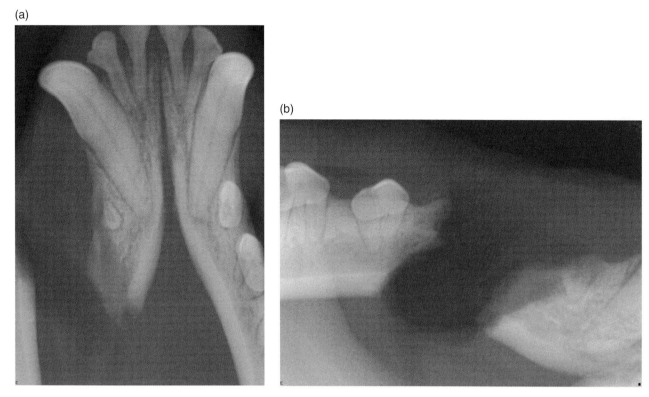

Figure 5.4 Intraoral ventral to lingual (a) and lateral (b) radiographic views of a displaced fracture of the rostral mandible between teeth 405 and 406.

(a)

(b)

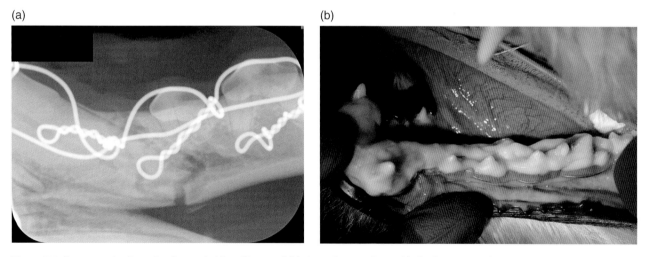

Figure 5.5 Postoperative lateral radiograph (a) and intraoral (b) view of a rostral mandibular fracture involving teeth 304 and 305 repaired using a Stout wire technique reinforced with acrylic. The wire and acrylic extend to the canine on the opposite side of the rostral mandibular fracture. There is a minimal amount of acrylic on the buccal side of the teeth distal to the mandibular first molar.

5.1.4 Temporomandibular Luxation

Patients with a TMJ luxation present with a dropped jaw appearance and an inability to properly close their mouth. When the TMJ luxates it is usually unilateral and in a rostrodorsal direction (Figures 5.8 and 5.9). The jaw appears dropped on the opposite side of the TMJ luxation. When the jaw is fractured, it drops on the same side as the fracture site. Rarely, the TMJ can luxate in a caudoventral direction. The prognosis for a caudoventral luxation is more serious as the retroarticular process is often fractured in this type of luxation.

Treatment of choice: TMJ luxation is reduced or closed by using a wooden dowel (a soft HB pencil works well). The pencil is placed into the mouth in the caudal-most

(a)

(b)

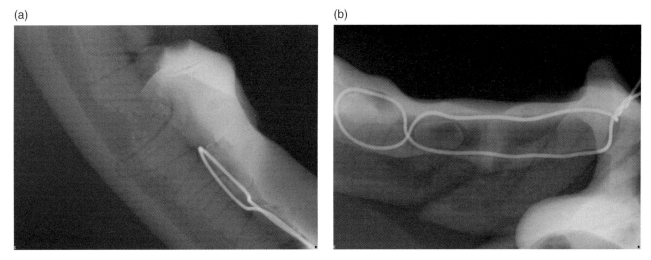

(c)

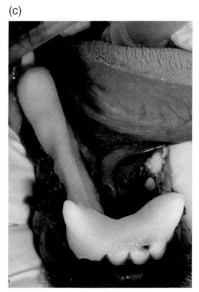

Figure 5.6 Lateral radiographs of the repair of a displaced fracture of the mandible between teeth 405 and 406 using interdental wiring and reinforced with acrylic extending two teeth distal to the fracture line (a). The right intraoral lateral oblique radiograph (b) and intraoral view (c) of the repair show the interdental wiring reinforced with acrylic and extending to and incorporating the opposite canine. It is important to include the contralateral canine to get suitable stability of the fracture site.

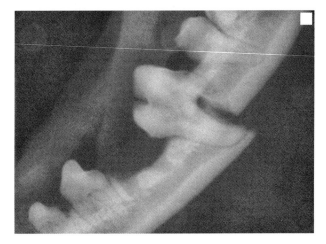

Figure 5.7 A left intraoral parallel lateral radiograph of an iatrogenic fracture of the left mandible that occurred during an extraction attempt of tooth 309.

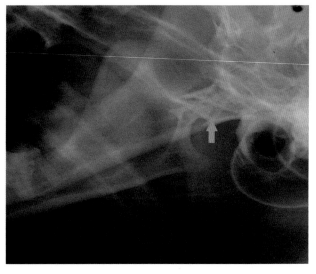

Figure 5.8 Radiograph of the left temporomandibular joint (TMJ) in its normal position (blue arrow), the mandibular condyle is in the mandibular fossa. *Source:* Used with permission of Loic Legendre DVM, DAVDC.

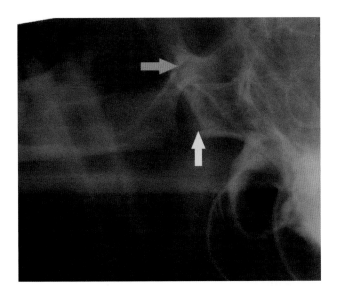

Figure 5.9 Radiograph of the right temporomandibular joint (TMJ) luxated in a rostral dorsal direction. Rostral dorsal displacement of the mandibular condyle (blue arrow), and the mandibular fossa (yellow arrow). *Source:* Used with permission of Loic Legendre DVM, DAVDC.

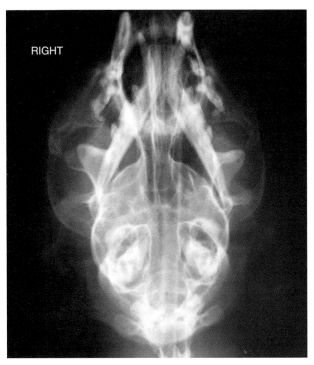

Figure 5.10 Radiograph of the right temporomandibular joint (TMJ) luxated in a rostral dorsal direction. The deviation of the mandible is opposite to the side of the dislocation. *Source:* Used with permission of Loic Legendre DVM, DAVDC.

aspect of the mouth on the dislocated side and then the jaw is closed, this will force the mandibular condyle back into its normal position. If necessary, the mandible is pulled slightly rostral on the side of the luxation to allow the articular eminence to clear the edge of the mandibular fossa. The mandible is then firmly and gently pushed caudally while turning it in a counter-clockwise motion to reduce the condyle into the mandibular fossa. This will allow reduction of the TMJ luxation.

Postreduction management: Postreduction radiographs must always be obtained (Figures 5.10 and 5.11). If the patient has concurrent mandibular fractures, then bonding of the canines is necessary to keep the TMJ joint reduced. If the canines need to be bonded to maintain occlusion, then a feeding tube should be placed in case the patient does not eat well during the first few days of recovery.

Prognosis: The prognosis is excellent with complete reduction and no caudal mandibular fractures or fractures of the retroarticular process. Immobilization of the TMJ joint for greater than 2–3 weeks will increase the risk of TMJ ankylosis, thus should be avoided. If the TMJ is not reducible, it may be because something else is fractured. Cases complicated with caudal mandibular fractures involving the TMJ are at high risk of TMJ ankylosis. Steroids such as prednisolone may be used in these cases for their catabolic effects in an attempt to decrease the likelihood of TMJ ankylosis. These cases are best handled by referral to a dental specialist.

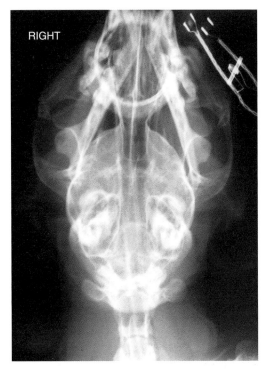

Figure 5.11 Postreduction radiograph of the right temporomandibular joint (TMJ) luxated in a rostral dorsal direction. There is no deviation of the mandible noted. *Source:* Used with permission of Loic Legendre DVM, DAVDC.

5.1.5 Other Mandibular Fractures

Fractures of the vertical ramus or below the condylar process are less common than fractures of the symphysis or the body of the mandible. They are often minimally displaced due to the enormous amount of musculature in the area. If non-displaced, they can be managed conservatively with a tape muzzle [2] (Chapter 24). If fractures are displaced or severely comminuted, referral should always be considered for the patient, as access to this area is difficult due to the amount of thick musculature involved.

A non-displaced fracture of the condylar process or fractures of the TMJ may be managed conservatively if all other fractures of the mandible are identified and stabilized [2]. Fractures in the TMJ area must be monitored carefully for ankylosis of the TMJ due to osteoarthritic changes during healing. This is a serious complication of fractures in this area and can be very painful. A non-functional TMJ will require a condylectomy to restore mobility and provide comfort for the patient [3]. A condylectomy is a procedure best left in the hands of a specialist due to the difficult access to this area.

5.2 Maxillary Fractures

5.2.1 Fracture and/or Avulsion of the Incisive Bone

Rostral maxillary fractures or avulsions of the incisive bone often occur near or through the alveolus of a maxillary canine (Figure 5.12). The maxillary canine tooth in a rostral maxillary fracture should not be removed unless it is periodontally affected. The maxillary canine tooth is a strategic anchor for the fracture repair (Figure 5.13).

Treatment of choice: This type of fracture can be repaired with interdental wiring using the Ivy loop, the Stout loop, or a modified interdental wiring technique reinforced with acrylic.

Postoperative management: The patient should be fed a gruel or soft food, if an esophageal feeding tube has not been placed, until the fracture has healed. Chew toys should also be avoided. The patient's mouth should be rinsed with saline twice daily to keep the repair site clean. The implants can be removed once the fracture has healed (approximately 8 weeks).

Prognosis: The prognosis for patients treated in this manner is excellent (Figure 5.14). Some patients with severe bone loss secondary to periodontal disease may not heal well. Teeth that are periodontally affected must be removed before the fracture repair is attempted. The teeth need to be monitored and endodontically treated if so indicated.

Patients with avulsed teeth, or fractures with necrotic bone may need aggressive debriding and require a partial removal of the rostral maxilla (Figure 5.15). Partial maxillectomy is a viable option when financial constraints are present or when patient/owner compliance is impossible. Amputation of part of the rostral maxilla is a preferred option rather than euthanasia (Figure 5.16). Patients do well postoperatively with a partial rostral maxillectomy (Figure 5.17).

5.2.2 Fractures of the Maxillary Bone

Fractures of the maxilla occur less frequently than fractures of the mandible. Maxillary fractures often present with a history of trauma and clinical signs of epistaxis, facial deformity, malocclusion, and patient discomfort. Maxillary fractures require repair if they cause a malocclusion, are unstable, communicate with the oral cavity, cause facial deformities, or obstruct the nasal cavity [1]. If the fracture is minimally displaced they too can be managed conservatively with a tape or nylon muzzle (Chapter 24).

If the mandible and the maxilla are both fractured, the mandible should be addressed first as it is easier to repair and then the maxilla can be aligned to the mandible [4].

5.3 Managing Expectations

Appropriate pain management is very important. The patient should have soft food only for 6 weeks. Chew toys should not be allowed until the fracture has healed. Activity should be controlled, thus restricted to leash walks until the fracture has healed usually for a minimum of 6 weeks. Gentle daily rinsing of the appliances with 0.12% chlorhexidine and daily cleaning of the face and the hair around the head and neck should be implemented until the appliances are removed.

5.4 Alternatives When the Treatment of Choice is Not an Option

A tape muzzle can always be tried if referral to a specialist is not an option. A tape muzzle will not help in a TMJ luxation and should not be considered an option for this condition. Reduction of the TMJ is not difficult and should always be attempted by a general practitioner before euthanasia. Owners need to be

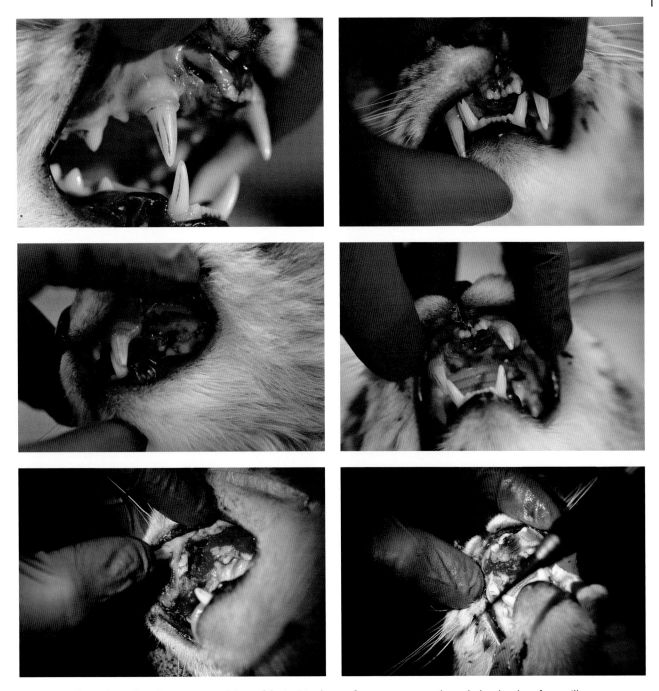

Figure 5.12 Rostral maxillary fractures or avulsions of the incisive bone often occur near or through the alveolus of a maxillary canine tooth.

encouraged to at least give a tape muzzle a try in cases of maxillofacial fractures if referral and more invasive repair techniques are not an option for the client. Chapter 24 contains tape muzzle instructions. If the patient cannot be managed by the client or if the patient cannot be cared for in a humane comfortable manner, then euthanasia may be considered an option for the patient.

5.5 Potential Complications of Maxillofacial Fracture Repair

- Soft tissue trauma.
- Iatrogenic trauma to tooth structures, soft tissues (e.g. the mandibular canal), and nasal sinuses.
- Malunion (may cause the patient to have a malocclusion, which may interfere with normal function).

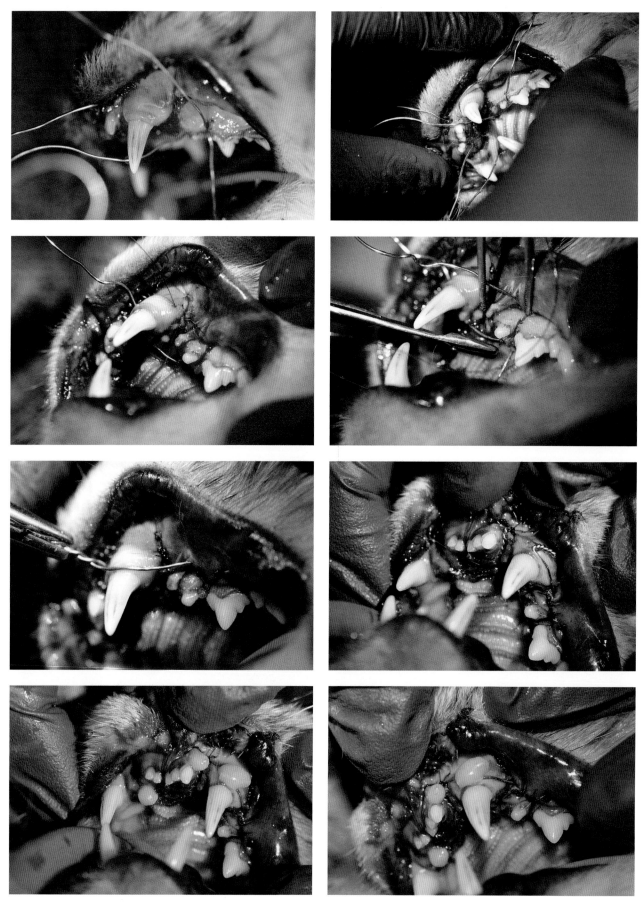

Figure 5.13 The maxillary canine tooth should not be removed unless it is periodontally affected. The maxillary canine tooth is a strategic anchor for the repair of a rostral maxillary fracture. Fractures in the rostral maxilla can be repaired with interdental wiring using the Ivy loop, the Stout loop, or a modified interdental wiring technique reinforced with acrylic.

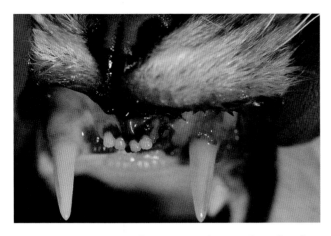
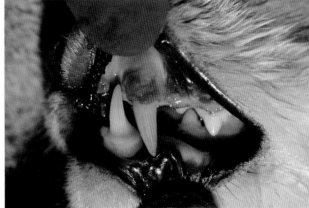

Figure 5.14 The prognosis for patients with a rostral maxillary fracture treated with interdental wiring using the Ivy loop, the Stout loop, or a modified interdental wiring technique reinforced with acrylic is excellent.

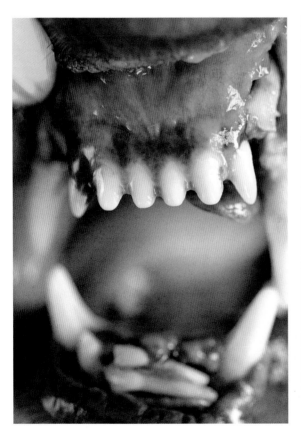
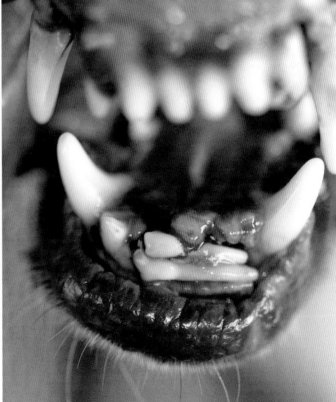

Figure 5.15 Patients with avulsed teeth, or fractures with necrotic bone, may need aggressive debriding and require a partial removal of the rostral maxilla.

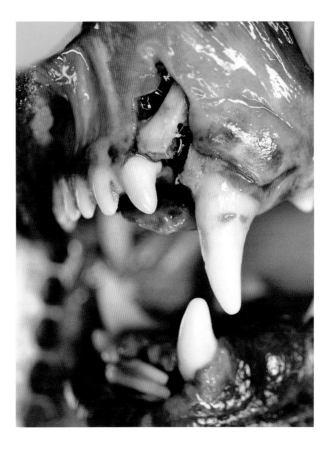

Figure 5.15 (Continued)

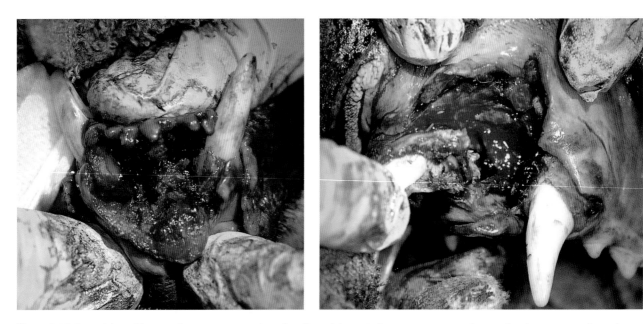

Figure 5.16 A partial maxillectomy is a treatment option when financial constraints are present or when patient/owner compliance is impossible. Amputation is acceptable when the only other option is euthanasia.

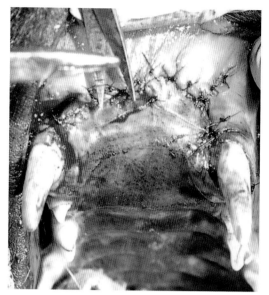

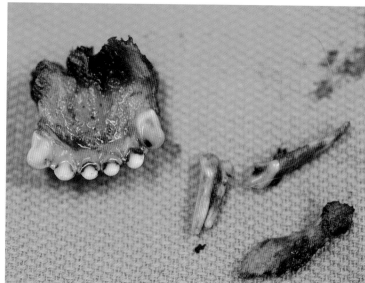

Figure 5.16 (Continued)

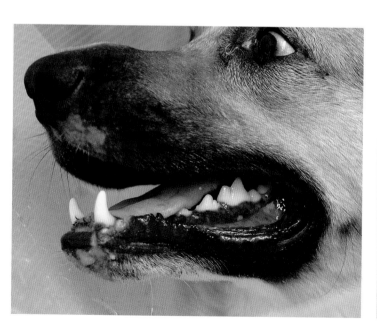

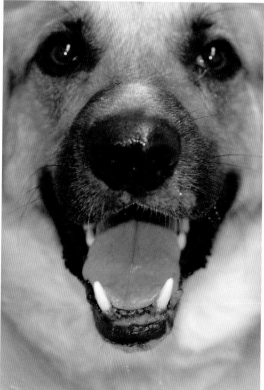

Figure 5.17 Patients treated with a partial rostral maxillectomy do extremely well and have very acceptable cosmetic results.

- Non-union (may cause mandibular drift leaving one or both of the mandibular canines to cause palatal trauma).
- Fibrous union (may cause the patient to have a malocclusion, which may be painful or interfere with normal function).
- Persistent infection of the soft tissues or osteomyelitis.
- Endodontic disease due to fractured teeth.

- Tooth death due to the initial trauma and/or iatrogenic disease due to the repair procedure or the hardware used [1].

Complications are always possible even in the best of hands after maxillofacial fracture repair. Referral to a trained dental surgeon or hands-on wet labs/courses to learn and perfect the techniques of maxillofacial fracture is strongly recommended.

References

1 Gorrel, C., Penman, S., and Emily, P. (1993). Jaw fractures. In: *Handbook of Small Animal Oral Emergencies* (ed. A.T.B. Edney), 37–45. New York: Pergamon Press.

2 Wiggs, R.B. and Lobprise, H.B. (1997). Oral fracture repair. In: *Veterinary Dentistry Principles and Practice* (ed. R.B. Wiggs and H.B. Lobprise), 259–279. Philadelphia, PA: Lippincott-Raven.

3 Verstraete, F.J. (1999). *Self-Assessment Colour Review of Veterinary Dentistry*, 21–22. Ames, IO: Iowa State University Press.

4 Legendre, L. (2005). Maxillofacial fracture repairs. In: *Veterinary Clinics of North American Small Animal Practice Dentistry* (ed. S.E. Holmstrom), 985–1008. New York: Elsevier Inc.

6

Scapula
Anne M. Sylvestre

Focus and Flourish, Cambridge, Ontario, Canada

Fractures of the scapula occur very infrequently in small animal patients [1]. Most scapular fractures occur secondary to vehicular trauma. Concurrent injuries to the chest (rib fractures, contusions, pneumothorax) or peripheral nerves or nerve roots are commonly observed, so careful evaluation of the patient, including chest radiographs and neurological examination, is important. The heavy musculature surrounding this bone aids to stabilize and bring blood supply to the fracture ends, which help with healing. Figure 6.1 identifies the important anatomical landmarks of the scapula.

6.1 Fractures

6.1.1 Fractures Through the Body and Spine of the Scapula (Figures 6.2 and 6.3)

Treatment of choice: Minimally displaced fractures will respond very well to treatment with a sling or splint. More complex, unstable fractures may recover faster with surgical correction using a bone plate or pins and wires. Surgical repairs of the scapula are best left in the hands of a trained surgeon because

(a)

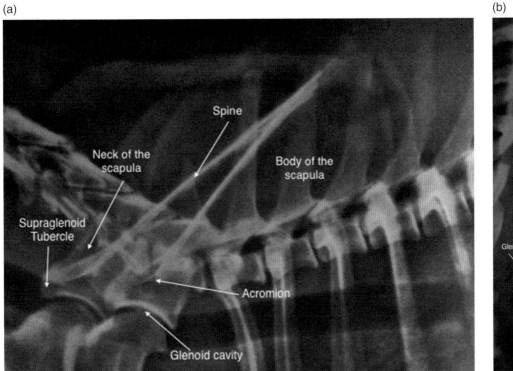

(b)

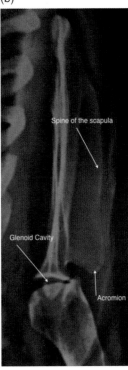

Figure 6.1 Mediolateral (a) and craniocaudal (b) views of the scapula identifying its anatomical landmarks.

Fracture Management for the Small Animal Practitioner, First Edition. Edited by Anne M. Sylvestre.
© 2019 John Wiley & Sons, Inc. Published 2019 by John Wiley & Sons, Inc.

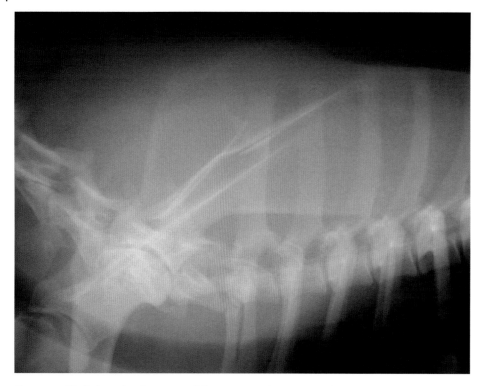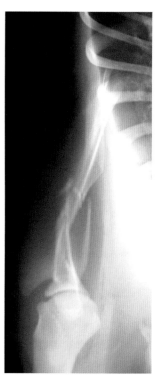

Figure 6.2 Mediolateral and craniocaudal projections of a minimally displaced fractured scapula through the body. This patient was treated conservatively. *Source:* Photos courtesy of Dr. M. Rochat.

the scapula is a thin, fragile bone, thus implants tend to readily pull out; also the heavy musculature surrounding the scapula makes the approach more difficult.

Postoperative management: A spica splint or Velpeau sling is used for 4 weeks whether treated surgically or managed conservatively. Proper splint/bandage care is imperative (Chapter 4).

Prognosis: Prognosis for return to function of the limb is excellent with fractures through the body and spine of the scapula.

6.1.2 Acromion Fractures (Figure 6.4)

These are avulsion type fractures and are very uncommon. A portion of the deltoid muscle originates from this tuberosity, which is what makes this a potentially significant fracture.

Treatment of choice: Surgery is necessary to reattach the muscular origin with a tension band wire system. The key is to stabilize the fragment, not to have perfect reduction. The small fragment and thinness of the bone make this repair difficult and it is best left in the hands of a trained surgeon.

Postoperative management: A Velpeau or carpal flexion bandage may be indicated for 2 weeks followed by activity restriction for another 2 weeks.

Prognosis: The outcome with surgery is very good. Without surgery, a chronic intermittent lameness may ensue [2].

6.1.3 Fractures of the Neck of the Scapula (Figure 6.5)

These are the most difficult of the non-articular scapular fractures to manage. The muscles pull the scapular neck in a medioproximal direction resulting in a poor alignment with the shoulder joint and, therefore, restricted range of movement.

Treatment of choice: Surgical stabilization with a T-plate or wires is indicated. This surgery is very challenging due to the heavy musculature in the area, inherently small distal fragment, and thin flat scapular structure, which does not offer good purchase for implants. This surgery is best left to the experienced surgeon.

Postoperative management: A non-weight bearing sling (Velpeau or carpal flexion sling) or spica splint may be recommended to help protect the repair site for 2 weeks.

Prognosis: Very good with surgical repair.

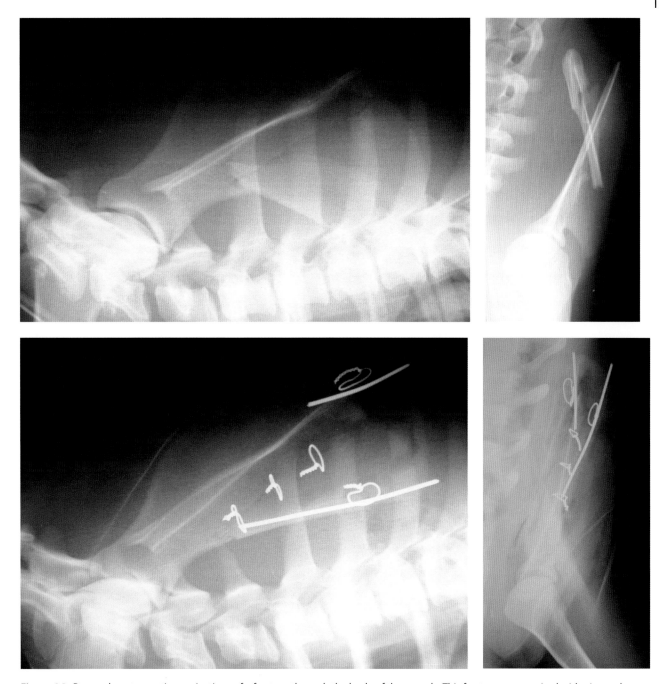

Figure 6.3 Pre- and postoperative projections of a fracture through the body of the scapula. This fracture was repaired with pins and cerclage wires. *Source:* Photos courtesy of Dr. M. Rochat.

(a) (b) (c)

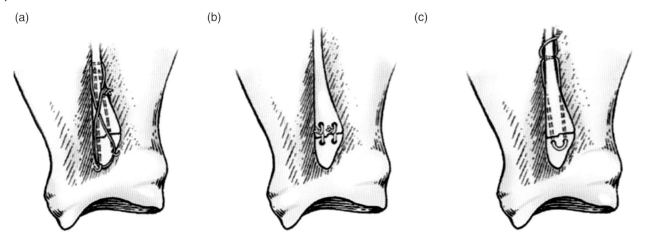

Figure 6.4 Fracture of the acromion process repaired using a tension band wire system (a); simple interfragmentary wire (b); interfragmentary wiring technique for the very small patient (c). *Source:* [2], p. 255, figure 9.4a and b.

(a) (b) (c)

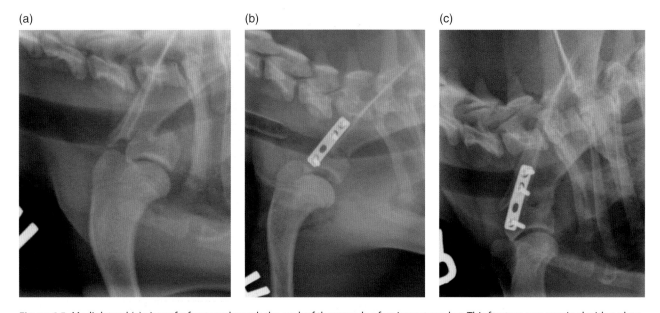

Figure 6.5 Mediolateral (a) view of a fracture through the neck of the scapula of an immature dog. This fracture was repaired with a plate and an inadequate number of screws in the distal fragment due to its small size. (b) The patient was placed in a spica bandage for 2 weeks. The fracture was healed on the radiograph taken 4 weeks postoperatively (c).

6.2 Managing Expectations with Recommended Treatments

Overall, the prognosis with scapular fractures is very good to excellent. Scapular fractures are not common and many are amenable to conservative management. The heavy musculature surrounding this bone aids with its stability and healing. Clients should be encouraged to seek proper treatment with the more difficult fractures as success rates are high and complications low.

Should a sling or bandage be applied to the patient, it should be properly cared for with weekly changes (Chapter 4).

6.3 Alternatives When Treatment of Choice is Not an Option

Many of the scapular fractures do not require surgery and may be treated with restricted activity with or without a bandage/sling. Acromion and neck fractures are definitely best treated with surgery as are complex, highly displaced fractures through the body. Should this not be possible, then conservative management is warranted with a spica splint for several weeks, until the fracture has healed or adequately stabilized itself with fibrous tissue (the acromion fracture or highly displaced fractures may not form a visible bony callus). A malunion will likely be evident on radiographs. Owners should be forewarned that a residual lameness or gait anomaly may be seen, especially with strenuous activity. Although this outcome may be suboptimal, it would still be considered acceptable by most owners. Euthanasia should not be a consideration for a scapular fracture.

References

1 Roush, J.K. (2015). Pet health by numbers: Prevalence of bone fractures in dogs and cats. Today's Veterinary Practice. Retrieved from: http://todaysveterinarypractice. navc.com/pet-health-by-the-numbers-prevalence-of-bone-fractures-in-dogs-cats.

2 DeCamp, C.E., Johnston, S.A., Déjardin, L.M., and Schaefer, S.L. (2016). Fractures of the scapula. In: *Brinker, Piermattei and Flo's Handbook of Small Animal Orthopaedics and Fracture Repair*, 5e, 412–421. St Louis, MO: Elsevier.

7

Shoulder Joint
Anne M. Sylvestre

Focus and Flourish, Cambridge, Ontario, Canada

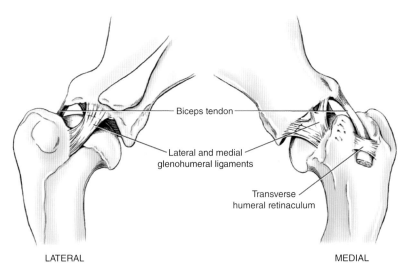

Figure 7.1 Left shoulder joint showing supporting structures. *Source:* From [1].

Biceps tendon

Lateral and medial glenohumeral ligaments

Transverse humeral retinaculum

LATERAL

MEDIAL

(a)

(b)

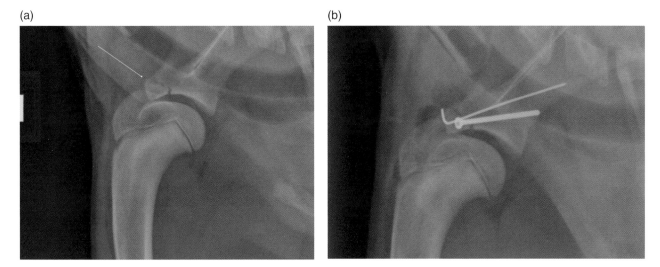

Figure 7.2 A lateral radiograph of the shoulder of an immature canine with an avulsion fracture of the supraglenoid tuberosity (a). The fracture was repaired with a screw and wire (b). *Source:* Photos courtesy of Dr. C. Popovitch.

The shoulder is a complex joint comprising a substantial humeral head creating the distal bony component of the joint and a relatively small scapular glenoid cavity creating the proximal boundary (Figure 7.1). The surrounding soft tissues provide a significant amount of support for the shoulder. The joint capsule and glenohumeral ligaments are its most important stabilizers. Fortunately, fractures and luxations of the shoulder joint are not very common.

7.1 Fractures and Luxations

7.1.1 Avulsion of the Supraglenoid Tuberosity (Figure 7.2)

This is the most common fracture of the shoulder joint. The biceps muscle originates from the supraglenoid tuberosity, making it an important structure. This fracture is seen most frequently in young, large breed dogs.

Treatment of choice: Acute fractures are best repaired by reducing the fragment and stabilizing with a lag screw or tension band wire system. The fragment is typically quite small making it difficult to insert implants, and the approach to this area can be challenging because of the heavy musculature and proximity of the suprascapular nerve. This surgery is best left in the hands of a trained surgeon. A chronic fracture may be best repaired by excision of the fragment and tenodesis (transposition) of the biceps brachii tendon.

Postoperative management: The patient is placed in a non-weight bearing sling (carpal flexion or Velpeau) for 10–14 days followed by restricted activity until the fracture has healed.

Prognosis: The prognosis is very good with the repair of an acute fracture. The acute, non-weight bearing lameness that ensues immediately after the trauma tends to quickly disappear. For this reason, owners may not seek veterinary care for their pet in a timely fashion. Prognosis for chronic cases treated with fragment excision and tendonesis has been reported to be very good [2]. Unfortunately, if the fracture is left untreated the patient will typically display chronic mild to moderate lameness with exercise.

7.1.2 T or Y Fractures of the Scapular Neck and Glenoid Rim (Figure 7.3)

These fractures, fortunately, are very rare.

Treatment of choice: The aim of this type of fracture repair will be to maintain the pieces in alignment and add a Velpeau sling or carpal flexion bandage to aid with stability. The surgery is challenging as the fragments are small and the neck and body of the scapula are

very thin, making it difficult to place implants in a manner that will reduce and stabilize the fragments adequately; the heavy musculature in the area and proximity of the suprascapular nerve make the approach challenging. This surgery is best left in the hands of a trained surgeon.

Postoperative management: The Velpea sling or carpal flexion bandage should be applied for 2 weeks; if external support is required for a longer period of time than a spica bandage can be used. Once the bandage is removed, activity restriction is continued until the fracture has healed (on average 6–8 weeks in total).

Prognosis: The prognosis is good for return to function but lameness may occur with exercise depending on the accuracy of the repair. As with all joint fractures, osteoarthritis will develop. This need not be a deterrent to pursuing appropriate treatment as it can be of minimal clinical significance with proper management.

7.1.3 Other Fractures Involving the Shoulder Joint

Fractures of the caudal or medial aspects of the glenoid rim and humeral head have been described. They are very uncommon.

Treatment of choice: Surgery is indicated for these rare fractures. The difficult approach to these areas, the need for accurate reconstruction of the articular surface, and small fragments make these fractures very challenging and they are therefore best left in the hands of the trained surgeon.

Postoperative management: A non-weight bearing bandage such as a Velpeau sling or carpal flexion bandage should be applied for 2 weeks; if external support is required for a longer period of time than a spica bandage can be used. Once the bandage is removed, activity restriction is continued until the fracture has healed (on average 6–8 weeks in total).

Prognosis: In general, shoulder fractures that are repaired have a favorable prognosis for return to function of the limb but residual osteoarthritis will need to be managed. One long-term study indicated that only 15% of patients were *completely free* of clinical signs after repair [3]. Some degree of lameness or stiffness may be seen, especially after exercise.

7.1.4 Medial Luxations

Traumatic luxations of the shoulder joint are uncommon. This is likely due to its heavy musculature and its proximity to the rib cage, which further helps to protect and stabilize the joint during a trauma. Most luxations, when they occur,

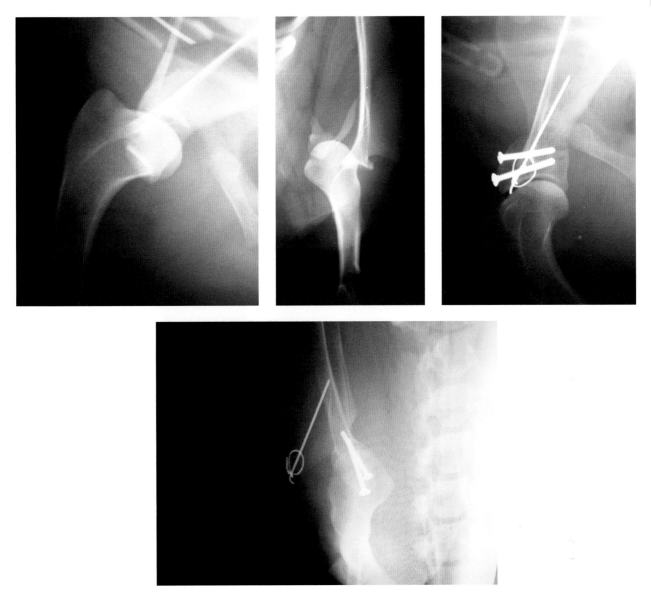

Figure 7.3 Pre and postoperative views of a "y" fracture of the scapular neck that was repaired with screws. The tension band system was used to repair the osteotomy for the acromion process to aid with the exposure of the fracture. *Source:* Photos courtesy of Dr. M. Rochat.

are medial (humerus moves medial to the scapula) with only a few being lateral and, very rarely, cranial. Acute luxations *without* a significant history of trauma are seen in the small dogs, especially toy poodles and shelties [4].

Treatment of choice: Acute, traumatic medial shoulder luxations are best treated with a closed reduction followed by immobilization with a Velpeau sling or spica splint for 2 weeks. The technique for reducing a medial shoulder luxation is as follows:

- Good analgesia and general anesthesia-induced muscle relaxation are essential.

- Suspending the patient by the paw once under general anesthesia may help further relax and stretch the muscles supporting the shoulder.
- The shoulder joint is held in extension.
- Digital pressure is applied to the medial aspect of the humeral head, pushing it laterally, back into position (Figure 7.4).

Postoperative management: A Velpeau sling or Spica bandage is applied for 10–14 days followed by a gradual return to regular activity.

Prognosis: The prognosis for success and return to normal function of the shoulder is very good [5].

(a) (b) (c)

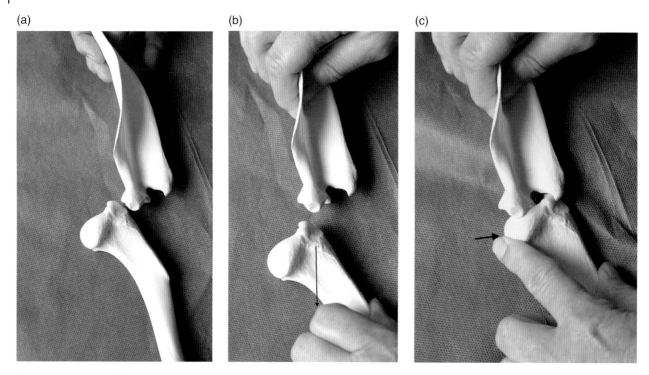

Figure 7.4 Bone models are used to demonstrate how to reduce a medially luxated shoulder. (a) Craniocaudal view of a left shoulder with a medial luxation. (b) To reduce the luxation distal tension is applied to the forelimb causing distraction at the shoulder joint. (c) Digital pressure is applied medially to the humeral head, moving it back into its normal position.

Congenital and chronic luxations, or those associated with structural malformations, are less likely to be successful with a closed reduction.

Additional treatment options: If closed reduction fails, then open reduction and stabilization is indicated. This surgery is best left in the hands of a trained surgeon as the approach and the repair itself can be very challenging. If the luxation is acute, then the stabilization may consist of imbricating the joint capsule and the torn tendon/ligament, if it can be identified. Chronic luxations, or those associated with a malformation, may require transposition of the bicipital tendon to a more caudal position (Figure 7.5).

Postoperative management: Postoperatively, the patient may be placed in a Velpeau or spica bandage for 10–14 days followed by activity restriction for an additional 10–14 days.

Prognosis: Surgical corrections of shoulder luxations have resulted in varied outcomes [6].

7.1.5 Lateral Luxations

Lateral luxations (humerus moves lateral to the scapula) are very rare and are handled in a similar manner to the medial ones. Lateral luxations are typically seen in larger breed dogs as a result of trauma. Following closed reduction it is better to place the limb in a spica splint and to avoid the Velpeau as the latter tends to turn the humeral head laterally [4]. The success with closed reductions of lateral luxations is very good to excellent.

7.2 Managing Expectations with Recommended Treatments

Trauma to the shoulder joint is not common so there is a paucity of specific information available for outcomes with various injuries and treatments. Having said that, what is available indicates that, overall, the prognosis is quite good. Shoulder fractures can be difficult to reconstruct and a residual lameness may be noted after strenuous activity, but oftentimes this can be managed with minor lifestyle changes. Owners are usually appreciative of the outcome, especially given the alternative, and should be encouraged to seek out the expertise of a trained surgeon for these repairs. General practitioners are encouraged to manage acute luxations.

If a bandage or splint is used after surgery, then it should be properly cared for and changed weekly (Chapter 4). Range of motion exercises are recommended (once the bandage is removed) to help maintain or re-establish proper function. As with all joint injuries, osteoarthritis

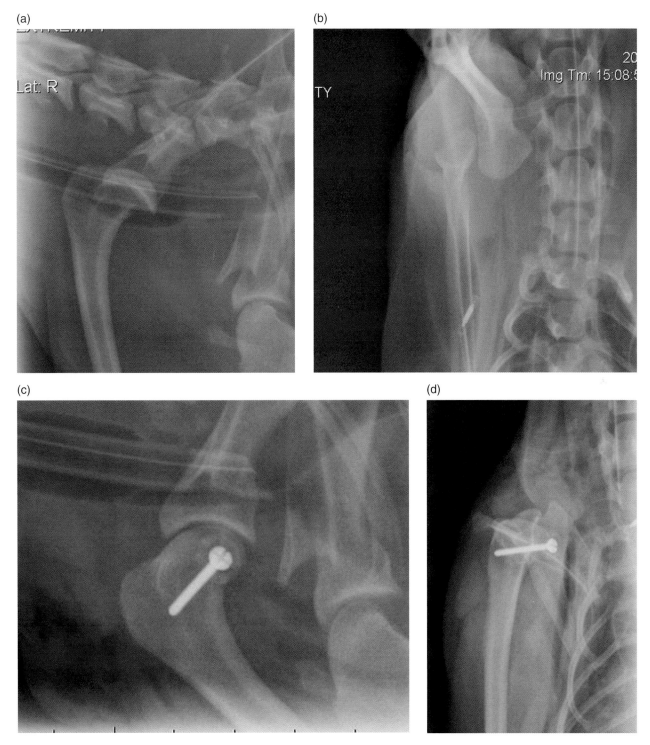

Figure 7.5 Mediolateral (a) and craniocaudal (b) projections of a canine shoulder joint with a medial luxation. The luxation was chronic and therefore surgically repaired by transposition of the bicipital tendon (c and d).

will develop. This need not be a deterrent to pursuing appropriate treatment as it can be of minimal clinical significance with basic osteoarthritis management (Chapter 3).

7.3 Alternatives When Treatment of Choice is Not an Option

7.3.1 Fractures

As with all joint fractures, surgical treatment is definitely the treatment method of choice. If referral or surgical repair are not options, then a Velpeau sling or spica splint can be used to immobilize the fracture and allow it to heal. A closed reduction to attempt to align the fragments is not in the realm of possibilities given the size and location of the pieces; therefore, a malalignment will likely ensue. The patient is likely to have a mild to moderate lameness that is exacerbated with strenuous activity.

7.3.2 Luxations

Limb function will be significantly impaired with a shoulder luxation that is not reduced. Over time, the pet will likely learn to use the now abnormal limb with reasonable success. The smaller the dog, the better the ambulation is likely to appear. Fortunately, traumatic shoulder luxations are rare. Owners should be encouraged to pursue a closed reduction of an acute luxation as this procedure has a high success rate and a good prognosis.

References

1 Evans, H.E. and de Lahunta, A. (2013). *Miller's Anatomy of the Dog*, 4e. St Louis, MO: Saunders/Elsevier.

2 Bergenhuyzen, A.L., Vermote, K.A., van Bree, H. et al. (2010). Long-term follow-up after arthroscopic tenotomy for partial rupture of the biceps brachii tendon. *Vet. Comp. Orthop. Traumatol.* 23: 51–55.

3 DeCamp, C.E., Johnston, S.A., Déjardin, L.M., and Schaefer, S.L. (2016). The shoulder joint. In: *Brinker, Piermattei and Flo's Handbook of Small Animal Orthopaedics and Fracture Repair*, 5e, 260–297. St Louis, MO: Elsevier.

4 Newton, C.D. (1985). Dislocations of the shoulder joint. In: *Textbook of Small Animal Orthopaedics* (ed. C.D. Newton and D.M. Nunamaker), 343. Phildelphia, PA: JB Lippincott Company.

5 Hohn, R.B., Rosen, H., Bohning, R.H., and Brown, S.G. (1971). Surgical stabilization of recurrent shoulder luxation in dogs. *Vet. Clin. North Am.* 1: 357–348.

6 Vasseur, P.B. (1983). Clinical results of surgical correction of shoulder luxation in dogs. *J. Am. Vet. Assoc.* 182: 503–508.

8

Humerus

Catherine Popovitch[1], Thomas W.G. Gibson[2], and Anne M. Sylvestre[3]

[1] *Veterinary Specialty and Emergency Center, Levittown, Pennsylvania, USA*
[2] *Ontario Veterinary College, University of Guelph, Guelph, Ontario, Canada*
[3] *Focus and Flourish, Cambridge, Ontario, Canada*

Humeral fractures account for approximately 10% of all long bone fractures seen in dogs and cats [1–3]. Figure 8.1 identifies the relevant bony landmarks of the humerus.

Nerve damage is possible with a humeral fracture as the radial nerve crosses the humerus in an area (mid- to distal third) where most fractures occur. One retrospective

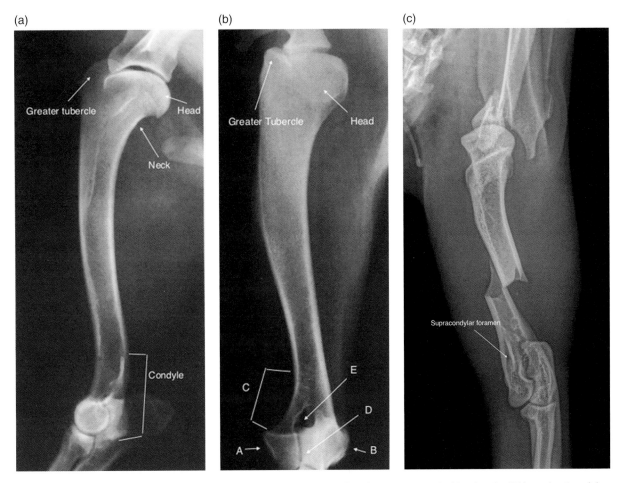

Figure 8.1 Mediolateral (a) and craniocaudal (b) views of the humerus identifying its anatomical landmarks. (A) lateral epicondyle; (B) medial epicondyle; (C) supracondylar area of the humerus; (D) trochlea; and (E) supratrochlear foramen. The cat has a supracondylar foramen on the medial aspect of the distal humerus through which pass the median nerve and brachial artery (c).

Fracture Management for the Small Animal Practitioner, First Edition. Edited by Anne M. Sylvestre.
© 2019 John Wiley & Sons, Inc. Published 2019 by John Wiley & Sons, Inc.

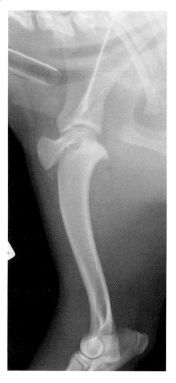
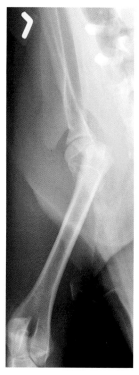
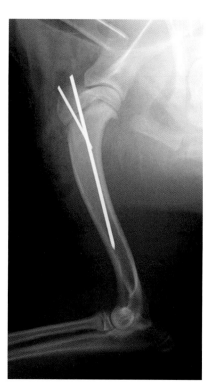
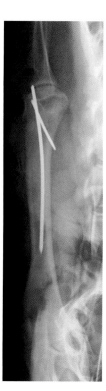

Figure 8.2 Pre- and postoperative mediolateral and craniocaudal radiographs of a Salter–Harris I fracture of the proximal humerus of an immature dog repaired with two Kirschner wires. *Source:* Photo courtesy of the Ontario Veterinary College.

study of 130 cases with humeral fractures identified two patients with nerve damage [4]. The abundant swelling as well as pain medications may prevent the patient from readily responding to a toe pinch, thus serial examinations may be necessary to accurately diagnose radial nerve damage.

The spica splint is recommended to immobilize the limb until the fracture can be treated surgically. Immobilization of the limb decreases further damage to muscles and nerves. If it is not possible to place a spica splint on the patient, then confinement to a small cage or crate is recommended to avoid further soft tissue injury.

8.1 Fractures

8.1.1 Physeal Fractures of the Proximal Humerus (Figure 8.2)

The proximal humerus contains the physes for both the humeral head and the greater tubercle. In the case of a traumatic event, these physes can separate independently or more commonly as a single entity in the growing animal resulting in a Salter–Harris I or II fracture.

Treatment of choice: This fracture is amenable to repair with parallel K-wires placed proximally to distally through the greater tubercle. Addition of a tension band wire can add to stability. Salter–Harris III and IV fractures involve the articular surface requiring accurate anatomic reconstruction and stabilization of the

joint surface and should only be attempted by the experienced surgeon.

Postoperative management: Exercise restriction is required until radiographic evidence of healing is present. These fractures should heal quickly in the young growing animal (4–6 weeks).

Prognosis: With adequate reduction and stabilization prognosis for a full return to function is very good.

8.1.2 Two-Piece Humeral Shaft Fractures

In the dog, the majority of humeral fractures involve the mid- to distal portions of the bone; where most humeral fractures in the cat are mid-shaft [4].

Treatment of choice: Transverse and short oblique fractures (Figure 8.3) are ideally repaired with a bone plate and screws; an intra-medullary (IM) pin and plate combination; or a pin and external fixator combination. An IM pin alone is not recommended as it lacks rotational stability.

Long oblique fractures, where the length of the fracture ends is at least twice the diameter of the bone, and spiral fractures can be repaired with an IM pin and full cerclage wires (Figure 8.4). Cats, small dogs, or younger dogs can do very well with this form of fixation. For large dogs, bone plate and lag screws may be a better choice. Surgery is the treatment of choice for most humeral fractures. It is strongly advised to send these cases to a trained surgeon as the approach to the humerus is challenging because of the position of the

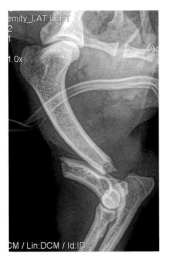
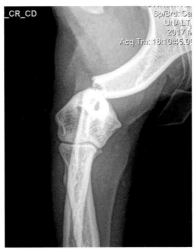
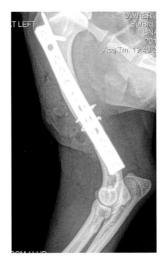
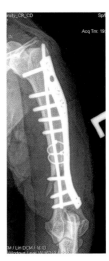

Figure 8.3 Pre- and postoperative mediolateral and craniocaudal radiographs of transverse fracture of the distal third of the shaft of a left humerus. The fracture was repaired with a pin and plate.

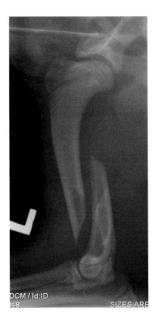
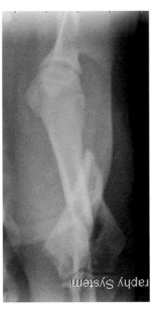
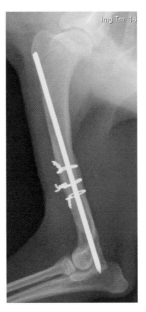
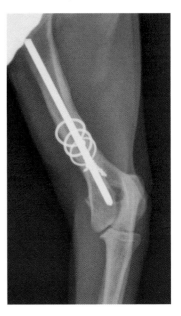

Figure 8.4 Pre-operative mediolateral and caudocranial radiographs of a long oblique mid- to distal left humeral shaft fracture of an immature dog. The length of the oblique fracture line is at least twice that of the width of the bone. The 5-week follow-up mediolateral and craniocaudal radiographs show the repair with a pin and cerclage wires and a fully healed fracture.

radial nerve and large brachialis muscle over the most commonly fractured area of the bone, and the difficulty of accurately contouring a bone plate to the humerus, which is necessary to achieve proper alignment. Even a simple (two-piece) mid-shaft fracture of the humerus is challenging to repair because of the anatomy. A general practitioner with appropriate equipment and some experience in fracture repair may prefer to send humeral fractures to a trained surgeon.

Postoperative management: These fractures rarely require a bandage or splint postoperatively but activity should restricted and the patient properly managed until the fracture has healed (Chapter 3).

Prognosis: The overall outcome with surgically repaired two-piece humeral shaft fractures is very good to excellent. This is not a commonly fractured bone, making it difficult to gain sufficient experience in general practice to become proficient.

8.1.3 Multifragmented Humeral Shaft and/or Supracondylar Fractures (Figure 8.5)

Multi-fragmented fractures are typically mid- to distal diaphyseal and often include the supracondylar area of the humerus.

Treatment of choice: These are best repaired with a bone plate and interfragmentary screws, an external fixator,

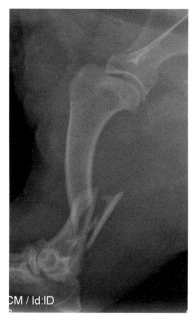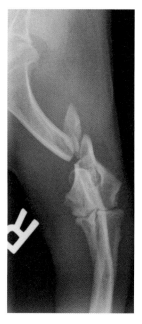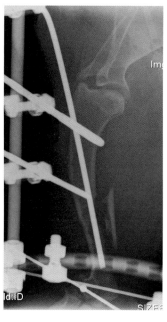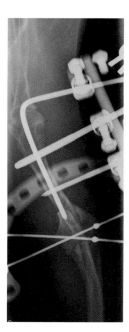

Figure 8.5 Pre- and postoperative mediolateral and craniocaudal radiographs of a comminuted fracture of the mid- to distal shaft of the humerus. This fracture was repaired with an intra-medullary (IM) pin tied into a hybrid external fixator.

or by using a combination of techniques such as pin–plate or pin–external fixator. Depending on the complexity of the fracture configuration and size of the patient, more than one bone plate may be necessary to stabilize the fracture. When a fracture is distally located on the humerus and/or comminuted, it is very challenging to place enough screws or pins to achieve sufficient rigidity. It is strongly advised to send these cases to a trained surgeon.

Postoperative management: Postoperative support with a spica splint (for 2–4 weeks) or carpal flexion bandage (for 2 weeks) may be recommended by the surgeon. Appropriate patient care as described in Chapter 3 is indicated.

Prognosis: 82 to 86% of the patients that undergo surgical repair for these fractures have good to excellent results [4]. The fair to poor results that occur in 14–18% of the patients are typically associated with complications such as osteomyelitis or implant failure due to inadequate rigidity [4, 5].

8.2 Managing Expectations with Recommended Treatments

Humeral fractures that are surgically repaired have a very good outcome overall. Even the more complex supracondylar fractures have a good prognosis. The more difficult fractures can carry a higher complication rate but these are still within the realm of acceptable in the hands of a trained surgeon. The humerus is a difficult

bone to repair and a general practitioner with appropriate equipment and some experience in fracture repair may still prefer to send humeral fractures to a board-certified surgeon. This is not a commonly fractured bone, making it difficult to gain sufficient experience in general practice to become proficient and enjoy high success rates. Clients who are hesitant to seek the services of a trained surgeon should be encouraged to do so.

If a bandage or splint is used afterward, then it should be properly cared for and changed weekly (Chapter 4). Range of motion exercises of the elbow are recommended (once the bandage is removed) to help maintain or re-establish proper function, especially with comminuted distal humeral fractures. As with all joint injuries, osteoarthritis will develop. This need not be a deterrent to pursuing appropriate treatment as it can be of minimal clinical significance with basic management (Chapter 3).

8.3 Alternatives When Treatment of Choice is Not an Option

A minimally displaced mid-shaft humeral fracture in an immature patient (Figure 8.6) can have a good outcome when managed with a spica splint alone. The reality is that most humeral shaft fractures are significantly displaced due to the muscular forces on the distal segment. A malunion is highly probable with non-surgical management. If surgery is absolutely not a possibility, then perhaps a properly managed spica splint (Chapter 4) is a viable option for patients with a mid-shaft two-piece

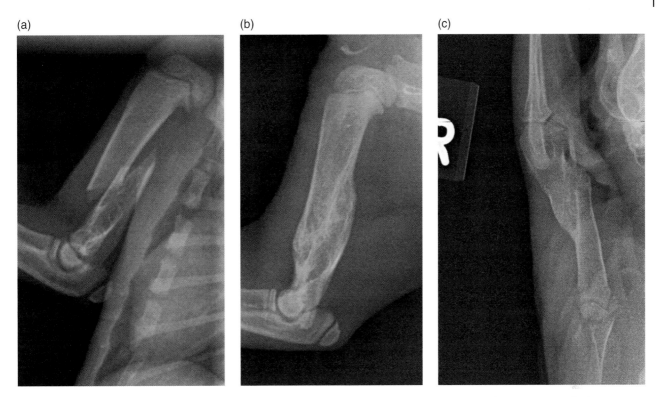

Figure 8.6 Mediolateral projection of a long oblique mid-shaft humeral fracture of a kitten at the time of presentation to the humane society (a). The kitten was given pain medication and confined to a cage. Mediolateral (b) and caudocranial (c) radiographs taken 4 weeks later show a fully healed fracture. Although a malunion is clearly visible on radiographs the kitten is asymptomatic. *Source:* Photos courtesy of the Kitchener Waterloo Humane Society.

fracture. Placing a spica splint on a very young animal (such as a 12-week-old kitten) may be very difficult. Placing this patient in a large crate with adequate pain management is often sufficient as they heal very quickly. Despite the malunion, the limb is often functional once healed. If an owner is contemplating a forequarter amputation rather than a repair, it might be worth noting that the cost difference between a forequarter amputation and the repair of a two-piece humeral fracture is small.

External coaptation (spica splint) is not a good alternative for the more distal supracondylar fractures because of the proximity of the elbow joint and high probability of a malalignment with the joint. Perhaps a forelimb amputation would be a better solution. The veterinarian's role is to ensure that the owner fully understands the consequences for the pet. A supracondylar fracture (non-articular) in the hands of a trained surgeon has a high likelihood of having a positive outcome. Given the high success rate and positive outcomes with surgical repair it is worth taking the time to properly educate the pet owner so that they can make an informed decision rather than an emotional one.

References

1 Unger, M., Montavon, P.M., and Heim, U.F.A. (1990). Classification of fractures of the long bones in the dog and cat: introduction and clinical application. *Vet. Comp. Orthop. Traumatol.* 3: 41–50.

2 Roush, J.K. (2015). Pet health by numbers: Prevalence of bone fractures in dogs and cats. Today's Veterinary Practice. Retrieved from: http://todaysveterinarypractice.navc.com/ pet-health-by-the-numbers-prevalence-of-bone-fractures-in-dogs-cats.

3 Miller, C.W., Sumner-Smith, G., Sheridan, C., and Pennock, P.W. (1998). Using the Unger system to classify 386 long bone fractures in dogs. *J. Small. Anim. Pract.* 39: 390–393.

4 Bardet, J.F., Hohn, R.B., Rudy, R.L., and Olmstead, M.L. (1983). Fractures of the humerus in dogs and cats. A retrospective study of 130 cases. *Vet. Surg.* 12: 73–77.

5 Kirby, K.A., Lewis, D.D., Lafuente, R.M. et al. (2008). Management of humeral and femoral fractures in dogs and cats with linear-circular hybrid external skeletal fixators. *J. Am. Anim. Hosp. Assoc.* 44: 180–197.

9

Elbow Joint
Anne M. Sylvestre

Focus and Flourish, Cambridge, Ontario, Canada

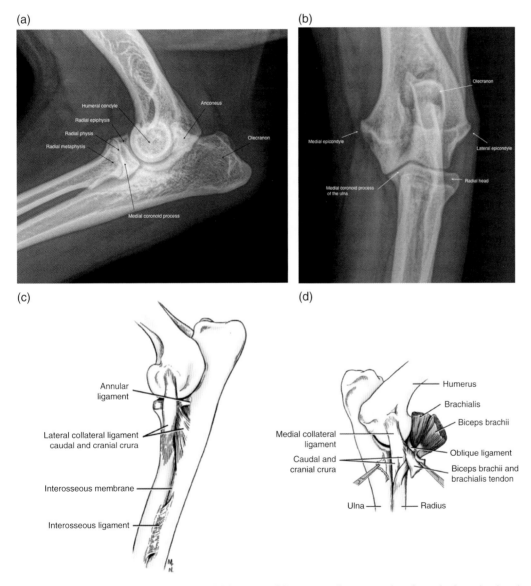

Figure 9.1 Mediolateral (a) and craniocaudal (b) views of the canine elbow joint identifying the bony landmarks. (c) left elbow, lateral aspect; (d) left elbow, medial aspect. *Source:* From [1].

The elbow is a composite joint formed by the humerus, radius, and ulna. Most of the weight is supported by the humoradial component while the humeroulnar part acts to stabilize the joint. Figure 9.1 shows the relevant soft tissue and bony structures of the elbow joint.

9.1 Fractures and Luxations

9.1.1 Condylar Fractures (Figure 9.2)

Condylar fractures are the most common type of fracture seen in the elbow joint. A fracture of the lateral condyle is much more common than of the medial one. Young dogs, especially small breeds, are more susceptible to this type of fracture. The fracture often occurs in association with a minor trauma such as jumping off of furniture or playing [2]. It is *very* important to take both the mediolateral and craniocaudal views in order to make the diagnosis as the fracture can be easily missed on the mediolateral view alone.

Treatment of choice: As with all joint surgeries, internal fixation is the only effective treatment for a good outcome. Condylar fractures are typically stabilized with a transcondylar screw and one or two Kirschner wire(s) that are placed while maintaining accurate reduction of the articular surface and sparing the physis. Many referral centers with fluoroscopic equipment will reduce the fracture closed and insert the implants through small stab incisions (minimally invasive osteosynthesis technique).

Postoperative management: Maintaining motion in the joint is important so these patients are typically not bandaged, and gentle passive range of motion (PROM) exercises are started immediately after surgery (Chapter 3). Exercise restriction is imperative until the fracture has healed.

Prognosis: The prognosis with internal fixation of the acute condylar fracture is very good [3]. One study showed that technical error accounted for many of the poor outcomes [4]. Therefore, referral to a trained surgeon for this procedure is recommended. If the fracture is chronic, a reduction in the range of motion of the elbow with occasional lameness is seen more frequently. Implants are not usually removed once the fracture has healed, unless they are causing problems. Pin migration or irritation of the soft tissues overlying the pins is a common complication. Pin removal is considered a minor procedure and its potential occurrence should not be viewed as a reason not to proceed with the repair. Other potential complications include implant failure before the fracture has healed (and hence failure of the repair),

reduced range of motion in the elbow joint, and osteoarthritis (OA).

Spaniels are known to be prone to incomplete ossification of the humeral condyle (IOHC), making them more susceptible to this type of fracture, at any age [5].

9.1.2 Bicondylar Fractures (Figure 9.3)

These are also known as the "Y" or "T" fractures. They tend to occur in mature animals [3].

Treatment of choice: Open reduction and internal fixation is the best option. The goal of surgery is to reconstruct the articular surface and stabilize the fragments using a transcondylar screw with a plate, or two, for added stability. A ring fixator is another repair choice that is especially useful in the more fragmented fracture. Bicondylar fractures are a very difficult fracture configuration to repair and are best left in the hands of a trained surgeon.

Postoperative management: Maintaining motion in the joint is important; however, preventing the animal from overstressing a difficult repair may be necessary. The surgeon may opt to place the patient in a carpal flexion bandage or spica splint for the early postoperative period. Diligent bandage care becomes crucial to prevent further issues from developing (Chapter 4). Once the spica splint is removed, gentle elbow PROM exercises can be started to help improve motion in the joint (Chapter 3). Implants are left in place unless they are associated with problems.

Prognosis: The prognosis for this type of fracture is less than ideal, with only 52% of patients returning to regular activity [4]. Loss of range of motion and ongoing lameness, especially after rigorous activity, are commonly cited as the reasons for the lower success rate.

9.1.3 Acute Luxations

Luxations of the elbow are not common as the three-bone configuration of this joint is inherently very stable. Good-quality radiographs, taken in the mediolateral and craniocaudal planes, are necessary to identify any associated fractures to the joint as this will alter the prognosis and treatment options. Most luxations are lateral (the radius and ulna move laterally, as one unit).

Treatment of choice: Closed reduction is the treatment of choice (Figure 9.4) and has a high success rate. Veterinarians are encouraged to do this. The technique for a closed reduction of a laterally luxated elbow is as follows:

- General anesthesia and good analgesia are required to allow for appropriate muscle relaxation.

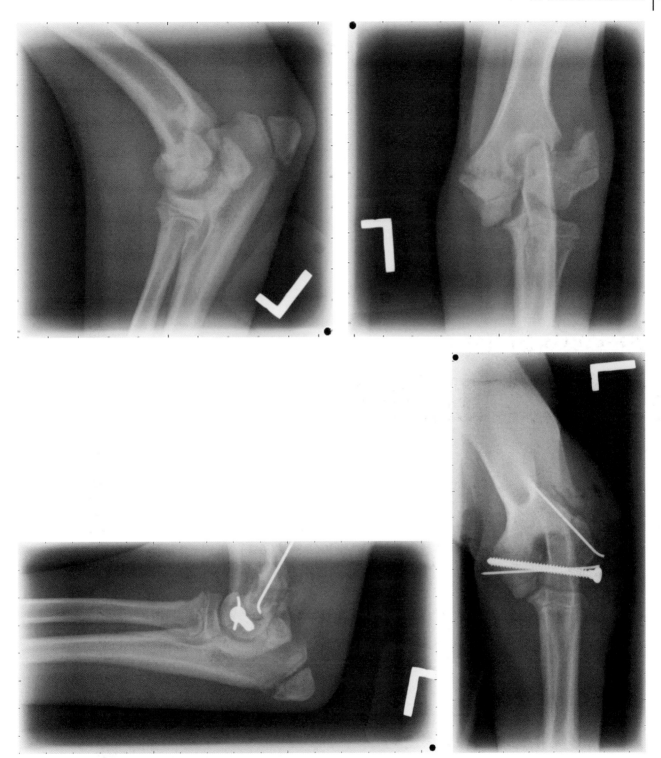

Figure 9.2 Pre- and postoperative mediolateral and craniocaudal radiographs of a lateral condylar fracture and repair. It is difficult to appreciate the fracture in the mediolateral projection. The fracture was repaired with a transcondylar lag screw and Kirschner wire and a supracondylar Kirschner wire.

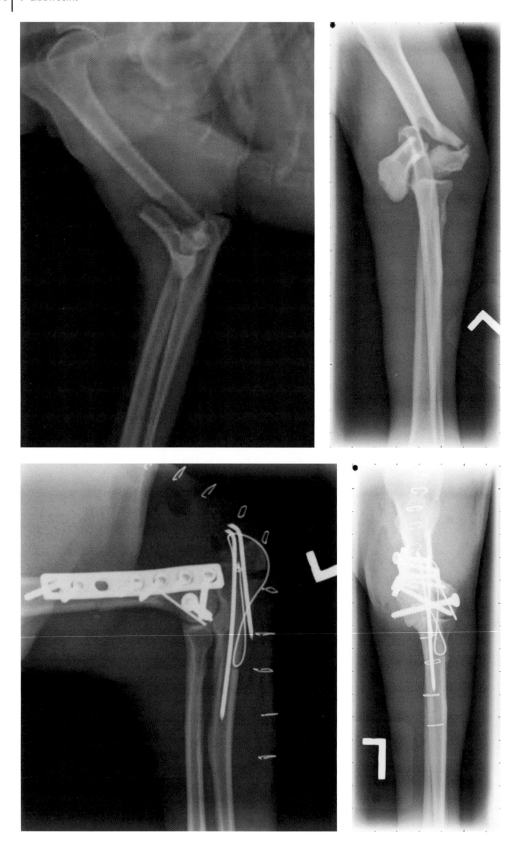

Figure 9.3 Pre- and postoperative mediolateral and craniocaudal radiographs of a canine elbow with a bicondylar ("Y") fracture. The fracture was repaired with a transcondylar lag screw, Kirschner wire, and a plate applied on the medial surface. An osteotomy of the olecranon was performed to improve exposure of the fracture and it was repaired with a tension band wire system.

- Hanging the limb with the patient under general anesthesia will help to relax the muscles.
- The anconeus is repositioned medial (inside) to the lateral epicondyle of the humerus by fully flexing the elbow joint and rotating the antebrachium inward (pronated).
- Digital pressure is applied to the anconeus to push it over the humeral condyle.
- With the anconeus now inside the lateral epicondyle, the elbow joint is extended slightly to lock it into place.
- Pressure is applied to the lateral aspect of the radial head to push it medially back into place.

- Flexing the elbow joint while pronating the antebrachium is often necessary to slip the radial head past the humeral condyle.
- Additional maneuverings with abduction of the elbow and adduction of the antebrachium may be helpful with this process.

Once the elbow joint has been reduced, the lateral and medial collateral ligaments are assessed to determine whether they are intact or not. To assess the collateral ligaments:

- The elbow and carpus are flexed to 90°.
- The paw is rotated in and out to evaluate the degree of pronation and supination (Figure 9.5).

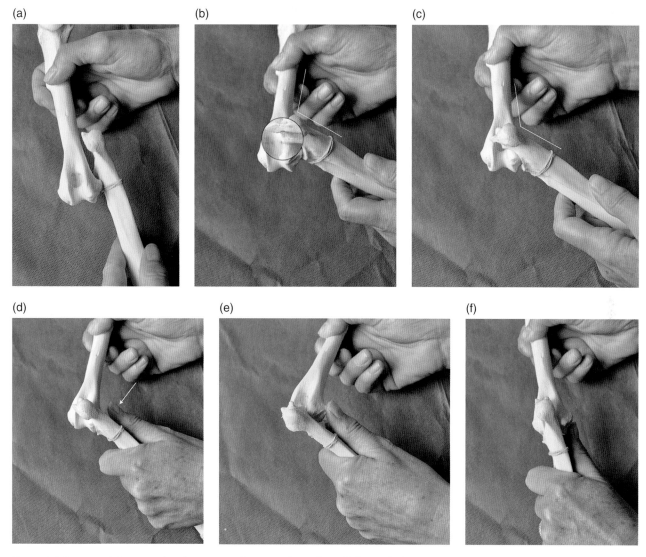

(a)   (b)   (c)

(d)   (e)   (f)

Figure 9.4 Bone models are used to demonstrate how to reduce a laterally luxated elbow. (a) Caudal view of a right elbow with the radius and ulna luxated laterally. (b) The anconeus is hooked over the lateral humeral condyle (circle) by flexing the elbow while internally rotating (pronating) the antebrachium and, if necessary, slightly abducting it. (c) The elbow is slightly extended to help anchor the anconeus in place. (d) Digital pressure is applied to the lateral aspect of the head of the radius (just in front of the ulna thus not visible in this picture) to push it into place, past the lateral humeral condyle. (e) A slight increase in flexion can assist with this maneuver. (f) The head of the radius "pops" back into place. A video of this demonstration is available at www.focusandflourish.com.

(a) (b)

(c) (d)

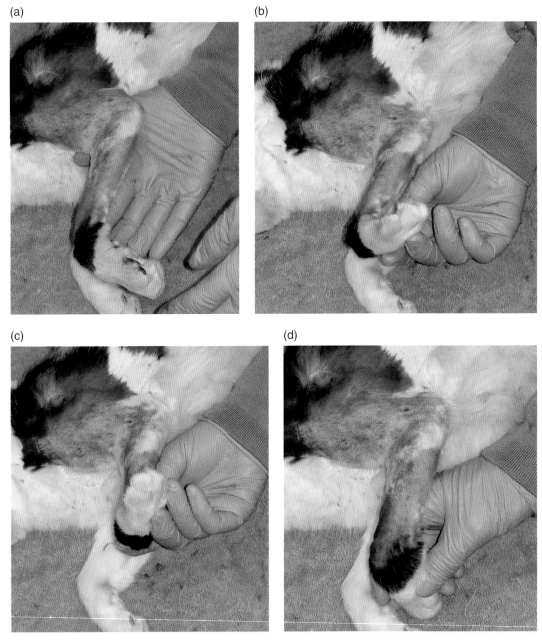

Figure 9.5 The lateral and medial collateral ligaments are assessed by rotating the paw with the elbow and carpus flexed to 90° (a). To check the medial collateral ligament, the paw is rotated laterally (b); if the medial collateral ligament is damaged then there is excessive pronation (c). To check the lateral collateral ligament, the paw is rotated inwardly (supinated) (d); if the supination is excessive then the lateral collateral ligament is damaged. It is best to compare the affected elbow to the normal, contralateral one. A video of this demonstration is available at www.focusandflourish.com.

- If there is excessive supination (increased medial rotation of the manus), the lateral collateral ligament is damaged.
- If there is excessive pronation (the paw can be excessively rotated laterally), the medial collateral ligament is damaged [6].
- The affected limb can be compared with the contralateral one.

Postoperative management: If there is no ligamentous damage identified, then the reduction tends to be quite stable and a spica bandage may be applied for 5–7 days. Once the bandage is removed, PROM exercises will help re-establish a normal range of motion and overall joint health. Restricted activity with controlled leash walks for an additional 2 weeks followed by a gradual return to regular activity is recommended. If there is damage to one or more collateral ligament then surgery is recommended (Section 9.1.4).

Prognosis: Prognosis for closed reduction of an acute luxation is excellent [7].

9.1.4 Chronic Luxations

These are luxations that are more than 4–5 days old. They are more difficult to reduce closed, although it is worth giving it a try.

Treatment of choice: If a closed reduction is not successful, then an open reduction and surgical stabilization are indicated. Surgery is also indicated after a successful closed reduction if ligamentous damage is identified. These surgeries are best left in the hands of a trained surgeon. The damaged ligament can be reconstructed with the use of bone anchors and heavy gauge suture material such as Prolene™ or nylon (Figure 9.6). If the ligament is simply avulsed from its

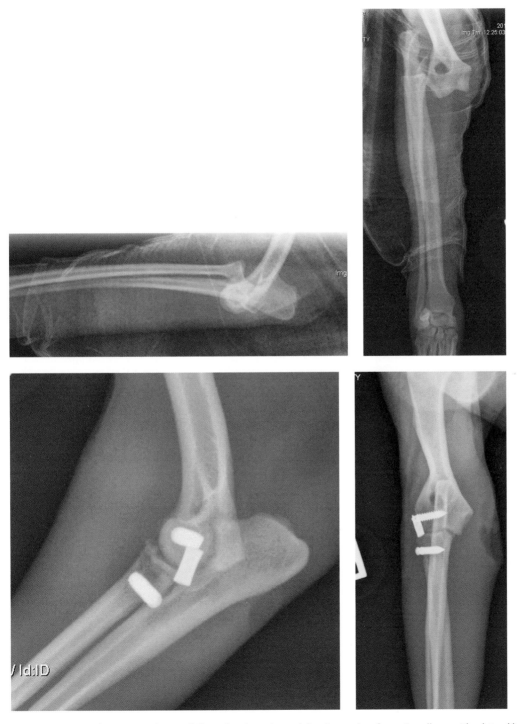

Figure 9.6 Pre- and postoperative mediolateral and craniocaudal radiographs of a canine elbow with a lateral luxation. The luxation was chronic therefore an open reduction was performed and the joint stabilized with bone anchors and crimped nylon.

origin or insertion, it can be re-anchored with a bone screw and washer.

Postoperative management: Patients with an open reduction or ligamentous reconstruction should be placed in a spica bandage for 2 weeks. Once the bandage is removed gentle PROM can be started to help re-establish range of motion (Chapter 3). Controlled, slow, short leash walks for 4 weeks are recommended followed by a gradual return to regular activity.

Prognosis: Prognosis with an open reduction is dependent on the chronicity of the luxation and difficulty of the open reduction. Patients with ligamentous damage and a relatively acute luxation generally have a very good to excellent prognosis [7]. Recurrence of luxation is a complication that occurs most frequently in patients with multiple orthopedic issues [7]. Other complications include decreased range of motion and OA of the elbow joint. Steps should be taken to properly manage the OA so that its clinical significance is minimized.

9.1.5 Proximal Ulnar Fractures (Figure 9.7)

Fractures of the proximal ulna can occur at the joint (semilunar notch) or just distal to it. Although the latter is technically not a joint fracture, its precise repair is crucial in order for the joint to function properly and it is therefore included in this section. The very strong triceps muscle group inserts on the olecranon; the pull of the triceps results in distraction forces being applied at the fracture line.

Treatment of choice: A proximal ulnar fracture can be repaired with a tension band wire mechanism, intramedullary pin, and cerclage wires or plate and screws;

the fracture configuration may dictate which option is best.

Postoperative management: Activity restriction until the fracture has healed and gentle PROM exercises are recommended (Chapter 3).

Prognosis: The prognosis is good with accurate reconstruction of the articular surface. Complications can include implant failure and hence failure of the repair; pin migration or breakage of the implants once the fracture is healed, which simply requires removal of the implants; decreased ROM of the elbow joint; and OA.

9.1.6 Monteggia Fractures (Figure 9.8)

A fracture of the proximal ulna that occurs in conjunction with a dislocation of the radial head is called a Monteggia fracture. This fracture may or may not be accompanied by a disruption of the annular ligament that stabilizes the radial head to the ulna.

Treatment of choice: Joint congruity is re-established and maintained with surgery. If the annular ligament is intact, then simply repairing the ulna with an intramedullary pin or a plate will serve to stabilize the luxation as well. If the ligament is ruptured, then a screw or cerclage wire securing the radial head to the ulna is also necessary [8].

Postoperative management: As with most joint fractures, re-establishing range of motion is imperative for proper function; therefore, immobilizing the joint with a splint is less desirable. However, the complexity of the fracture and the patient's personality may dictate if postoperative support is necessary. A spica

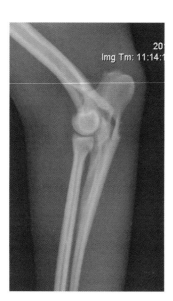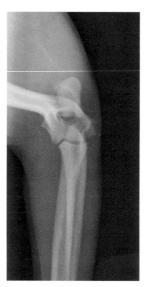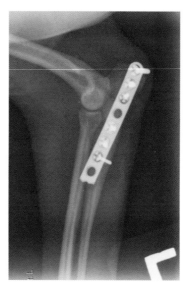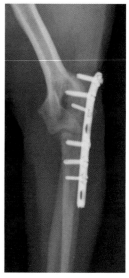

Figure 9.7 Pre- and postoperative mediolateral and craniocaudal radiographs of a canine elbow with an articular fracture of the ulna. The fracture was repaired with a plate applied on the lateral surface of the ulna.

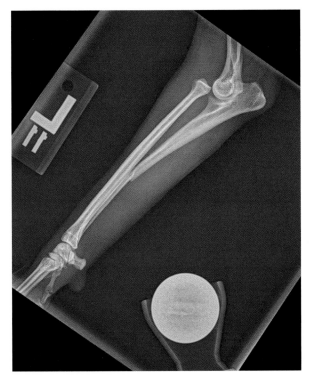 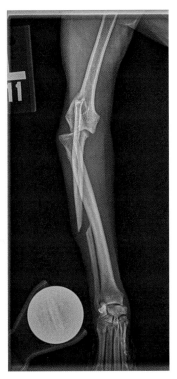

Figure 9.8 Mediolateral and craniocaudal radiographs of a Monteggia fracture. A luxated radius and fractured ulnar shaft are present in this type of fracture. *Source:* Photos courtesy of Dr. M. Rochat.

splint may be used for the immediate postoperative period. A carpal flexion bandage is not useful because the ulna is not a significant weight bearing bone.

Prognosis: Prognosis is dependent on the complexity and chronicity of the fracture as well as the amount of soft tissue damage. Patients who receive a repair within a few days of the trauma tend to have a very good outcome [8, 9]. Complications include implant failure and hence failure of the repair; pin migration or breakage of implants with the fracture healed requiring implant removal; decreased ROM of the elbow joint; and OA.

9.2 Managing Expectations with Recommended Treatments

Most elbow injuries have a very good outcome when surgically managed. Because of the complexity and precision required to achieve a positive outcome, these surgeries are best left to the trained surgeon. The most common complication associated with elbow repairs is pin migration; removal of the pin(s) is a minor procedure so should not be viewed as a deterrent to seeking repair.

General practitioners are encouraged to reduce acute luxations when there are no associated fractures present. Some chronic luxations and the more complex "Y"

fracture may be associated with a residual lameness seen after exercise and a decreased range of motion in the joint.

Clients may wish to consider the use of a chest harness to help assist their pet in the postoperative period. If a bandage or splint is used after surgery, then it should be properly cared for and changed weekly (Chapter 4). Range of motion exercises are recommended (once the bandage is removed) to help maintain or re-establish proper function. As with all joint injuries, OA will develop. This need not be a deterrent to pursuing appropriate treatment as it can be of minimal clinical significance with basic OA management (Chapter 3).

9.3 Alternatives When Treatment of Choice is Not an Option

9.3.1 For Patients with a Fracture

The elbow joint is a complex three-bone system that requires structural integrity to function properly. Also, a fracture through the olecranon will be subject to the strong upward distraction forces from the triceps muscle group. The distractive forces will prevent the olecranon from healing and the animal will be unable to fix the elbow joint during weight bearing. Without surgical reconstruction, this complex joint will not function

(a)   (b)

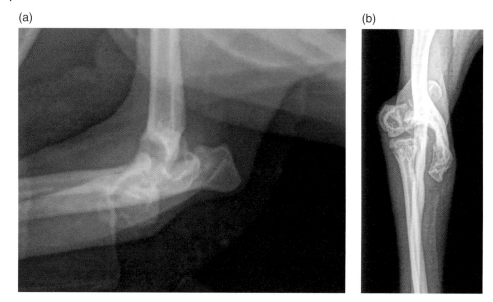

Figure 9.9 Mediolateral (a) and craniocaudal (b) projections of a canine elbow with a non-repaired lateral condylar fracture that healed with a significant malunion. The dog used the limb in a very limited fashion. *Source:* Photo courtesy of the VCA Canada Mississauga Oakville veterinary emergency Hospital and referral group.

properly and ongoing discomfort to the patient will ensue; this outcome often being considered undesirable (Figure 9.9). Having said that, the author has seen several *toy breed* dogs with lateral condylar fractures managed only with a spica splint have outcomes that are *acceptable* to the owners with consideration of the pet's lifestyle. For mid- to large breed dogs, where reconstruction is not an option, then perhaps a forelimb amputation should be considered.

9.3.2   For Patients with a Luxation

A non-reduced luxated elbow will not have a satisfactory outcome and will be painful to the patient for several months. The patient will likely never use the limb very well. Fortunately, a closed reduction is often successful and carries an excellent prognosis. It is therefore definitely worth attempting.

If ligamentous damage is identified once the luxation has been reduced but surgical stabilization is not a possibility, then a spica splint for at least 4 weeks is a reasonable alternative. The prognosis for a small, non-athletic patient with a ligamentous damage that has not been surgically repaired can be good to very good, but may be less optimal in a larger, or more active dog.

If a closed reduction is not successful but the open reduction and surgical reconstruction is not possible, then a forelimb amputation may be the alternative choice.

References

1 Evans, H.E. and de Lahunta, A. (2013). *Miller's Anatomy of the Dog*, 4e. St Louis, MO: Saunders/Elsevier.
2 Perry, K.L., Bruce, M., Woods, S. et al. (2015). Effect of fixation method on postoperative complication rates after surgical stabilization of lateral humeral condylar fractures in dogs. *Vet. Surg.* 44: 246–255.
3 Vannini, R., Smeak, D.D., and Olmstead, M.L. (1988). Evaluation of surgical repair of 135 distal humeral fractures in dogs and cats. *J. Am. Anim. Hosp. Assoc.* 24: 537–545.
4 Bardet, J.F., Hohn, R.B., Rudy, R.L., and Olmstead, M.L. (1983). Fractures of the humerus in dogs and cats. A retrospective study if 130 cases. *Vet. Surg.* 12: 73–77.
5 Marcellin-Little, D., DeYoung, D.J., Ferris, K.K., and Berry, C.M. (1994). Incomplete ossification of the humeral condyle in spaniels. *Vet. Surg.* 23: 475–487.
6 Farrell, M., Draffan, D., Gemmill, T. et al. (2007). In vitro validation of a technique for assessment of canine and feline elbow joint collateral ligament integrity and description of a new method for collateral ligament prosthetic replacement. *Vet. Surg.* 36: 548–556.

7 Sajik, D., Meeson, R.L., Kulendra, N. et al. (2016). Multi-centre retrospective study of long-term outcomes following traumatic elbow luxation in 37 dogs. *J. Sm. Anim. Pract.* 57: 422–428.

8 Schwarz, P.D. and Schrader, S.C. (1984). Ulnar fractures and dislocation of the proximal radial epiphysis (Monteggia lesion) in the dog and cat, a review of 28 cases. *J. Am. Anim. Hosp. Assoc.* 185: 190–194.

9 Vallone, L. and Schulz, K. (2011). Repair technique of Monteggia fractures using an Arthrex tightrope system and ulnar plating. *Vet. Surg.* 40: 734–737.

10

Radius and Ulna

Catherine Popovitch[1], Thomas W.G. Gibson[2], and Anne M. Sylvestre[3]

[1] *Veterinary Specialty and Emergency Center, Levittown, Pennsylvania, USA*
[2] *Ontario Veterinary College, University of Guelph, Guelph, Ontario, Canada*
[3] *Focus and Flourish, Cambridge, Ontario, Canada*

Figure 10.1 identifies the relevant anatomical landmarks of the radius and ulna. Fractures of the diaphysis of the radius and ulna are the most frequently seen fractures in small animal general practices [1]. Banfield hospitals noted that fractures of the radius accounted for 36.5% of all the fractures and 43.1% of the long bones fractures seen in 2014 [1]. In academic referral practices however, fractures of the radius have been reported to have a

(a)

(b)

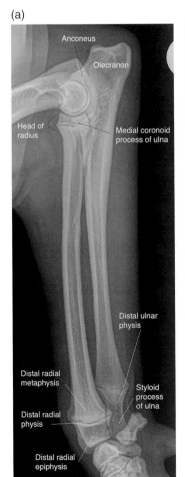
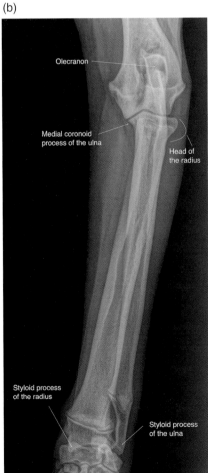

Figure 10.1 Mediolateral (a) and craniocaudal (b) views of the radius and ulna identifying its anatomical landmarks.

lower prevalence than those of the femur [2, 3]. The vast majority (63–75%) of all radial fractures are located in the diaphysis [2, 4].

10.1 Fractures

10.1.1 Fractures of the Proximal Ulna (Figure 10.2)

Fractures through the proximal-most aspect of the ulna (the olecranon), whether in the mature animal or through the proximal ulnar physis of an immature patient, are extremely rare.

Treatment of choice: A surgical repair of this fracture has to counteract the pull of the triceps muscle, making a pin and tension band repair ideal.

Postoperative management: Postoperatively, a soft padded bandage is placed for 2–3 days for compression of the soft tissues. Activity restriction is recommended until radiographic signs of healing have occurred. Controlled activity in the form of on-leash walks and formal physical therapy is recommended.

Prognosis: The outcome is good with a stable repair. Complications include pin migration or pin and/or wire failure particularly if the patient is not adequately exercise restricted.

10.1.2 Fractures of the Proximal Radius

Isolated fractures of the proximal radius are rare, as the anatomy of the elbow joint predisposes to fractures of the lateral portion of the humeral condyle, sparing the radius. Fractures of the radial head usually involve the articular surface and these require meticulous anatomical reconstruction.

Treatment of choice: Accurate repair is essential as the radiohumeral joint carries the majority of load during weight bearing essential for normal walking. Repair should not be attempted without expertise and experience. Immature patients may suffer a Salter–Harris type I physeal injury. Fractures of the radial neck are infrequent and usually are comminuted fractures involving the proximal radius and ulna. Chronic fractures with severe articular damage or non-reconstructable severely comminuted fractures may necessitate a salvage procedure.

Postoperative management: Postoperative immobilization using a lateral splint or Robert Jones bandage may be required for 2–6 weeks to augment internal fixation of comminuted fractures. Serial radiographs to monitor bone healing will determine when splint removal is appropriate.

Prognosis: Prognosis for a successful outcome depends upon the fracture type and the stability and accuracy of the repair particularly with articular fractures. Radial head fractures will commonly result in development of osteoarthritis. As with all young patients with a Salter–Harris type I injury, the owner must be warned that growth disturbances may occur even after an apparently successful surgical repair. Premature closure of the physis and shortening of the radius are possible sequelae.

10.1.3 Fractures of the Radius in Toy Breed Dogs

These fractures are by far the most common fracture seen in small animal practices [2, 3]. They are most prevalent in young, toy breed dogs and are usually the result of a jump down from a height. One study reported that they occurred bilaterally in 26% of the cases [4].

10.1.3.1 Isolated Fracture of the Radius, with the Ulna Intact (Figure 10.3)

These account for approximately 18% of radius–ulnar fractures [2]. The intact ulna acts as an internal splint providing stability.

Treatment of choice: A splint placed on the palmar aspect of the antebrachium is used to treat fractures involving only the radius.

Patient management: The limb should be splinted until the fracture has healed, which should take between 4 and 8 weeks, based on the patient's age and amount of displacement.

Prognosis: These fractures typically heal quickly and the prognosis is excellent.

10.1.3.2 Complete Fracture of the Mid- to Distal Third of the Radius (Toy Breed Dogs)

These are most often transverse or short oblique fractures and the majority of them have significant displacement (Figure 10.4).

Treatment of choice: Bone plating is the best fixation method and is the best choice for these fractures. The cranial approach to the distal portion of the radius is straightforward and a two-piece mid-diaphyseal fracture configuration is one a general practitioner with the appropriate equipment and training in fracture fixation can readily handle.

Postoperative management: Postoperatively these patients may require a soft padded bandage to control swelling for 3–5 days. A splint is not routinely required. Only the fracture of the radius is repaired; the ulna is left without fixation.

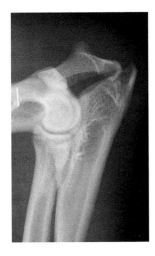

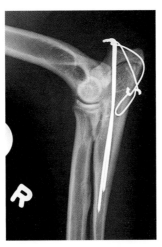

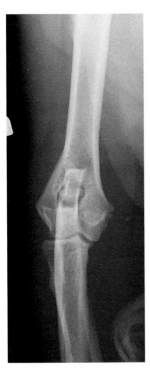

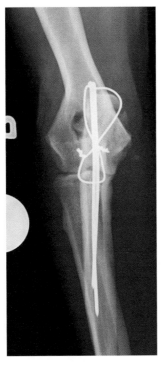

Figure 10.2 Pre- and postoperative mediolateral and craniocaudal radiographs of a fracture through the proximal ulna. This is technically an articular fracture but serves well to demonstrate the repair principle of using a tension band wire system. A non-articular fracture of the proximal-most ulna is very rare. *Source:* Photo courtesy of the Ontario Veterinary College.

Prognosis: The prognosis for return to normal function with these fractures is excellent and the complication rate low [4–7]. The radius must never be repaired with an intra-medullary pin; a major complication rate of up to 80% has been reported with this technique [5]. Complications with plating of diaphyseal

fractures in toy breed dogs are relatively uncommon and include:

- Thermal conduction, where the pet will be lame when out in cold weather. This is a concern in colder climates where the pet may be in temperatures well below 0°C. The reality is that most toy breed dogs are not out on very cold days for any significant duration of time. Plate removal or alterations to the pet's lifestyle during cold spells can resolve this issue.
- Stress protection (Figure 10.5) is seen more frequently with a fracture of the radius and ulna in the toy breed dogs than with any other type of fracture. If the plate is too rigid for the small bone, then most of the stress applied to the antebrachium will be transferred to the plate, rather than the bone, resulting in disuse atrophy (resorption) of the bone. To prevent this problem, the plate can be removed once the bone has healed. Another option is to follow the patient radiographically (6 months after healing has occurred and perhaps again 12 months later) over time and remove the plate if thinning of the radius is observed. Consideration can be given to selecting a repair technique that is less rigid over one that is stronger and more rigid (more screws, thicker plate) for stabilizing the fracture. The less rigid repair can be augmented, if necessary, by applying a short palmar splint postoperatively for 2 weeks (Chapter 4).
- Failure of the repair (Figure 10.6) where the plate breaks or the screws pull out of the bone. A revision surgery is necessary for these patients. Appropriate selection of implants, adhering to the principles of plating and good surgical technique are all instrumental in decreasing the chance of such a failure occurring. This is not a common occurrence.

10.1.4 Fractures of the Radius and Ulna in Non-Toy Breed Dogs and Cats (Figures 10.7 and 10.8)

Fractures of the radius in non-toy breed dogs and in cats are usually a result of a mid- to high-velocity trauma, such as a vehicular accident. These fractures are often located in the distal and mid-portions of the radius with a small percentage found in the proximal diaphysis. They are often multi-fragmented and may be open due to the lack of soft tissues covering the area. In some open fractures the bone will protrude through the skin at the time of the impact but the fracture ends will then recede back under the skin as the limb settles into its post-impact position. The patient must be examined carefully for skin wounds located close to the fracture site. Open fractures

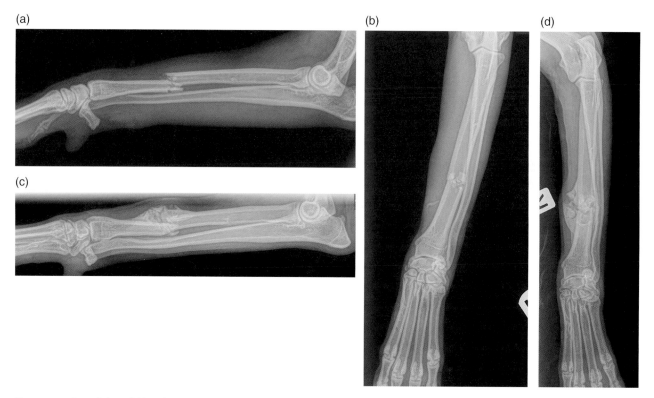

Figure 10.3 A mediolateral (a) and craniocaudal (b) projections of a toy breed dog with an isolated fracture of the radius (intact ulna). The fracture was treated with external coaptation. Follow-up radiographs (c and d) were taken 6 weeks later showing the formation of a bony callus.

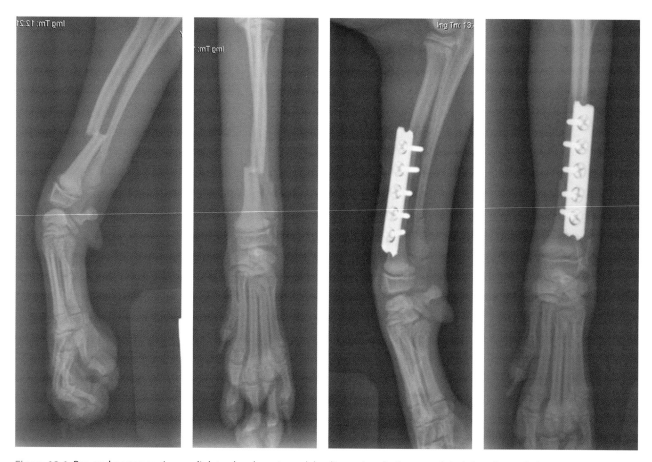

Figure 10.4 Pre- and postoperative mediolateral and craniocaudal radiographs of a fracture of the left radius and ulna in an immature Yorkshire terrier. This fracture was repaired with a cuttable plate and screws.

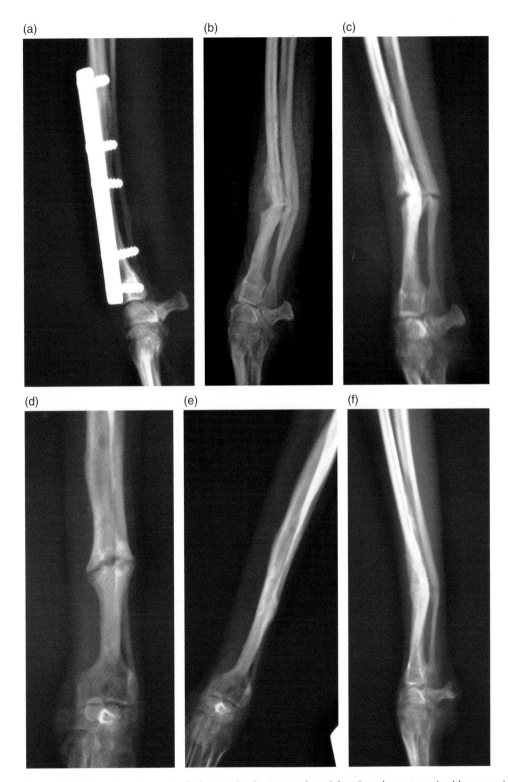

Figure 10.5 Mediolateral view (a) of a fractured radius in a toy breed dog, 5 weeks post-repair with an oversized plate. The plate was removed and the limb was splinted. Eight weeks after the plate was removed one can still appreciate the atrophy and a re-fracturing through the previous site with a mild malalignment (b). Clinically the dog was doing well so splinting was continued. Mediolateral (c) and craniocaudal (d) projections of the limb 6 weeks later. The bone atrophy appears to have progressed so the rigidity of the splint was reduced. Four months later the craniocaudal (e) and mediolateral (f) views show that the fractures have healed and the bone density/thickness has improved. The splint was replaced with a soft padded bandage. Eleven months after the initial fracture the dog was bandage free. Several years postoperatively the dog is still doing well on the limb and has not re-fractured. This case is quite extreme but illustrates well the importance of weight bearing and transference of stresses along a bone, as well as the importance of appropriate selection of implants.

(a)

(b)

(c)

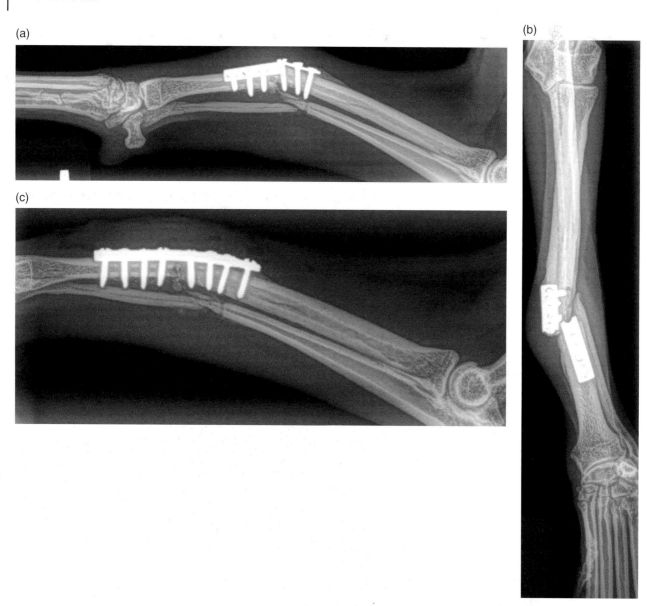

Figure 10.6 Mediolateral (a) and craniocaudal (b) projections of a fractured plate on the radius, which occurred 3 weeks after the initial repair. A mediolateral view of the revision (c) shows that a thicker and longer plate was used. The fracture healed well after the second surgery.

must be treated accordingly to decrease the potential for osteomyelitis (Chapter 2).

Treatment of choice: As with fractures in the toy breeds, if the ulna is intact, then a splint is sufficient to stabilize the fracture. However, when the radius and the ulna are both fractured then fixation with a bone plate or an external fixator are the techniques of choice. The external fixator may be a preferred technique in patients with severely comminuted and/or second- and third-degree open fractures. Typically, only the fracture of the radius is stabilized and the ulna is allowed to heal on its own. Fractures of the radius in the non-toy breed dogs are often more complex, and may involve the proximal portion of the radius, which is more challenging to approach. These repairs can be more difficult and are best left in the hands of the trained surgeon.

Postoperative management: A bandage may be placed on the limb to help reduce swelling for 3–5 days. However, patients with a more complex fracture configuration may require a palmar splint for 2–4 weeks after surgery.

Prognosis: Patients with a fracture of the radius and ulna that is surgically repaired with a plate or external fixator have a very good to good outcome (greater than 90%) with few complications [5]. The poorer outcomes

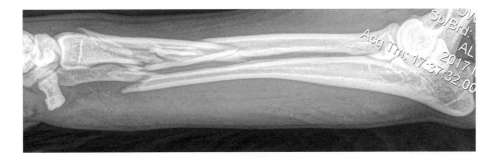

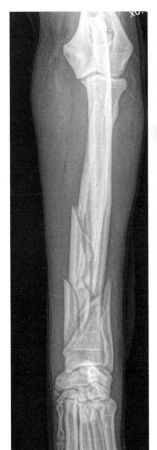
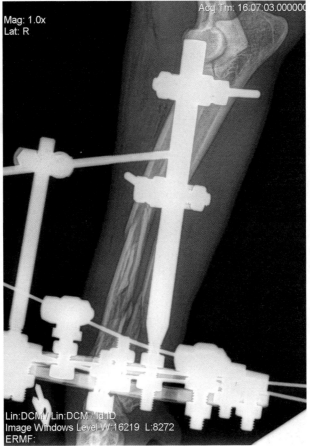
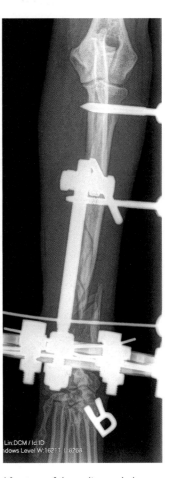

Figure 10.7 Pre- and postoperative mediolateral and craniocaudal radiographs of a multi-fragmented fracture of the radius and ulna that was repaired with a hybrid fixator. *Source:* Photo courtesy of VCA Canada Mississauga Oakville veterinary emergency Hospital and referral group.

and complications were often associated with a failed previous repair attempt with an intra-medullary pin. The radius *must never* be repaired with an intra-medullary pin; a major complication rate of up to 80% has been reported with this technique [5].

The potential types of complications are similar to those described for the toy breed dogs except that stress protection is less common in the larger dogs. However, angular limb deformities +/− elbow subluxation can occur in the non-toy breeds. Around 17.6% of very young large breed dogs (less than 6 months) with fractures of the radius and ulna may suffer from growth abnormalities as they mature skeletally [5]. The conical configuration of the distal ulnar physis makes it more prone to being damaged at the time of the trauma. Damage to this growth plate is typically not visible on the acute radiographs. As the dog grows, a valgus deviation and cranial bowing of the distal radius may become evident (Figure 10.9).

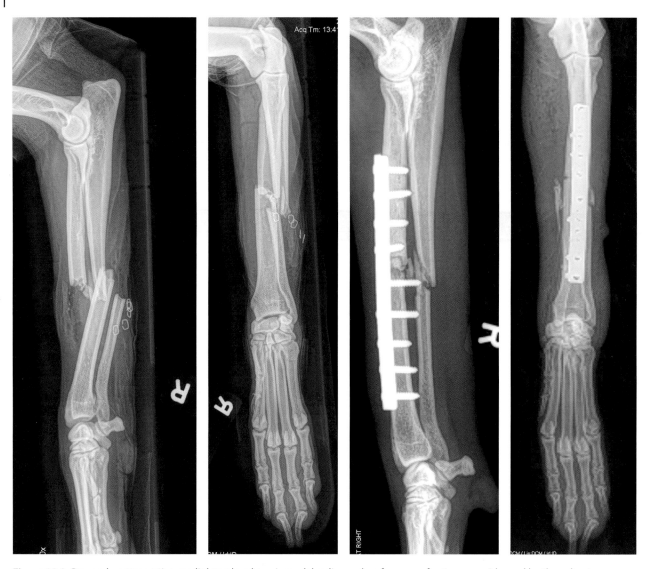

Figure 10.8 Pre- and postoperative mediolateral and craniocaudal radiographs of an open fracture, as evidenced by the subcutaneous pockets of air in the right radius and ulna of a golden retriever. This fracture was repaired with a 3.5 broad compression plate and screws.

There is not much information in the literature on cats with fractures of the radius and ulna. Subjectively, we have found that cats tend to have very good outcomes with plating of a diaphyseal fracture of the radius.

10.1.5 Isolated Fractures of the Shaft of the Ulna (Figure 10.10)

These occur rarely. It is important to emphasize fractures of the diaphysis of the ulna are described here, not ones that are close to the elbow joint. These fractures usually are a result of blunt trauma.

Treatment of choice: A soft padded bandage or palmar splint.

Management: Four to six weeks in a bandage or splint should be sufficient.

Prognosis: The prognosis is excellent.

10.1.6 Physeal Fractures of the Distal Radius (Figure 10.11)

Treatment of choice: Fractures of the distal physis have little soft tissue coverage and may be repaired in a closed fashion with fluoroscopic guidance. Open reduction and repair with cross pins may require small bilateral incisions.

Postoperative management: Repairs should be augmented with placement of a caudal splint for 2–3 weeks and recheck radiographs should be performed at 3–4 weeks

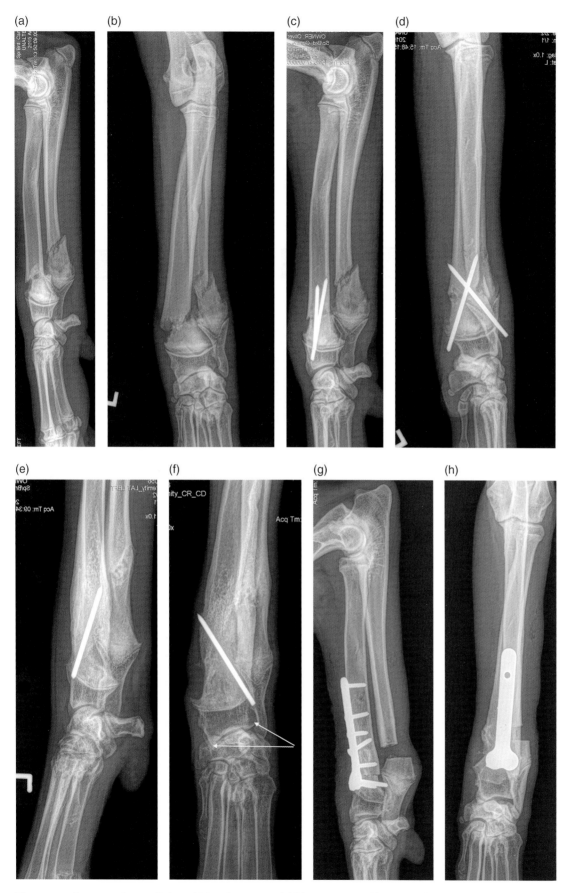

Figure 10.9 Pre-operative mediolateral (a) and craniocaudal (b) projections of fractures of the radius and ulna in a 4-month-old German shepherd dog. The radial fracture was stabilized with cross pins as seen in the postoperative views (c and d). The follow-up radiographs taken 4 weeks later (e and f) show significant valgus angulation (arrows) of the distal radius due to premature closing of the ulnar physis; one pin had loosened and had been removed previously. The problem was rectified with a corrective osteotomy (g and h). *Source:* Photo courtesy of VCA Canada Mississauga Oakville veterinary emergency Hospital and referral group.

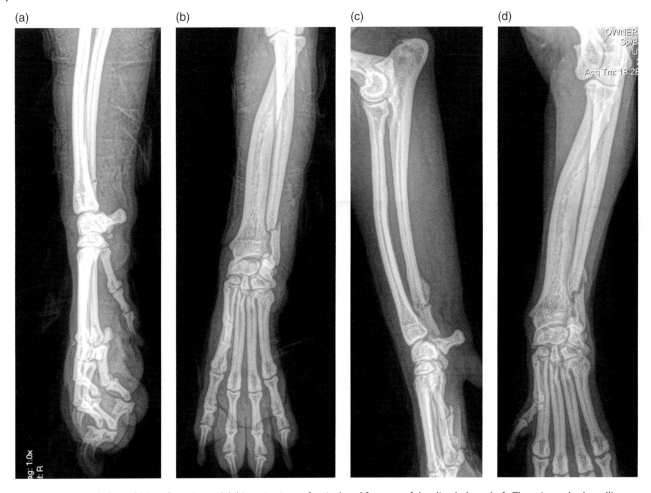

(a) (b) (c) (d)

Figure 10.10 Mediolateral (a) and craniocaudal (b) projections of an isolated fracture of the distal ulnar shaft. There is marked swelling associated with the trauma that caused the fracture. The carpus was stable and the limb was placed in a short caudal splint for 4 weeks. The follow-up radiographs (c and d) show that a bridging callus is forming.

with expectation of rapid and complete healing. Once evidence of radiographic healing has occurred, pins may be removed.

Prognosis: The prognosis with this repair is very good. Owners should be warned of the possibility of pin migration, and, potentially but not commonly, premature closure of growth plates resulting in angular limb deformities, including elbow incongruity.

10.2 Managing Expectations with Recommended Treatments

The outcomes with most fractures of the radius/ulna seen in small animal practices carry a very high success rate with few complications when managed surgically. Owners should be strongly encouraged to seek appropriate surgical management for their pet rather than relying on an alternative treatment method. A general practitioner with the appropriate equipment and *training in plating*

techniques can expect a high success rate in two-piece mid- to distal diaphyseal fractures of the radius in toy breed dogs. Because of potential stress protection issues in toy breeds, some surgeons will routinely remove the plates from the radius once healing is complete. Others may choose to use a less rigid fixation and place the patient in a splinted bandage for a few weeks.

10.3 Alternatives When Treatment of Choice is Not an Option

There is no doubt that the best treatment option for most fractures of the radius is stabilization with a plate or external fixator. However, should this not be an option for a pet or owner, then external coaptation using a splint or bivalve cast can be attempted. In most cases of radius and ulnar fracture the ends of the bones are displaced. Closed reduction should be attempted in order to try and realign the fracture ends if the fracture is transverse in configuration.

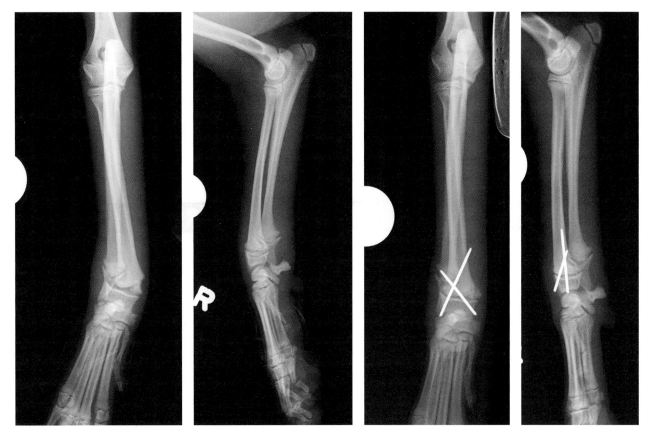

Figure 10.11 Pre- and postoperative craniocaudal and lateral radiographs of a laterally displaced Salter–Harris I fracture of the distal radius in a dog repaired with K-wires using a crossed pin technique.

External coaptation may be more successful with a less prolonged healing time if there is cortical contact between the fracture ends. Closed manipulation is done using traction and digital manipulation. Hanging the limb from a height places traction on the fracture helping to displace the fragments and making reduction easier. This is especially helpful in larger dogs. Closed reduction can be challenging when the distal fragment is too small to grasp and maneuver into place. Reduction is considered adequate when there is a minimum of 25% contact between the two fracture ends, with no angulation [5]. Oblique and multifragment fracture configurations are inherently less stable and will fall out of alignment in a splint or cast.

A full encircling fiberglass cast is the most stable external coaptation. The disadvantage is the inability to evaluate the limb for any cast related sores; also, these can be quite heavy for the toy breeds. A palmar splint or bivalve cast may be a better option for management purposes (Chapter 4 has more details on bandages and splints). It is best to avoid using a large amount of cast padding as this allows the bones to shift within the splint once the padding has become compressed. This can lead to a malalignment, delayed healing, or non-union.

A 1983 study [5] indicated that mid-sized (10–65 lb) and immature dogs had the best outcomes with fractures of the radius and ulna treated with a splint or cast. The success rate declined as the age of the patients increased. The toy breeds treated with a cast or splint had a high nonunion rate [8]; the immature toy breed dogs had better outcomes with splinting than did the older ones. The message is that external coaptation for fractures of the radius and ulna in toy breeds is not a great choice, but perhaps the following guidelines might help manage that risk:

- A palmar splinted bandage that *excludes* the elbow can be applied. These fractures are located in the distal third of the bone and the support is adequate with the shorter splint (not so for fractures located in the proximal radius). Not incorporating the elbow makes the splinted bandage lighter, more comfortable, and precludes the formation of skin lesions over the olecranon and distal biceps area (Chapter 4 has more information).
- Splinting material that is not heavy should be used; for example, a tongue depressor cut to appropriate size may be adequate for a toy breed dog; a heavy custom fiberglass splint should be avoided.

- The paw can be incorporated within the splint for the first 4–6 weeks. After that, the splint can be shortened (a tongue depressor works well for this) so that it extends from the mid-metacarpals to the proximal third of the antebrachium. The patient can now walk on the paw of the splinted limb so that the stresses transmitted to the bone can help with healing.
- The splinted bandage must fit the antebrachium well enough to prevent motion and malalignment, avoiding excessive padding. If using stirrups, they should not "hold up the bandage," but rather, the bandage should stay in place because of appropriate tensions. A well-fitted splinted bandage should maintain the fragments in a functional alignment while minimizing the formation of sores over the bony prominences.
- Excellent care of the splinted bandage by the owner and veterinary staff is key to maximizing success (weekly changes are recommended).
- Caution should be exercised when changing the splinted bandage so as not to allow the patient to walk on the limb and to ensure that the antebrachium is always supported in order to prevent motion at the fracture site while the splint is off.
- Once there is radiographic evidence that the fracture has healed, the splint should be replaced by a soft padded bandage for 2 weeks. Jumping from heights should be prevented for several more weeks to allow the bone to develop more strength.
- If the patient is mature (over 12 months), the owner should be strongly encouraged to pursue surgery. It is important to properly educate the client regarding the high success rate and low complication rate with surgery in contrast to the lower success rate and higher complication rate with splinting.

In summary, a fracture of the radius and ulna addressed conservatively can have a good outcome, especially if the patient is young and of mid-size and the owners are compliant in terms of bandage care. Caution must be exercised with the toy breed dogs as a higher rate of malunions and non-unions can be expected (Figure 10.12). It is important to appreciate the potential frustrations, difficulties, and costs associated with long-term splinting; this is not to dissuade the client from proceeding but to ensure that they will participate in their pet's care. Given the high success rate and positive outcomes with repair of these fractures, it is worth taking the time to ensure that the clients truly understand the likelihood that their pet will do well rather than let fear of

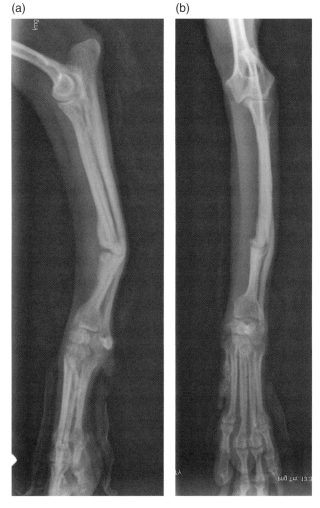

(a)   (b)

Figure 10.12 Mediolateral (a) and craniocaudal (b) projections of a healing fractured radius and ulna treated with a splint for 10 months because of delayed healing. Notice: (1) the thick callus that has formed, indicative of micromotion at the fracture site; (2) the callus is starting to bridge medially and laterally indicating that the delayed union is progressing to a union; (3) the ulna is complete at this time; (4) the significant radiographic caudal malalignment was only slightly clinically apparent; and (5) the slight decrease in density of the carpal bones is common in antebrachii splinted for long periods of time. The splinted bandage was replaced by a soft padded bandage for 2 weeks after these radiographs were taken. This patient had a very good outcome and the owners were satisfied despite the delayed union and mild malunion.

a potential complication and financial concerns be the basis for their decision making.

The alternative to splinting would be a forelimb amputation. The cost of this procedure would be only marginally less than that of a fracture repair. Again, given the high success and low complication rates with repair of these fractures, amputation should not be a primary consideration.

References

1 Roush, J.K. (2015). Pet health by numbers: Prevalence of bone fractures in dogs and cats. Today's Veterinary Practice. Retrieved from: http://todaysveterinarypractice. navc.com/pet-health-by-the-numbers-prevalence-of-bone-fractures-in-dogs-cats.

2 Unger, M., Montavon, P.M., and Heim, U.F.A. (1990). Classification of fractures of the long bones in the dog and cat: introduction and clinical application. *Vet. Comp. Orthop. Traumatol.* 3: 41–50.

3 Miller, C.W., Sumner-Smith, G., Sheridan, C., and Pennock, P.W. (1998). Using the Unger system to classify 386 long bone fractures in dogs. *J. Small Anim. Pract.* 39: 390–393.

4 Larsen, L.J., Roush, J.K., and McLaughlin, R.M. (1999). Bone plate fixation of distal radius and ulna fractures in small- and miniature-breed dogs. *J. Am. Anim. Hosp. Assoc.* 35: 243–250.

5 Lappin, M.R., Aron, D.N., Herron, H.L., and Malnati, G. (1983). Fractures of the radius and ulna in the dog. *J. Am. Anim. Hosp. Assoc.* 19: 643–650.

6 Waters, D.J., Breur, G.J., and Toombs, J.P. (1993). Treatment of common forelimb fractures in miniature- and toy-breed dogs. *J. Am. Anim. Hosp. Assoc.* 29: 442–448.

7 Pozzi, A., Hudson, C.C., Gauthier, C.M., and Lewis, D.D. (2013). Retrospective comparison of minimally invasive plate osteosynthesis and open reduction and internal fixation of radius-ulna fractures in dogs. *Vet. Surg.* 42: 19–27.

8 Vaughan, L.C. (1964). A clinical study of non-union fractures in the dog. *J. Small Anim. Pract.* 5: 173–177.

11

Carpal Joint
Anne M. Sylvestre

Focus and Flourish, Cambridge, Ontario, Canada

The carpus is a very complex joint. It is composed of seven bones and one small spherical sesamoid (Figure 11.1). It has three joint levels: the antebrachiocarpal joint, the middle carpal joint, and the carpometacarpal joint. Properly identifying the fractures and ligamentous instabilities that can occur in the carpus can be a challenge.

Stress radiographic views and/or computed tomography are often necessary to accurately image this joint. Radiographic interpretation can be difficult because of its complexity. Fortunately, the widespread use of digital radiography has made it easy to engage the expertise of a board-certified radiologist to help with these cases.

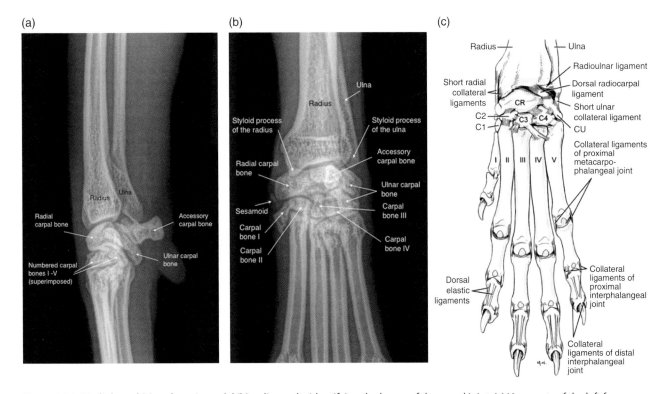

Figure 11.1 Mediolateral (a) and craniocaudal (b) radiographs identifying the bones of the carpal joint. (c) Ligaments of the left forepaw, dorsal aspect. (d) Tendons and ligaments of the carpus, palmar aspect. (e) Deep ligaments of the left forepaw, palmar aspect. CI to CIV, first, second, third, fourth carpals; CR, radial carpal; CU, ulnar carpal; I to V, metacarpals; CA, accessory carpal. *Source:* From [13].

Fracture Management for the Small Animal Practitioner, First Edition. Edited by Anne M. Sylvestre.
© 2019 John Wiley & Sons, Inc. Published 2019 by John Wiley & Sons, Inc.

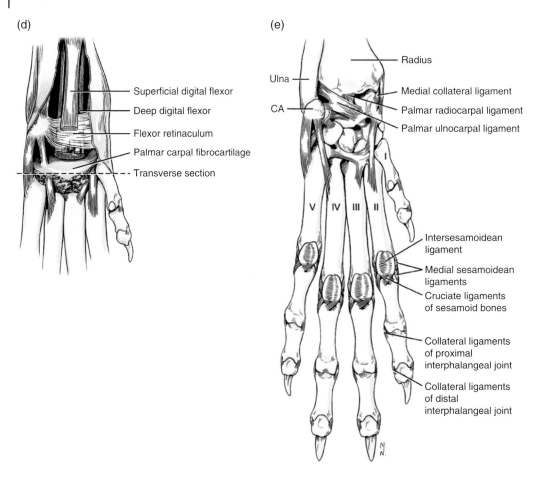

(d)

Superficial digital flexor
Deep digital flexor
Flexor retinaculum
Palmar carpal fibrocartilage
Transverse section

(e)

Ulna
CA

Radius
Medial collateral ligament
Palmar radiocarpal ligament
Palmar ulnocarpal ligament

V IV III II I

Intersesamoidean ligament
Medial sesamoidean ligaments
Cruciate ligaments of sesamoid bones

Collateral ligaments of proximal interphalangeal joint

Collateral ligaments of distal interphalangeal joint

Figure 11.1 (Continued)

11.1 Fractures and Ligamentous Injuries

11.1.1 Fractures of the Styloid Process of the Radius or Distal Ulna

The styloid processes are the distal-most points of the ulna and medial radius. The medial collateral ligament originates on the radial styloid process and the lateral collateral ligament originates from the ulnar styloid process; therefore, a fracture of either styloid can lead to an instability of the carpal joint. Section 11.1.5 below describes how to diagnose collateral ligament instability of the carpal joint. Fractures of the radial styloid process (medial) are more common than fractures of the ulnar styloid process (Figure 11.2).

Treatment of choice: These fractures are best repaired with Kirschner wires +/- tension band wires or with a lag screw. A fracture of the styloid process of the radius is also considered an articular fracture and therefore requires accurate reduction as well as rigid fixation.

Postoperative management: Additional support with a short palmar splint is usually recommended for 4–6 weeks following surgery.

Prognosis: The prognosis with a repaired styloid fracture is very good to excellent in the hands of a trained surgeon. The wires may need to be removed once the healing process is complete as there is little soft tissue coverage over the implants so they may irritate the skin.

A fracture of the ulnar styloid process that is *without* a lateral collateral instability of the carpal joint can occur (Figure 11.3). Such a fracture can be treated conservatively with restricted activity and a splinted bandage for 4 weeks.

11.1.2 Fractures of the Radial Carpal Bone (Figure 11.4)

These are very difficult to diagnose as they are easily missed on routine radiographs. Slab or chip fractures can occur on this large cuboidal bone directly below the radius as a result of a jump or fall, but, more commonly, this fracture presents as a chronic intermittent lameness in sporting dogs, with no history of trauma. These dogs will have soft tissue swelling over the carpus.

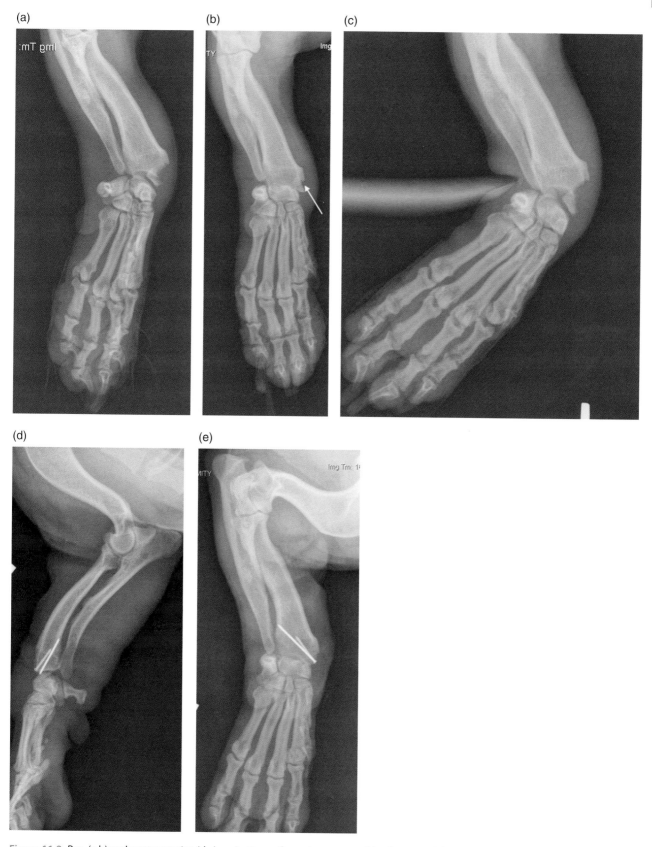

Figure 11.2 Pre- (a,b) and postoperative (d,e) projections of a canine carpus with a fracture of the medial styloid process that was repaired with a screw and wire. The stress view (c) shows the instability in the carpal joint as a result of this fracture. *Source:* Photos courtesy of Dr. M. Rochat.

(a)

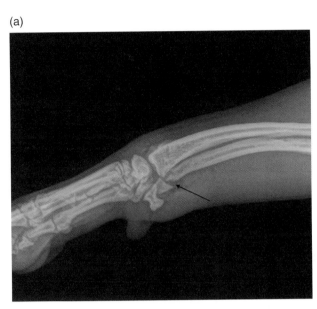

(b)

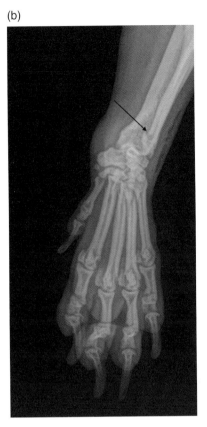

Figure 11.3 Mediolateral (a) and craniocaudal (b) projections of canine carpus with a fracture of the ulnar styloid process without instability of the lateral collateral ligament to the carpal joint. The dog was treated with a soft padded bandage for 2 weeks.

Treatment of choice: The most appropriate treatment method is unclear for these chronic non-traumatic fractures. Methods that have been used include: reattaching the fragment with a countersunk bone screw; excision of smaller fragments; external coaptation and rest; and pancarpal arthrodesis.

Postoperative management: Patients that have had surgery are typically placed in a short palmar splint for 2–4 weeks.

Prognosis: Varying degrees of lameness, exacerbated by exercise, have been reported with all treatment methods [1–3]. A more recent study reported that the patients were free of lameness after internal repair with a low profile screw [4].

11.1.3 Fractures of the Accessory Carpal Bone

These fractures are most commonly seen in racing greyhounds. Fractures of the accessory carpal bones in non-racing dogs occur infrequently. When they do they are usually comminuted fractures of the body of the accessory carpal bone (Figure 11.5), or avulsion fractures of the proximal tip of the accessory carpal bone, where the tendon of the flexor carpi ulnaris muscle inserts.

Treatment of choice: For the racing dog, surgical repair (usually with a lag screw) is preferred in order for them to successfully race again [5]. This surgery is best left to the trained surgeon. The non-racing dog with the comminuted fracture of the body of the accessory carpal bone can be treated conservatively, with external coaptation until there is radiographic evidence that the fracture has healed (approximately 6–8 weeks). In the case of an avulsion fracture, the small fragment can be excised [5].

Postoperative management: After surgery, the patient is placed in a splint for 2 weeks. Once the splint is removed, a soft padded bandage is applied for 2 more weeks and then continued activity restriction for another month before gradually returning to regular activity.

Prognosis: The outcome for these patients is good [5].

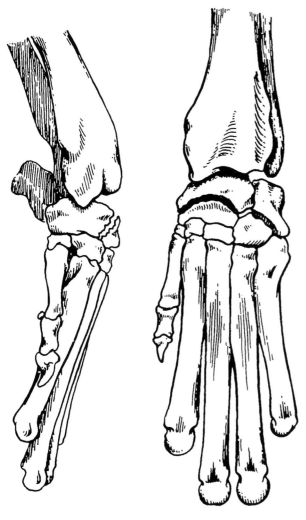

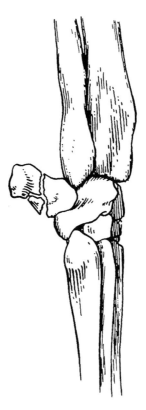

Figure 11.5 Schematic representation of a comminuted fracture of the body of the accessory carpal bone. *Source:* From [14].

Figure 11.4 Schematic representation of a fracture of the radial carpal bone. *Source:* From [14].

11.1.4 Fractures of the Ulnar Carpal Bone

These are very rare fractures. The location of the ulnar carpal bone makes it difficult to access and the small nature of the bone makes reconstruction challenging. There is one report of a dog with a multi-fragmented fracture of the ulnar carpal bone. The smaller fragments were surgically excised and the limb was splinted postoperatively. The dog had an acceptable outcome according to the owners, with lameness after exercise and when first rising after rest [6].

11.1.5 Collateral Ligament Injuries

Ligamentous injuries to the carpal joint are more frequent than fractures. Damage to the medial radial collateral ligament is one of the more common injuries

to the carpus. Exaggerated valgus deformity can be observed due to the medial instability.

Diagnosis: Damage to the medial collateral ligament is made by placing the carpus straight or in slight extension, and applying pressure on the lateral surface of the carpus with the thumbs while trying to "crack" the medial surface of the joint open (Figure 11.6). It is helpful to compare the injured carpus to the normal contralateral one.

Treatment of choice: The damaged ligament is reconstructed by drilling tunnels into the radius and radial carpal bones, or by using bone anchors at the appropriate landmarks, through which a strong, heavy-gauge suture material is threaded. The repair of a medial collateral ligament injury is best left in the hands of a trained surgeon.

Postoperative management: Postoperatively, the limb is placed in a short caudal splint for approximately 4 weeks followed by a soft padded bandage for 2 weeks and continued restricted activity for a total of 8 weeks. Commercially available braces may also be helpful for these cases. Activity restriction and appropriate patient care, as described in Chapter 3, are indicated.

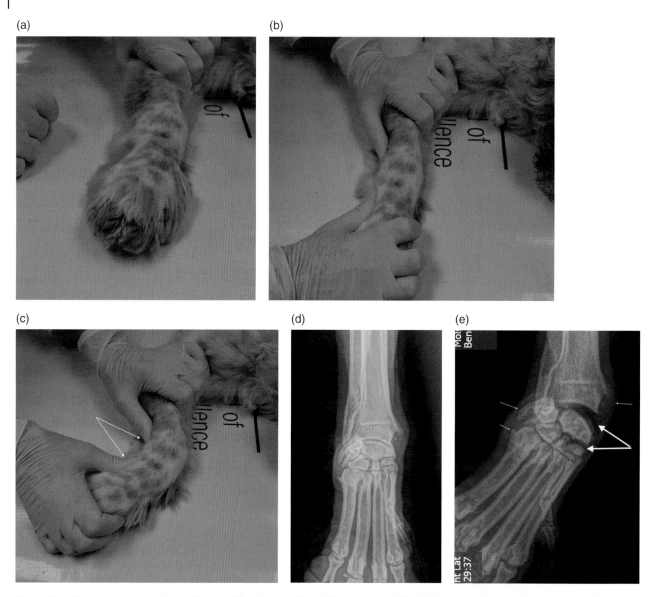

Figure 11.6 To assess the carpus for medial instability due to collateral ligament or radial styloid process damage, the patient should be heavily sedated or anesthetized. The paw and antebrachium are aligned in a natural, straight position (no flexion) (a). The clinician's hands are placed on the metacarpals and the antebrachium with the thumbs on the lateral aspect of the carpus (b) and pressure is applied (arrows c), via the thumbs, to the lateral aspect of the carpus to "crack" the medial side "open." In subtle cases, it is best to compare the injured side to the contralateral, normal, limb. Craniocaudal radiographs are taken of the limb in the "normal" (d) and "stressed" position (e) to demonstrate where the opening is located (thick arrows). The patient in this radiograph has other incidental chronic abnormalities in that carpus (thin arrows).

Prognosis: Patients with a damaged collateral ligament can have a very good outcome with surgical stabilization. Osteoarthritis will ensue and the patient should be managed accordingly (Chapter 3). Damaged collateral ligaments treated with splinting alone do not have favorable outcomes.

11.1.6 Shearing Injuries

The collateral ligaments can also be damaged by a shearing injury. These typically occur as a result of an automobile accident. There is often significant loss of skin, soft tissue, and bone associated with this injury.

Treatment of choice: The initial treatment is to manage the wound by debriding the exposed tissues, and stabilizing the joint with a short palmar splint. Surgical stabilization of the joint is often delayed until the wound bed is clean and showing healthy granulation tissue. The joint can be surgically stabilized by reconstructing the collateral ligament (as described in Section 11.1.5) or with a pancarpal arthrodesis. The choice may depend on the extent of the injury.

Postoperative management: Postoperatively the carpus is supported with an external fixator or a palmar splint. Some surgeons will argue that wound management is easier with an external fixator. The decision whether to use a palmar splint or an external fixator is one of personal preference. Either way, ongoing management of the initial wound with regular bandage changes will likely be necessary.

Prognosis: The prognosis is dependent on the degree of damage to the carpus and surrounding soft tissues; but overall, an appropriately managed patients can expect good outcome. Many of these cases will benefit from the expertise of an experienced surgeon.

11.1.7 Hyperextension Injuries

Hyperextensions are among the more common injuries to the carpus. They usually occur as a result of a fall or jump from a significant height and imply that there has been disruption of palmar ligaments and/or the fibrocartilaginous plate. The animal may start to weight bear within a week of the trauma but the stance will be plantigrade, in varying degrees, depending on the extent of the injury.

Diagnosis: A mediolateral radiograph is taken with the joint hyperextended to its maximum as well as the standard mediolateral and dorsopalmar views. Heavy sedation is required for the hyperextended radiographic view. The carpometacarpal joint (Figure 11.7) is the most commonly affected location (46%), followed by the middle carpal (Figure 11.8) (28%), the

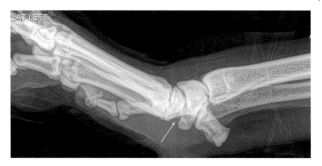

Figure 11.8 Mediolateral projection of a carpus with a hyperextension injury centered at the mid-carpal level. The increased space between the ulnar carpal bone and numbered carpal bones is evident (arrow). The injury was repaired with a partial carpal arthrodesis. *Source:* Photos courtesy of VCA Canada Mississauga Oakville veterinary emergency Hospital and referral group.

middle carpal and carpometacarpal combined (16%), and finally the least frequently injured is the antebrachiocarpal joint (10%). Severe disruption of the palmar ligaments and fibrocartilaginous plate can lead to hyperextension on multiple levels including a luxation of the accessory carpal bone (Figure 11.9) [5].

Treatment of choice: Proper identification of the level of the hyperextension is paramount in order to use the appropriate treatment option. Hyperextension of the carpometacarpal joint as well as for that of the middle carpal joint (or a combination of the two) are managed with a partial carpal arthrodesis (Section 11.5 has more details including postoperative management and prognosis). A pancarpal arthrodesis is performed with a hyperextension injury of the antebrachiocarpal joint (see Section 11.4 for more details).

11.1.8 Luxation of the Antebrachiaocarpal Joint (Figure 11.10)

Luxation of the antebrachial joint is an extremely rare problem. It implies severe damage to all the supportive structures of this joint.

Treatment of choice: A pancarpal arthrodesis is the best treatment for this injury (Section 11.4 has more details).

11.1.9 Luxation of the Accessory Carpal Bone (Figure 11.9)

This luxation is a rare occurrence [5]. With this injury, the accessory bone is angled proximally and there is increased space between the distal portion of the accessory carpal bone and ulnar carpal bone. It may be associated with a mid-carpal hyperextension injury.

Treatment of choice: This injury can be repaired with a partial carpal arthrodesis or a pancarpal arthrodesis (Sections 11.4 and 11.5 have more details).

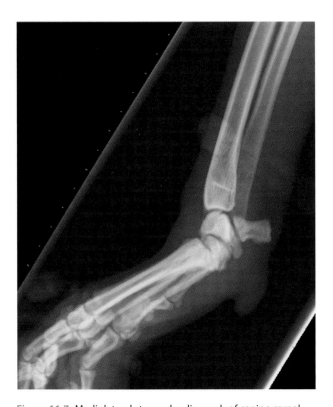

Figure 11.7 Mediolateral stressed radiograph of canine carpal hyperextension at the intercarpal and carpometacarpal level. The proximal carpal bones override the distal row. *Source:* Mark Bush, East of England Vets.

(a)

(b)

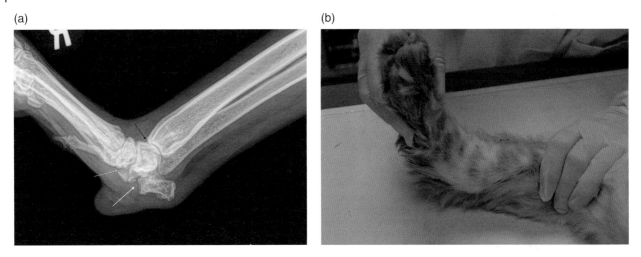

Figure 11.9 Mediolateral projection (a) of a carpus with a luxation of the accessory carpal bone; the proximal angle and increased space between the base of the accessory carpal bone and the ulnar carpal bone (thick arrow). This patient also has a mid-carpal hyperextension injury (thin arrow) and excessive motion in the antebrachiocarpal joint (black arrow). (b) The extent of hyperextension of the carpus noted on physical exam under heavy sedation. *Source:* Photo courtesy of VCA Canada Mississauga Oakville veterinary emergency Hospital and referral group.

(b)

(a)

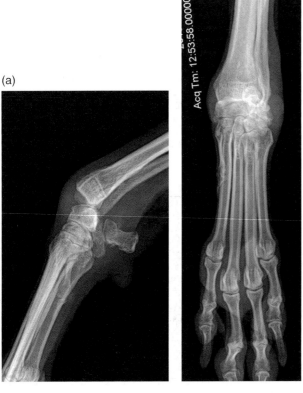

Figure 11.10 Mediolateral (a) and craniocaudal (b) projections of canine carpus with a luxation of the antebrachiocarpal joint. The injury was successfully treated with a pancarpal arthrodesis.

11.1.10 Luxation of the Radiocarpal Bone (Figure 11.11)

This is also a rare trauma. The large cuboidal bone just below the radius can luxate following a fall or jump.

Treatment of choice: A large dog will benefit from surgical repair with a transarticular K-wire and reconstruction of the radial ligament [5]. This surgery is best left in

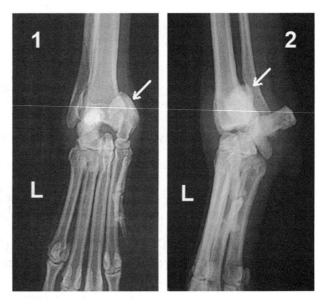

Figure 11.11 Luxation of the radiocarpal bone. *Source:* [7].

the hands of a trained surgeon. A small breed dog may have an acceptable outcome with a closed reduction and a splint.

Postoperative management: The carpus is immobilized with a short palmar splint for 4–6 weeks postoperatively followed by a soft padded bandage for 1–2 weeks.

Prognosis: There is little information on the outcome of patients with this injury because there are so few reported cases.

11.2 Managing Expectations with Recommended Treatments

Overall success with surgical management of carpal injuries is very good so owners should be encouraged to seek appropriate treatment for their pet. Many of the carpal injuries and repairs will be protected with a short palmar splint for 4–6 weeks. Proper bandage care with weekly changes will be necessary (Chapter 4).

The implants, especially pins and some bone anchors, may be a source of irritation of the overlying skin given the lack of soft tissue coverage in that area. They can be removed once the fracture has healed or once there is sufficient fibrosis following ligamentous reconstruction.

Osteoarthritis (OA) will develop in any joint that has sustained a significant trauma; therefore, owners must be counseled on how to manage OA. The eventuality of OA need not be a deterrent for pursuing surgical repair as pets can still have an active life with appropriate management.

Partial carpal arthrodesis carries a good prognosis and low complication rate. The overall function of the carpal joint will be only slightly altered. Pancarpal arthrodesis is a much more involved and detail-oriented surgery, and the function of the carpus will be completely altered; having said that, the outcome for the patient is good. Both these surgeries should be performed by a trained surgeon; owners should be encouraged to seek the appropriate care.

11.3 Alternatives When Treatment of Choice is Not an Option

11.3.1 For Patients with a Fracture

In general, there are no good alternatives to surgery for fractures of the articular surfaces of the carpus, unless the fragment is minimally displaced. Should

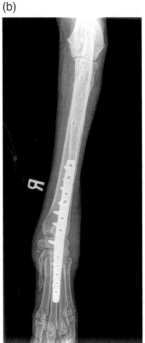

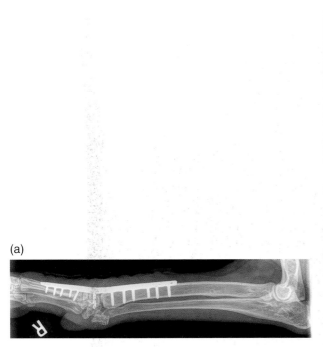

Figure 11.12 Mediolateral (a) and craniocaudal (b) projections of canine carpus with a pancarpal arthrodesis. These are the postoperative radiographs of the patient in Figure 11.9. *Source:* Photos courtesy of VCA Canada Mississauga Oakville veterinary emergency Hospital and referral group.

surgery not be a possibility at all then conservative management with external coaptation until the fracture has healed (6–8 weeks) can be attempted. The outcome will depend on the fracture type, severity of displacement, and location. The best outcome that can be expected would be a lameness that occurs after strenuous activity, while the worst would be a constant moderate lameness.

11.3.2 For Patients with Ligamentous Injuries

When there is a significant instability in a joint, non-surgical treatment options that will result in a pet returning to a reasonable level of activity do not exist. Clients can be reassured that their pet can have a good outcome with surgery and be encouraged to seek the appropriate care. Without surgery the instability will remain causing difficulties for the patient. A carpal brace can be purchased, which will help the pet ambulate more comfortably, but it will not solve the instability or hyperextension problem. Some dogs can enjoy a reasonably good level of activity that includes daily walks and some gentle off-leash activity with a brace. A custom-made brace is far superior to the commercially available type. The pet tends to be more comfortable in a custom-made brace and will experience fewer sores created from an inappropriate fit. Owners are more likely to use the brace if their pet is comfortable and it is easy to apply. A custom-made brace is worth the extra expense.

11.4 About Pancarpal Arthrodesis (Figure 11.12)

A pancarpal arthrodesis implies that the entire carpal joint is surgically fused. The plate will span from the distal third or quarter of the radius to approximately the mid-third metacarpal bone. At surgery, the cartilage between each bone is removed using a high-speed burr. Once that process is complete a plate is applied, typically to the dorsal surface of the limb. Cancellous bone graft is inserted between all the bones and the site is closed. The carpus can no longer be flexed or extended. This procedure is indicated for patients with antebrachiocarpal hyperextension, antebrachiocarpal luxations, articular fractures that cannot be repaired, and severe osteoarthritis of the carpal joint.

Postoperative management: The repair is typically protected with a short palmar splint until there is radiographic evidence of bony union of the major carpal joints (approximately 6–8 weeks) followed by a soft padded bandage for another 2 weeks.

Prognosis: The long-term outcomes have been reported to be good (occasional lameness) to excellent (return to regular activity without lameness). The major complication rate has been reported to be as high as 17% and examples of complications include: fractures of the third metacarpal bone, draining tracts necessitating removal of the implants, implant breakage, and osteomyelitis [8–11]. This surgery is best left in the hands of the trained surgeon.

11.5 About Partial Carpal Arthrodesis (Figure 11.13)

The partial carpal arthrodesis implies that only some of the joints of the carpus are surgically fused, typically the middle and/or distal joints, leaving the main, antebrachiocarpal joint fully mobile. Together, the middle and distal joints account for only

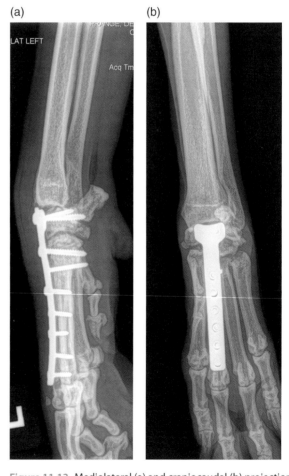

Figure 11.13 Mediolateral (a) and craniocaudal (b) projections of canine carpus with a partial carpal arthrodesis using a T-plate. These are the postoperative radiographs of the patient in Figure 11.8. *Source:* Photos courtesy of VCA Canada Mississauga Oakville veterinary emergency Hospital and referral group.

approximately 10–20% of the normal motion of the carpus. Therefore, a partial carpal arthrodesis does not significantly affect the patient's overall carpal range of motion. This procedure is indicated for injuries to the middle carpal and carpometacarpal joints. At surgery, the cartilage between each bone of the middle and distal rows is removed using a high-speed burr. Once that process is complete a T-plate is typically applied to the dorsal surface of the middle and distal carpal bones and the third metacarpal bone. Some surgeons prefer to stabilize using pins or a tension band system. A cancellous bone graft is inserted between all the bones that were denuded of their cartilage and the site is closed.

Postoperative management: The limb is placed in a palmar splint until there is radiographic evidence of bony union.

Prognosis: Prognosis is very good to excellent (no lameness or mild lameness after vigorous activity) in 82% of patients [12]. Complications include: pin migration, implant failure, and osteomyelitis. OA has been reported to occur radiographically in the adjacent antebrachiocarpal joint in 16% of patients [12].

References

1 Tomlin, J.L., Pead, M.J., Langley-Hobbs, S.J., and Muir, P. (2001). Radial carpal bone fracture in dogs. *J. Am. Anim. Hosp. Assoc.* 37: 173–178.

2 Li, A., Bennett, D., Gibbs, C. et al. (2000). Radial carpal bone fractures in 15 dogs. *J. Small Anim. Pract.* 41: 74–79.

3 Gnudi, G., Mortellaro, C.M., Bertoni, G. et al. (2003). Radial carpal bone fracture in 13 dogs. *Vet. Comp. Orthop. Traumatol.* 16: 178–183.

4 Perry, K., Fitzpatrick, N., Johnson, J., and Yeadon, R. (2010). Headless self-compressing cannulated screw fixation for treatment of radial carpal bone fracture or fissure in dogs. *Vet. Comp. Orthop. Traumatol.* 23: 84–101.

5 DeCamp, C.E., Johnston, S.A., Déjardin, L.M., and Schaefer, S.L. (2016). Fractures and other orthopedic conditions of the carpus, metacarpus and phalanges. In: *Brinker, Piermattei and Flo's Handbook of Small Animal Orthopaedics and Fracture Repair*, 5e, 400–403. St Louis, MO: Elsevier.

6 Vedrine, B. (2013). Comminuted fracture of the ulnar carpal bone in a Labrador retriever dog. *Can. Vet. J.* 54: 1067–1070.

7 Pillard, P., Bismuth, C., and Viguier, E. (2014). Luxation palmairo-mediale de l'os radial du carpe chez un chien. *Revue Me Vet* 5–6: 150–159.

8 Parker, R.B., Brown, S.G., and Wind, A.P. (1981). Pancarpal arthrodesis in the dog: A review of forty-five cases. *Vet. Surg.* 10: 35–43.

9 Clarke, S.P., Ferguson, J.F., and Miller, A. (2009). Clinical evaluation of pancarpal arthrodesis using a CastLess plate in 11 dogs. *Vet. Surg.* 38: 852–860.

10 Ramirez, J.M. and Macias, C. (2016). Pancarpal arthrodesis without rigid coaptation using the hybrid dynamic compression plate in dogs. *Vet. Surg.* 45: 303–308.

11 Whitelock, R.G., Dyce, J., and Houlton, J.E.F. (1999). Metacarpal fractures associated with pancarpal arthrodesis in dogs. *Vet. Surg.* 28: 25–30.

12 Willer, R.L., Johnson, K.A., Turner, T.M., and Piermattei, D.L. (1990). Partial carpal arthrodesis for third degree carpal sprains. A review of 45 carpi. *Vet. Surg.* 19: 334–340.

13 Evans, H.E. and de Lahunta, A. (2013). *Miller's Anatomy of the Dog*, 4e. St Louis, MO: Saunders/ Elsevier.

14 DeCamp, C.E., Johnston, S.A., Déjardin, L.M., and Schaefer, S.L. (2016). *Brinker, Piermattei and Flo's Handbook of Small Animal Orthopedics and Fracture Repair*, 5e. St Louis, MO: Elsevier.

Section 3

The Hindquarter

12

Pelvis

Anne M. Sylvestre

Focus and Flourish, Cambridge, Ontario, Canada

Fractures to the pelvic bones account for 20–30% of traumatically induced fractures [1]. They commonly occur as a result of a vehicular accident. The abundant muscles that envelope the pelvis provide good blood supply and inherent stability to the fractured bones; both these attributes contribute to healing. The box-like structure of the pelvis is such that when it fractures, it must do so in more than one location. Common combinations of pelvic fractures include the pelvic floor (pubis) with an ilial shaft or sacroiliac (SI) or acetabular fracture. The bones of the pelvis are identified in Figure 12.1.

(a)

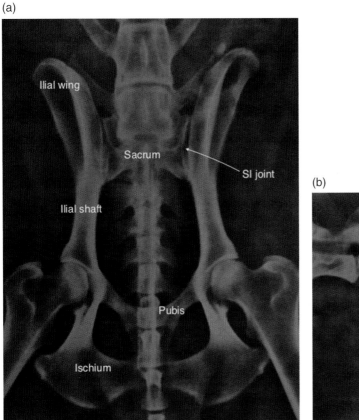

(b)

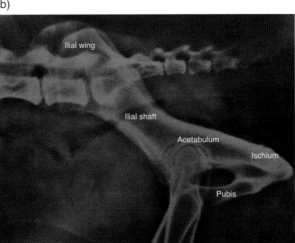

Figure 12.1 Ventrodorsal (a) and lateral (b) projections of a pelvis identifying the various components.

12.1 Co-morbidities

Nerve damage: Patients with a fractured pelvis must be carefully assessed for nerve damage. It can be very difficult to properly assess their neurological status because of the presence of marked pain and/or opiates for pain control. These patients can be naturally reluctant to stand; supporting them to stand can cause pain, making them uncooperative. The use of narcotics will make the patient much more comfortable but may significantly affect the neurological exam. Therefore, clinical acumen and several examinations within the first few days may be necessary to make an accurate assessment. Patients with pelvic fractures that are neurologically intact should be able to place their paws and able to stand, perhaps with some support. They should display purposeful movement and flex the stifle and hock when the toes are pinched. They should also have anal and tail tone. One retrospective study found that 81% of the patients with peripheral nerve injury secondary to a pelvic fracture regained good to excellent limb function [2].

Abdominal trauma: Pelvic fractures can also be associated with abdominal injuries, such as hemoabdomen, a ruptured bladder, or a urethral tear. Intra-abdominal injuries have been reported in to occur in 37% of dogs with pelvic, especially sacral, fractures [3]. Injuries to the pelvic floor can also be associated with an abdominal wall hernia as the attachment of the prepubic tendon (abdominal wall attachment to the pelvis) becomes disrupted.

Urethral tears: Urethral tears are more frequently associated with fractures of the pubis. The patient's ability to fill and properly empty the bladder should be monitored as well as other clinical signs such as: anemia, depression, metabolic imbalances, marked bruising, and swelling in the inguinal/pubic area.

Rectal tears: Fortunately these occur much less commonly than other co-morbidities. Again, clinical acumen and multiple examinations of the patient within the first 24–36 hours may be necessary to make an accurate assessment. Rectal tears are associated with significant mortality and morbidity [3].

Any associated problem can affect the management protocol and prognosis for the patient. The treatment of these co-morbidities usually takes precedence over that of the fractured pelvic bones.

12.2 Fractures

More than one fracture will be seen concurrently in the pelvis because of its "box-like" configuration. Not all fractures need to be addressed surgically.

12.2.1 SI Luxations/Fractures (Figure 12.2)

SI luxations can occur unilaterally or bilaterally and with marked or subtle displacement. The close proximity of the nerve roots to the SI joint means that nerve damage and marked pain are more frequently associated with SI trauma than with other pelvic fractures. Careful assessment of the patient's neurological status is imperative.

Diagnosis: On the ventrodorsal radiographic projection, the smooth regular contour of the pelvic "ring" is interrupted with a step at the level of the luxation. It is important to carefully evaluate the pelvic radiograph of a patient that has sustained a major trauma because a bilateral SI luxation without other pelvic fractures can be misinterpreted as normal at first glance (Figure 12.3). With a unilateral luxation, the acetabulum on the affected side will appear further proximal than the contralateral one.

Treatment of choice: Surgical stabilization with a lag screw or a lag screw and pin to the sacrum is the treatment of choice. If there is nerve damage, the need to strongly recommend surgery to the pet owner is greater. The preferred method for many SI luxations is to do a closed repair, using minimally invasive surgical techniques [4, 5]. Fluoroscopy equipment and appropriate training are necessary to perform this type of surgery. The surgery, whether closed or open, is best left in the hands of the trained surgeon as reduction can be difficult to achieve, the landmarks are elusive, and the accurate placement of the implants is technically challenging.

Postoperative management: Pain is usually easier to manage once the SI luxation/fracture has been reduced and stabilized. Basic after care for orthopedic patients is indicated with activity restriction for 4 weeks after surgery followed by a gradual return to regular activity (Chapter 3 has more information on this topic).

Prognosis: The prognosis for surgically repaired SI luxations is very good but the patient's outcome may be influenced by co-morbidities.

12.2.2 Fractures of the Ilial Shaft or Wing (Figure 12.4)

Ilial shaft fractures are seen commonly with pelvic trauma. It is important to take both the lateral and ventrodorsal radiographic views as the fractures can be elusive on one view. On the ventrodorsal projection, the coxofemoral joint on the fractured side can appear more proximal than the intact contralateral one. Ilial shaft fractures can be associated with nerve damage and with narrowing of the pelvic canal.

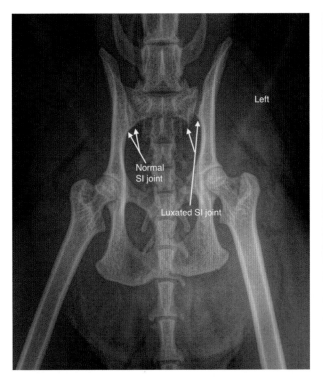
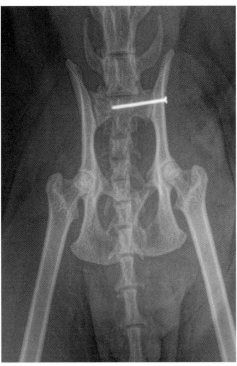

Figure 12.2 Pre- and postoperative ventrodorsal projections of a pelvis with a left sacroiliac luxation. The step between the ilial wing and the sacrum where the luxation has occurred can be compared with the smooth contour on the contralateral side. The luxation was reduced and stabilized with a lag screw. Fracture of the left pubic bone is visible.

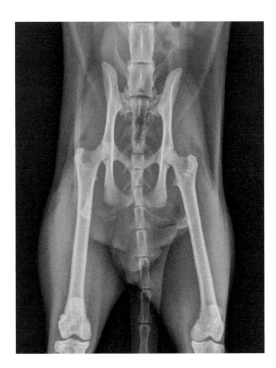

Figure 12.3 Ventrodorsal projection of a cat pelvis with bilateral sacroilial luxations.

Treatment of choice: A repair with a lateral plate is a popular technique. Locking plates may be preferred to the non-locking dynamic compression plates as they help to prevent screws from pulling out of the bone [6]. Surgical repair of pelvic fractures is best left in the hands of a trained surgeon.

Postoperative management: Basic after care for orthopedic patients is indicated with activity restriction for 4 weeks after surgery followed by a gradual return to regular activity (Chapter 3 has more information on this topic). Supporting the patient with a sling may be useful as well as offering stool softeners to aid with bowel movements.

Prognosis: The outcome for repaired ilial shaft fractures is very good to excellent providing there are no detrimental co-morbidities or surgical complications. A high rate of screw loosening has been reported in the cat and the dog, resulting in a loss of reduction and potentially, further narrowing of the pelvic canal (Figure 12.5) [7, 8]. This can be more significant in the cat, which has a narrower pelvic ring when compared with the dog. Cats with pelvic canal narrowing of 45% or more are prone to suffer from constipation or obstipation within 12 months of the trauma [5]. Constipation, although a possibility, is not a reported sequelae in the dog [9].

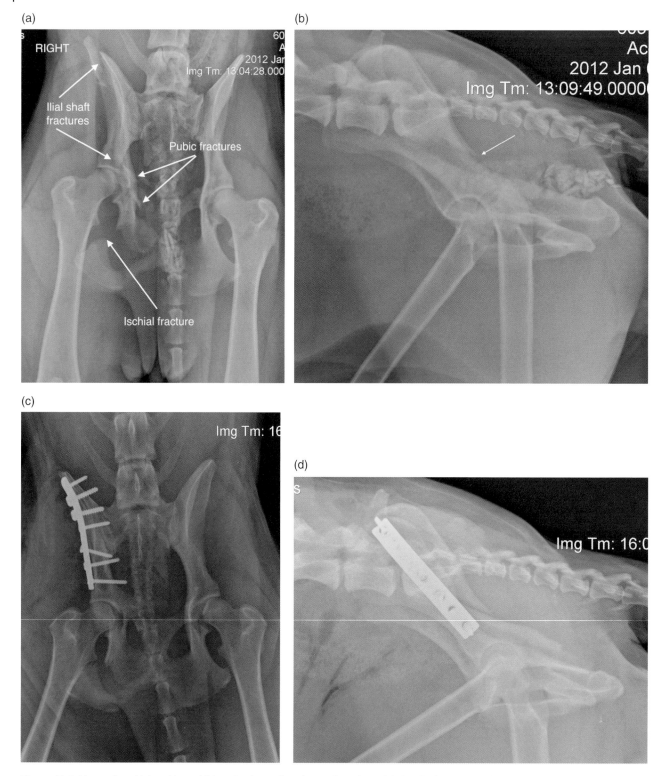

Figure 12.4 Ventrodorsal (a) and lateral (b) projections of a pelvis with ipsilateral ilial, ischial, and pubic fractures. The right coxofemoral joint is further proximal than the left one because of the overriding ilial shaft fragments. On the lateral view (b) a sharp edge of the ilial shaft fracture line is readily visible (arrow). The ilial shaft fracture was repaired with a plate and screws (c and d).

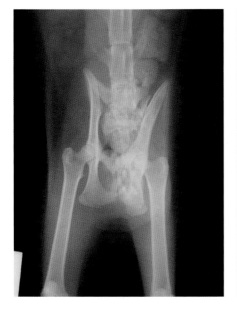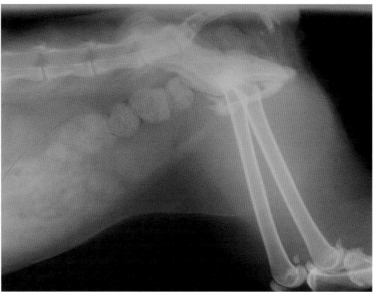

Figure 12.5 Ventrodorsal projection of a feline pelvis with a narrowed canal secondary to trauma that occurred 2 years prior. This cat presented for constipation, which is evident on the radiograph.

Ilial wing fractures can sometimes be seen in isolation, but most frequently occur in conjunction with other pelvic fractures. The ilial wing is a non-weight bearing portion of the pelvis where the iliocostalis and longissimus lumborum muscles insert. These muscles create a cranial pull on the wing; however, the middle gluteal muscle covers a large portion of the lateral surface of the wing, aiding to counteract the cranial pull and therefore preventing the wing from distracting completely.

Treatment of choice: Isolated fractures of the ilial wing are best managed conservatively with activity restriction and pain control.

Patient management: Restricted activity for 4 weeks followed by a gradual return to regular exercise is indicated.

Prognosis: The prognosis for an isolated ilial wing fracture is excellent.

12.2.3 Acetabular Fractures

Acetabular fractures are discussed with other hip trauma in Chapter 13.

12.2.4 Ischial Fractures (Figure 12.6)

Ischial fractures can occur in isolation but more commonly are seen in conjunction with other fractures of the pelvis. The hamstring muscles (semitendinosus and semimembranosus) originate from the ischial tuberosity, which tends to pull the fragment distally.

Treatment of choice: In most cases, the displacement is mild to moderate and surgical repair is not required. Even if a bony callus is not evident on radiographs, a strong fibrous union is sufficient to allow for proper function of the limb.

Patient management: Conservative management consists of pain control and marked activity restriction for 4–6 weeks followed by a slow, progressive return to exercise.

Prognosis: Isolated ischial fractures have an excellent outcome. The author has seen one case remain with a mild to moderate gait abnormality 8 weeks post-trauma. The patient was a large breed dog with a severe, unilateral, ventral displacement of the ischial tuberosity. Such a marked displacement is uncommon but perhaps this patient would have benefited from having the fracture repaired with a tension band system.

12.2.5 Fractures of the Pelvic Floor (Figure 12.7)

Fractures of the pubis, or pelvic floor, do not commonly occur in isolation. The abdominal wall inserts on the cranial border of the pubis via the prepubic tendon, and the urethra lies just dorsal to the pubic symphysis. Therefore, fractures in this area can be associated with a disruption of the lower urinary tract and/or a caudal abdominal wall herniation. Repair of these soft tissue injuries is of prime importance to the patient's wellbeing.

Treatment of choice: Fractures of the pelvic floor (pubis) are typically managed conservatively. The repair of the

(a)

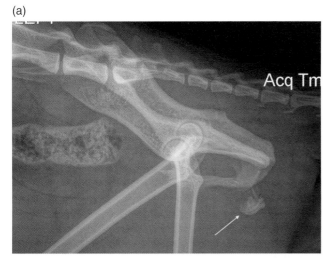

(b)

(c)

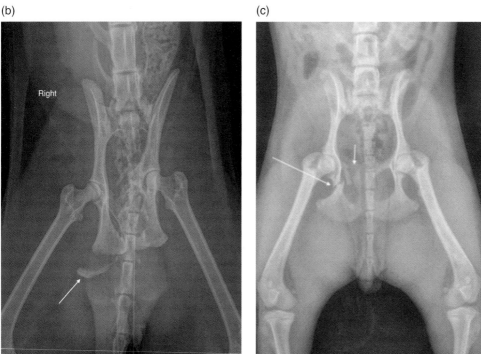

Figure 12.6 Mediolateral (a) and ventrodorsal (b) projections a feline pelvis with a left sacroilial luxation and an ischial fracture on the right. The arrow points to the distracted ischial fragment. (c) A ventrodorsal projection of a canine pelvis with ischial (long arrow) and pubic (short arrow) fractures.

concurrent fractures (ilial shaft, SI luxation) is often sufficient to stabilize the pelvic floor.

Patient management: Fractures of the pelvic floor, without co-morbidities, are managed with pain control and restricted activity until the fractures have healed (6–8 weeks) followed by a gradual increase in exercise.

Prognosis: The prognosis is usually determined by the associated injuries (e.g. ilial fracture or urethral tear); if there are none, then the prognosis is excellent.

12.2.6 Summary of Indications for Surgical Repair of Pelvic Fractures

The pelvis is stabilized by surgically repairing SI luxations/ fractures and ilial shaft fractures. Ischial and pubic fractures are typically allowed to heal conservatively. Surgical repair of pelvic fractures should be strongly recommended in animals with the following radiographic and clinical observations:

- A significantly narrowed pelvic canal (>45% in cats; >50% in dogs) (Figure 12.5).

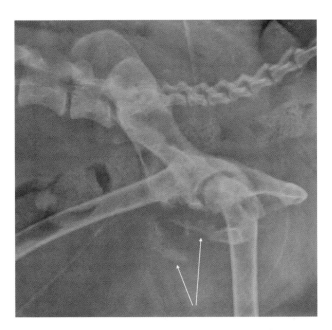

Figure 12.7 Mediolateral projection of a pelvis with multiple fractures. The arrows point to the free-floating pubic bones.

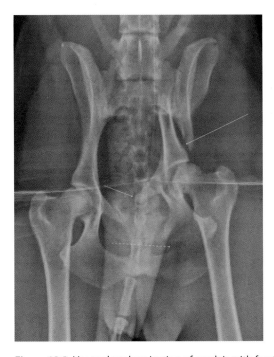

Figure 12.8 Ventrodorsal projection of a pelvis with fractures through the ilium (long arrow), pubis (short arrow), and ischium (dotted arrow) creating a "free-floating" or unstable acetabular component.

- Fractures involving the acetabulum (discussed in Chapter 13).
- Fractures through the ipsilateral ilium, pubis, and ischium creating a free-floating (unstable) acetabular fragment (Figure 12.8).

- Difficult-to-manage pain such as can be seen with SI fractures/luxations.
- Markedly unstable pelvis due to numerous, significantly displaced fragments (Figure 12.9).
- Damage to a sciatic nerve.

12.3 Managing Expectations with Recommended Treatments

Patients that present with pelvic fractures often have significant other issues that require attention. They may need intensive care and perhaps extensive rehabilitation, depending on the severity of the co-morbidities; having said that, many patients do very well after suffering from pelvic fractures. Surgical repair will hasten their recovery and improve their overall ability to properly ambulate, especially where significant pelvic trauma has been sustained. Owners should be encouraged to pursue appropriate care in cases where the co-morbidities are not life-threatening or altering. The surgical repair of pelvic fractures is best left in the hands of the trained surgeon.

The client often needs to become implicated in their pet's rehabilitation. Stool softeners and a harness or sling are often required, and the owner may need to help lift the patient in the early postoperative, post-trauma period. However, these patients tend to heal well given the great muscle mass and blood supply to the pelvic bones. This is encouraging for the owners. Cats with a reduced (>45%) pelvic canal diameter may suffer from constipation or obstipation as a consequence to the pelvic trauma. Owners of these cats should be strongly encouraged to seek appropriate surgical care. If not they need to be managed appropriately with stool softeners. Should this fail and the cat suffers from chronic recurring obstipation, then a colonectomy or segmental pelvectomy may be necessary. These procedures are less desirable than an initial fracture repair. Although this same concern exists for the dog, severe constipation is not a common occurrence [9].

Patients with peripheral nerve damage noted at the initial examination may be given the benefit of the doubt as many will improve with time [2].

12.4 Alternatives When Treatment of Choice is Not an Option

Those patients that would greatly benefit from surgery (as indicated above) but where surgery is simply not an option can be managed with crate rest and a closely monitored pain control regime. A stool softener may be

(a) (b)

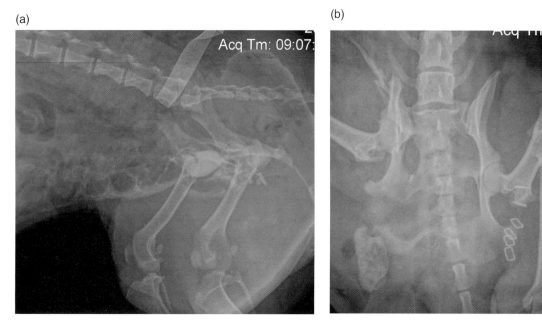

Figure 12.9 Mediolateral (a) and ventrodorsal (b) projections of a pelvis with a large number of significantly displaced pelvic fractures. A contrast study is being performed to confirm the presence of a bladder rupture (a).

helpful as these patients can be reluctant to position themselves for bowel movements. If the patient is not very mobile, then good, clean, dry bedding should be provided and the patient turned from side to side frequently and regularly throughout the day to help prevent formation of decubital sores. Providing the patient does not have significant co-morbidities, a functional outcome can be expected. A clinical study on pelvic fractures in 15 dogs showed that all dogs in whom surgery was indicated, but who were managed conserva- tively, had an intermittent or consistent, mild to moder- ate lameness 4–87 months post-trauma [10]. Six of these dogs did have an acetabular fracture, which may account for the more pronounced lameness. Euthanasia should be considered for patients where surgery is not a possi- bility and they have significant co-morbidities, intracta- ble pain, or non-responsive neurologic damage. Owners of cats with marked stenosis of the pelvic canal should be forewarned of the possibility of constipation/obstipation and the cat should be appropriately supported.

References

1 Bookbinder, P.F. and Flanders, J.A. (1992). Characteristics of pelvic fractures in the cat. *Vet. Comp. Orthop. Traumatol.* 5: 122–127.

2 Jacobson, J. and Schrader, S.C. (1987). Peripheral nerve injury associated with fracture of fracture-dislocation of the pevis indigos and cates: 34 cases (1978–1985). *J. Am. Vet. Med. Assoc.* 5: 569–572.

3 Hoffberg, J.E., Koenigshof, A.M., and Guiot, L.P. (2016). Retrospective evaluation of concurrent intra-abdominal injuries in dogs with traumatic pelvic fractures: 83 cases (2008–2013). *J. Vet. Emerg. Crit. Care.* 26: 288–294.

4 Tomlinson, J.L., Cook, J.L., Payne, J.T. et al. (1999). Closed reduction and lag screw fixation of sacroiliac luxations and fractures. *Vet. Surg.* 28: 188–193.

5 Tonks, C.A., Tomlinson, J.L., and Cook, J.L. Evaluation of closed reduction and screw fixation in lag fashion of sacroiliac fracture-luxations. *Vet. Surg.* 37: 603–607.

6 Schmierer, P.A., Kirchen, P.R., Hartback, S., and Knell, S.C. (2015). Screw loosening and pelvic canal narrowing after lateral plating of feline ilial fractures with locking and nonlocking plates. *Vet. Surg.* 44: 900–904.

7 Breshears, L.A., Fitch, R.B., Wallace, R.J. et al. (2004). The radiographic evaluation of repaired canine ilial fractures. *Vet. Comp. Orthop. Traumatol.* 17: 64–72.

8 Hamilton, M.H., Evans, D.A., and Langley-Hobbs, S.J. (2009). Feline ilial fractures: assessment of screw loosening and pelvic canal narrowing after lateral plating. *Vet. Surg.* 38: 326–333.

9 Averill, S.M., Johnson, A.L., and Schaeffer, D.J. (1997). Risk factors associated with development of pelvic canal stenosis secondary to sacroiliac separation: 84 cases (1985–1995). *J. Am. Vet. Med. Assoc.* 211: 75–78.

10 Vassalo, F.G., Rahal, S.C., Agostinho, F.S. et al. (2015). Gait analysis in dogs with pelvic fractures treated conservatively using a pressure-sensing walkway. *Acta Vet. Scand.* 57: 68–71.

13

Coxofemoral Joint

Thomas W.G. Gibson[1] and Anne M. Sylvestre[2]

[1] Ontario Veterinary College, University of Guelph, Guelph, Ontario, Canada
[2] Focus and Flourish, Cambridge, Ontario, Canada

Fractures of the hip joint can involve the acetabulum and/or the femoral head or neck. If the patient is immature then a physeal fracture may be seen. Coxofemoral luxations are also commonly seen. The trauma endured by the patient may have caused significant problems in other parts of the body as well. A thorough examination of the patient, including chest and abdomen, is paramount. Figure 13.1 shows the relevant anatomical structures associated with the hip joint.

13.1 Fractures and Luxations

13.1.1 Acetabular Fractures

Acetabular fractures can be seen in isolation or in conjunction with other pelvic fractures. A good neurological assessment is indicated as damage to the sciatic nerve, although not common, can occur with these fractures. Fractures of the acetabulum can have a variety of

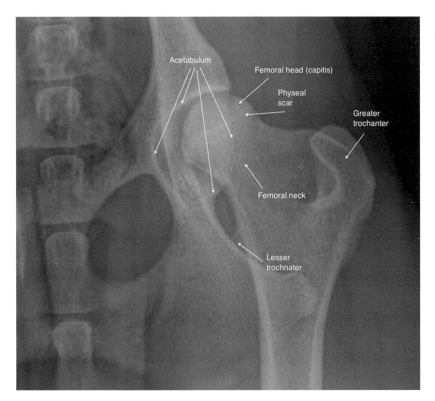

Figure 13.1 Ventrodorsal projection of a canine coxofemoral joint identifying the relevant bony landmarks.

Fracture Management for the Small Animal Practitioner, First Edition. Edited by Anne M. Sylvestre.
© 2019 John Wiley & Sons, Inc. Published 2019 by John Wiley & Sons, Inc.

configurations but the most common are the centrally located ones [1] (Figure 13.2).

Treatment of choice: The best option, especially for large breeds of dogs, is to surgically reconstruct the acetabulum and stabilize with a plate or pins and polymethyl methacrylate (bone cement). These fractures are very challenging to repair and are best left in the hands of a trained surgeon. The approach is difficult and often requires an osteotomy of the greater trochanter; the sciatic nerve is in close proximity and special instrumentation is required to assist with retraction of muscles as well as manipulation of the fragments. It is difficult to accurately contour a plate to the acetabular rim even with specialized plates, such as the "c-shaped" plate and the reconstruction plates that can be bent in several planes. The key to a successful outcome is an accurate reconstruction of the articular surface. A femoral head osteotomy (FHO) can also be considered as a treatment of choice for patients with an acetabular fracture, especially in small and medium-sized animals. Section 13.4 has more information on this procedure. Multi-fragmented acetabular fractures (Figure 13.3) may be better managed with an FHO or total hip replacement because accurate reconstruction is often not possible.

Postoperative management: The surgeon may choose to place the patient in a non-weight bearing sling or to recommend the use of an abdominal or pelvic sling for 2 weeks after reconstruction of the acetabulum.

Prognosis: The prognosis is highly dependent on the complexity of the fracture and the accuracy of the reconstruction. One study indicated that dogs with a fracture stabilized with an acetabular plate had an excellent to good return to function in 69% of cases. Those that did not do well had implant failure (screws breaking or backing out) or had multiple other injuries that contributed to a poorer outcome [2].

Immature animals with minimally displaced acetabular fractures, especially those located in the caudal third, can be treated conservatively with good results. It is advised to place the patient in a non-weight bearing sling (Robinson or 90-90) for 2–4 weeks to prevent displacement of the fragments [1]. However, in the adult patient, the outcome with a conservative approach, even in the caudal acetabulum, can be disappointing [3]. A patient with trauma to the acetabulum will develop osteoarthritis (OA) in the hip joint, even with a repair. Osteoarthritis need not be a devastating problem but the owner should be counseled on how to manage a pet with OA (Chapter 3 has more detail on this topic).

13.1.2 Hip Luxations

The femoral head can luxate in several directions although craniodorsal luxations are by far the most common [4]. Craniodorsal luxations occur in 78% of dogs and 73% of cats with a hip luxation [5]. There may be significant soft tissue trauma associated with a hip luxation. The round ligament and a portion of the joint capsule will be torn; in severe cases some of the gluteal muscles may also be damaged.

Treatment of choice: Closed reduction of a luxated hip should be attempted if the trauma occurred within 4–5 days, providing the patient is stable enough for general anesthesia, and there are no contraindications such as fractures [4]. Surgical correction as the primary treatment method may also be preferred for patients with concurrent orthopedic issues since they would benefit from a rapid return of function of the limb without the need for a postoperative Ehmer sling [5, 6]. The techniques for reducing a luxated hip are described below.

13.1.2.1 Craniodorsal Luxations (Figure 13.4)

- The patient must be well managed for pain and the muscles relaxed with general anesthesia.
- The patient is placed in lateral recumbency with the affected limb up.
- An assistant is necessary to apply counter-traction by standing along the dorsum of the patient and holding onto a soft rope or towel placed around the groin area.
- The surgeon can place one hand on the stifle (left hand for left hip and right hand for right hip) to externally rotate the femur and then apply caudoventral traction on the limb (Figure 13.5).
- Once the femoral head has "cleared" the acetabular rim, the femur is rotated inward to help redirect the head into the acetabulum.
- It can be helpful to place the fingers of the other hand in front of the femoral head and help push or guide it over the acetabular rim and back into the socket. This technique works best in the smaller patients.
- A "popping" sensation can be felt when the head falls into the acetabulum. At this point, pressure is applied to the greater trochanter and the hip is placed through a full range of motion to move soft tissues and blood clots out of the acetabulum.
- The stability of the reduction is then tested by placing the hip joint through a full range of motion without applying pressure on the greater trochanter. If the hip pops out readily, then surgical intervention may be necessary.

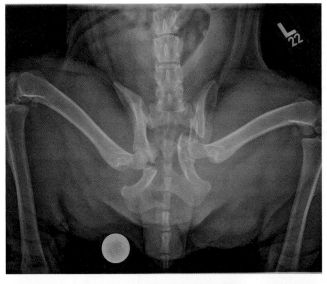
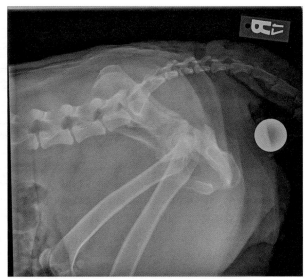
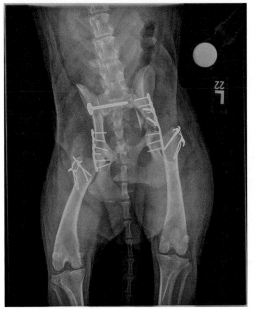
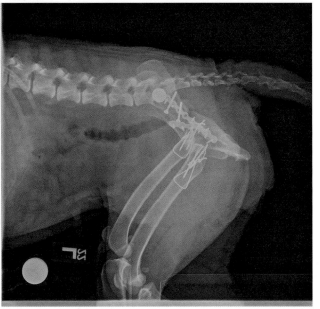

Figure 13.2 Pre- and postoperative projections of a canine pelvis with bilateral acetabular fractures that were repaired using string of pearl plates. Adequate reduction was not possible on the left and therefore a femoral head ostectomy was performed. An osteotomy of the greater trochanter was performed bilaterally to help improve the exposure. The osteotomies were repaired with a tension band wire system.

13.1.2.2 Caudodorsal Luxations (Figure 13.6)

Closed reduction can be attempted by (1) first placing the luxated femoral head into a craniodorsal position and proceeding as described in Section 13.1.2.1. If this is not successful then the steps below are followed:

- The patient must be well managed for pain and the muscles relaxed with general anesthesia.
- The stifle is externally rotated while distal traction is applied to the limb.

- The femoral head now can clear the caudal acetabular rim.
- Pressure is then applied to the proximal femur, greater trochanter area to push it forward over the acetabular rim.
- The femur is internally rotated to drop the femoral head into the socket.
- A "popping" sensation can be felt when the head falls into the acetabulum. At this point, pressure is applied to the greater trochanter and the hip is placed through

(a)

(b)

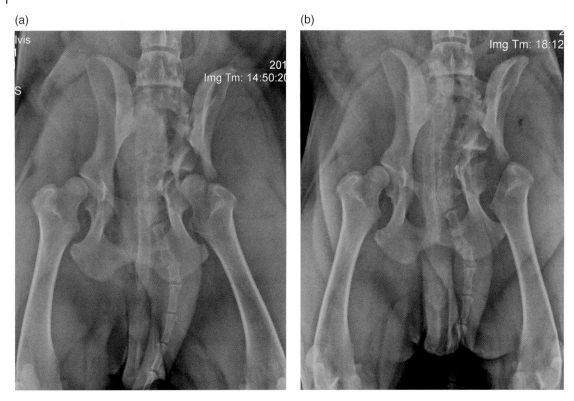

Figure 13.3 A ventrodorsal projection (a) of a canine pelvis with a multi-fragmented acetabular fracture. The fracture was managed with a femoral head ostectomy (b).

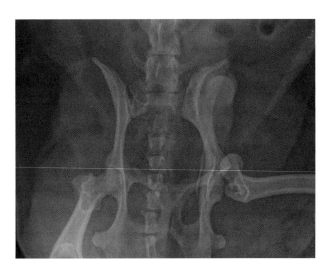

Figure 13.4 Ventrodorsal projection of a pelvis with a craniodorsal luxation.

a full range of motion to move soft tissues and blood clots out of the acetabulum.

- The stability of the reduction is then tested by placing the hip joint through a full range of motion without applying pressure on the greater trochanter. If the hip

pops out readily, then surgical intervention may be necessary.

13.1.2.3 Ventral Luxations (Figure 13.7)

Ventral luxations can be cranioventral or caudoventral to the acetabulum. The author has seen ventral luxations occur spontaneously in patients with moderate to severe ataxia.

If the femoral head is located cranioventral to the acetabulum:

- The patient must be well managed for pain and the muscles relaxed with general anesthesia.
- Traction is applied along with an upward pressure to reposition the head craniodorsal to the acetabulum.
- It can be reduced from this position as described in Section 13.1.2.1.

A caudoventral luxation is reduced in the following manner:

- The patient must be well managed for pain and the muscles relaxed with general anesthesia.
- Slightly abducting the stifle and applying distal traction to the limb.
- An assistant applies counter-pressure on the pubic and/or ischial bones.

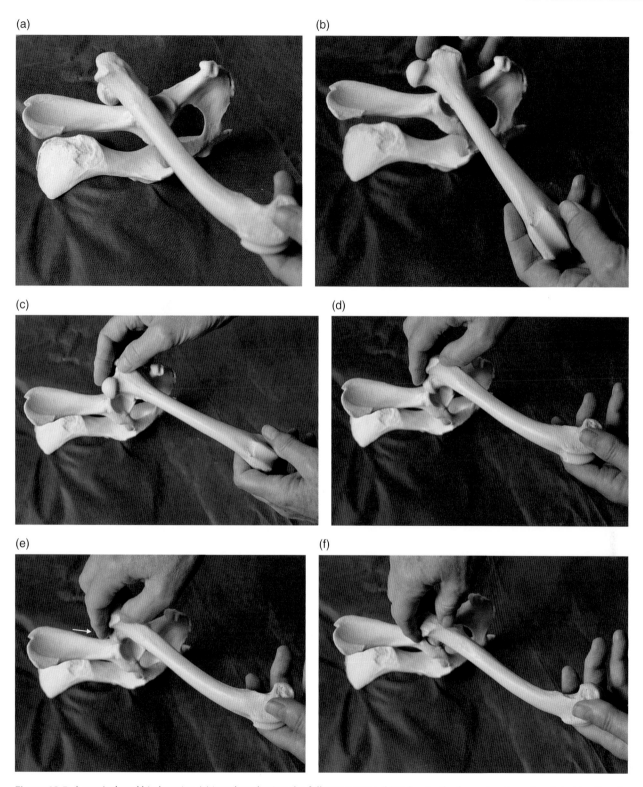

Figure 13.5 A craniodorsal hip luxation (a) is reduced using the following steps. (b) To begin, the femur is externally rotated to allow the femoral head to "clear" the acetabular rim when traction is applied (note the position of the trochlear groove as compared with that in (a)). (c) Ventral and caudal traction are simultaneously applied to the femur (an assistant standing on the dorsal aspect of the patient would create counter-pressure along the pubis with hands or a rolled towel). (d) The femur is then internally rotated to help push the femoral head into the acetabulum. (e) Digital pressure can be applied to the femoral head to help push it back into the acetabulum; this can be especially useful in the smaller patients. (f) The femoral head will "pop" back into the acetabulum. (g) Once the head is in position, pressure is placed onto the greater trochanter while the hip is placed through a range of motion. A video of this demonstration is available at www.focusandflourish.com.

(g)

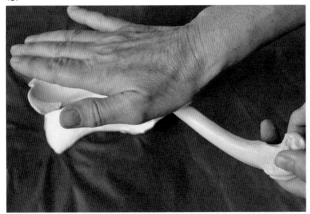

Figure 13.5 (Continued)

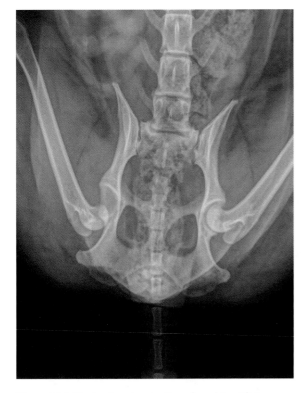

Figure 13.6 Ventrodorsal projection of a pelvis with a caudodorsal luxation.

- With a hand on the medial aspect of the femur, close to the femoral neck, upward pressure is applied to lift the femoral head back into the acetabulum.
- A "popping" sensation can be felt when the head falls into the acetabulum. At this point, pressure is applied to the greater trochanter and the hip is placed through a full range of motion to move soft tissues and blood clots out of the acetabulum.

- The stability of the reduction is then tested by placing the hip joint through a full range of motion without applying pressure on the greater trochanter. If the hip pops out readily, then surgical intervention may be necessary.

Post-reduction care: Once the hip has been successfully reduced, the limb should be placed in an Ehmer sling for approximately 10 days (more information on the Ehmer sling is available in Chapter 4). At this time it is important to note that keeping an Ehmer sling on a cat is very difficult, maybe impossible. Therefore, in cats one may wish to omit the use of an Ehmer sling; however, if the hip does not feel stable in reduction, it may be best to proceed immediately with a definitive surgical procedure. Patients that have had a ventral luxation may be placed in hobbles (rather than an Ehmer) for 7–10 days to protect against recurrence. Excellent pain management and activity restriction are necessary as well as avoiding slippery surfaces and stairs. A follow-up radiograph should be taken at the time of sling removal to document that the femoral head is still properly seated in the acetabulum. Gentle hip passive range of motion PROM exercises and stretches, continued restricted activity, and exercises geared toward rebuilding the muscle mass are indicated for 1 month post sling removal (Chapter 3). Gradual, incremental, slow return to normal activity should occur over the following 4 weeks.

Prognosis: Success rate with a single (first attempt) closed reduction treatment was reported in a 1965 study to be 85% [7]. However, subsequent reported success rates with a closed reduction tend to be low (35–53%) [4, 8]. Most studies look at cases from referral institutions only where patients are often referred by a primary care hospital. Clearly those that had a successful closed reduction performed by the general practitioner were not referred in, and therefore not included in the studies. The inherent population bias in these studies can skew the outcomes toward an erroneous higher failure rate. Factors identified that tend to contribute to failure of a closed reduction include: pre-existing hip dysplasia, fractured acetabular rim, fracture of the femoral head (usually an avulsion fragment from the round ligament; Figure 13.8), failed previous closed reduction, and chronic luxation (greater than approximately 1 week) [5]. A surgical correction of the luxation as the primary treatment method is likely the better choice for these patients.

13.1.3 Alternative Treatment of Choice: Open Reduction

Several open reduction techniques have been described for surgical reduction of a luxated hip and include: suturing

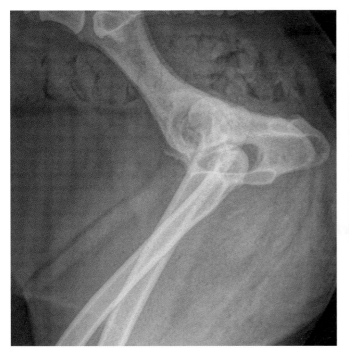
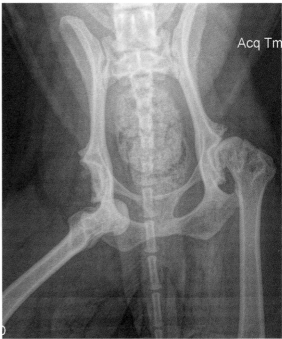

Figure 13.7 Mediolateral and ventrodorsal projections of a pelvis with a right caudoventral luxation and bilateral severe osteoarthritis secondary to hip dysplasia.

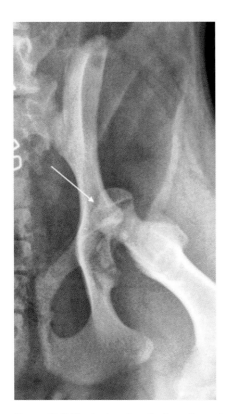

Figure 13.8 Ventrodorsal projection of a canine hip with a craniodorsal luxation and avulsion fracture of the round ligament.

the joint capsule (capsulorrhaphy), toggle pin fixation, prosthetic capsular reconstruction, repositioning of the greater trochanter, and an iliofemoral band (Figure 13.9). These open reduction procedures are best left in the hands of a trained surgeon. An FHO is also an excellent choice for small to medium-sized patients with a luxated hip that cannot be reduced in a closed manner. The key to success with this procedure is diligent postoperative rehabilitation (Section 13.4 has more details). Large and giant breed dogs, where a closed reduction has failed or is not possible due to underlying disease, may be best treated with an open reduction or total hip replacement.

Postoperative care: The patient may or may not be placed in an Ehmer sling (depending on the chosen technique and level of stability). Good pain management and gentle hip PROM exercises will be helpful to the patient. Activity should be markedly restricted for the first 2 weeks post-repair followed by short, slow, controlled leash walks for another month before proceeding with a gradual return to regular activity.

Prognosis: Outcomes with an open reduction are reported to be good to excellent for limb use but complications, especially reluxation, can occur within a week or two after the surgery in 5–23% of cases [5, 6, 8, 9]. Complications will vary depending on the chosen technique, but reluxation, implant failure, and the development of significant OA are the most common.

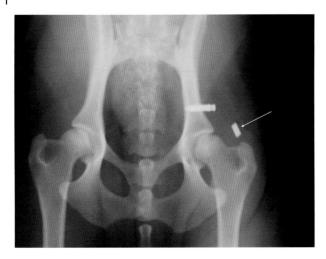

Figure 13.9 Postoperative ventrodorsal projection of an open reduction of a craniodorsal hip luxation repaired with an iliofemoral band technique. A bone anchor (Everost™) was used to secure the heavy suture (nylon) to the iliopubic eminence and a bone tunnel was created to secure it to the femur. A crimp was used to "tie" the nylon (arrow).

Spontaneous, Idiopathic Hip Luxation: This is a syndrome that has been reported in dogs. This usually occurs in mature, overweight dogs. They will present with an acute craniodrosal luxation of one or both hips but without any history of trauma. The treatment of choice for these patients is an FHO as the prognosis with closed or open reduction is poor [10]. The author has seen this condition in two Cavalier King Charles spaniels, one of which was bilateral at presentation, and one beagle, which luxated both hips but 1 year apart. All three dogs (five hips) did very well with an FHO.

13.1.4 Capital Physeal Fractures of the Proximal Femur (Figure 13.10)

A Salter–Harris I fracture of the capital physis of the proximal femur or "slipped capital physis" is a traumatic injury seen in immature animals. This fracture often results in minimal displacement of the femoral head. It is therefore essential to have good-quality orthogonal radiographs of the coxofemoral joint when the potential for this fracture is being investigated. "Frog-legged" positioning is often required to confirm this fracture, as this position will often result in displacement of the femoral capitis making the fracture line visible. Immature animals with a non-weight bearing lameness, with a history of trauma, and palpable crepitus of the hip joint should be carefully evaluated for presence of this fracture.

Treatment of choice: Repair of this fracture as soon as it is safe to anesthetize the patient is essential, as delaying the repair will make adequate reduction difficult resulting in poorer outcomes. Conservative management of this fracture is contraindicated, and open and closed repair techniques have been described most commonly utilizing K-wires placed in a normograde fashion. In cases where the fracture is chronic or the animal may be considered too small for implant placement, a salvage procedure such as a femoral head and neck ostectomy could be considered. In larger patients with a chronic fracture, a total hip arthroplasty could also be considered. Closed reduction and stabilization is typically reserved for situations where fluoroscopy can be utilized for accurate pin placement ensuring pins do not enter the coxofemoral joint. A high degree of skill and expertise is required.

Postoperative management: Restricted activity protocols should be followed until radiographic healing is present and recheck radiographs should be performed at 4 weeks to evaluate healing and implant position.

Prognosis: Prognosis is generally good with this type of stabilization. Pin migration does occasionally occur, warranting pin removal.

Feline Proximal Femoral Physeal Dysplasia: This is a condition that affects the proximal femoral growth plate of cats and results in fractures through the physis [11, 12] (Figure 13.11). This condition is comparable with the slipped capital femoral epiphysis seen in humans. Affected cats are typically male, young (from 8 months to 2 years) and often heavy (overweight or a large breed cat such as the Maine coon). The onset of clinical signs is typically not acute but rather quickly progressive over several days to a few weeks [11]. The cat may show a lameness or behavioral changes due to the discomfort in the hip(s). As the disease progresses and the fracture occurs, the pain becomes very pronounced. Because of the quick progression of the problem, owners may miss the early signs and give a history of acute onset. There is no associated trauma. The problem is more often unilateral but can be bilateral. The cats are very painful in the affected hip joint(s). The bilaterally affected cats can be mistaken for a neurological or saddle thrombus patient as they tend to drag their hind limbs rather than stand on the painful hips. Radiographically there is a thinning of the proximal femoral neck and a physeal fracture may be present. Patients with this condition do very well with an FHO; if bilateral then both hips can be done simultaneously. It is very difficult to manage the pain on these cats without surgery therefore conservative management may not be an appropriate alternative to surgery.

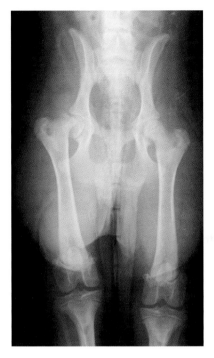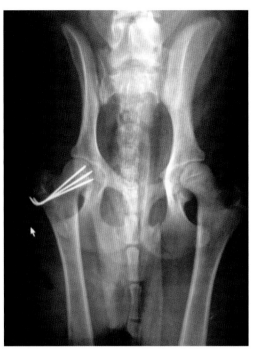

Figure 13.10 Pre- and postoperative ventrodorsal radiograph of the pelvis showing repair of a capital physeal fracture of the proximal femur of an immature dog using diverging K-wires. (*Source:* Photos courtesy of the Ontario Veterinary College).

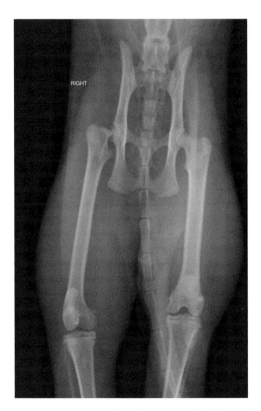

Figure 13.11 Ventrodorsal projection of a feline pelvis with proximal femoral physeal dysplasia of the right hip joint. The thinness of the femoral neck and resulting fracture are evident.

13.1.5 Fractures of the Femoral Neck (Figure 13.12)

These are most often seen in dogs and cats less than 1 year of age.

Treatment of choice: The fracture can be repaired with a compression (lag) screw or with K-wires. Many referral centers have fluoroscopy and can do this type of fixation closed, using minimally invasive osteosynthesis techniques. The fluoroscopy is very helpful to ensure that the implants are properly positioned and not entering the joint. The accuracy of this repair can be much more difficult to accomplish in the small dog and cat. An FHO may be a better alternative for these patients.

Postoperative management: The patient is placed in an Ehmer or Robinson sling to prevent weight bearing for 2 weeks. Activity is restricted until the fracture has healed. Gentle rehabilitative exercises (such as PROM exercises) are recommended during this time period (Chapter 3).

Prognosis: The success of this repair is dependent on early surgical intervention, accurate reduction, and implant placement, as well as closely monitored follow-up care. An 11% failure rate has been reported with surgical stabilizing, meaning that the patients had to undergo an FHO within days of the primary repair. Postoperative complications can be reduced by

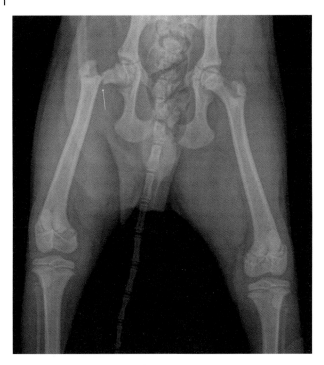

Figure 13.12 A ventrodorsal projection of an immature dog with a fracture of the right femoral neck (arrow).

inserting the screw or wires along the angles of inclination and anteversion of the femoral neck [13]. However, excellent to very good clinical outcomes have been found in 77–100% of the patients that had a successful primary repair of a femoral head or neck fracture [14]. Very good success rates have also been reported in cats [15]. Complications include: implant failure (necessitating FHO), resorption of the femoral neck (which is often asymptomatic), OA of the coxofemoral joint, especially if the reduction has inaccuracies, pin migration after healing, and sepsis.

13.2 Managing Expectations with Recommended Treatments

Trauma to the coxofemoral joint is quite common; fortunately, the overall success rate with reduction and repair is very good. Owners should be encouraged to seek appropriate surgical management for their pet. The patient will develop OA in the affected hip joint but this need not be a deterrent to seeking appropriate care and making the financial commitment, as many dogs and cats can still have a very active lifestyle with basic management of hip OA (Chapter 3).

FHO should always be considered as a viable alternative to surgical reconstruction, especially in the small to mid-size patients. More details on this procedure can be found below.

13.3 Alternatives When Treatment of Choice is Not an Option

13.3.1 Acetabular Fractures

Fractures in the acetabular component of the coxofemoral joint that are not repaired can be surprisingly well tolerated by many animals, especially the smaller patients with minimally displaced fractures. Appropriate pain management is required until such time as there has been sufficient healing. Some patients may return to near-normal ambulation with time. Upon closer examination of these patients, however, decreased range of motion with loss of extension of the hip joint and a decrease in muscle mass are likely to be present. Lameness is likely to be noted after activity. The pet may be reluctant to jump or climb stairs. OA will be present and will require appropriate management (Figure 13.13). This is not to say that conservative management of an acetabular fracture is a recommended treatment choice, but rather to state that conservative management may be a viable alternative to euthanasia.

13.3.2 Luxations

If a closed reduction is not successful (or financially feasible for a client), then there are no good alternatives for patients with a luxated hip. Without surgical treatment,

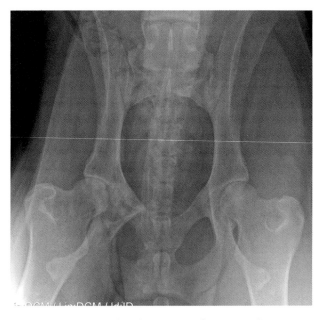

Figure 13.13 A ventrodorsal projection of a canine pelvis 3 months after sustaining an acetabular fracture that was not repaired surgically. The patient was a giant breed dog. Although he ambulated well, he had a decreased range of motion in that hip and would be lame after prolonged walks.

the discomfort of the luxated hip will eventually dissipate but this may take many months. The patient will learn to ambulate with the altered limb, in time. A residual lameness/abnormal gait will likely remain. Smaller animals seem to adapt to the altered limb function better than larger ones. If the surgical expertise is not available locally for open reduction or FHO, then a disarticulation amputation may be a more suitable option than conservative management. A disarticulation amputation is more challenging than a mid-femoral one. The veterinarian who is performing this procedure for the first time is strongly encouraged to become very familiar with the regional anatomy and position of the femoral artery before attempting this surgery. It is this author's opinion that a disarticulation amputation is a more difficult procedure than an FHO.

13.3.3 Femoral Head and Neck Fractures

There are no good alternatives to surgery in these cases. Non-surgically managed femoral head or neck fractures tend to remain painful and the patient is likely to endure a significant lameness. Therefore, conservative management is not a good alternative for this type of fracture. Owners should be encouraged to pursue surgery given the high odds for a good to excellent outcome with a repair or an FHO, and the very poor outcome without. If a fracture repair or total hip replacement is not possible for a large or giant breed dog, then an FHO is a viable alternative to euthanasia. Many private practitioners are comfortable with this procedure so hopefully that expertise is available locally. Amputation could be an alternative but should be a disarticulation rather than mid-shaft to relieve the pain in the coxofemoral joint. It is this author's opinion that a disarticulation amputation is a more difficult procedure than an FHO. The veterinarian who is performing a disarticulation amputation for the first time is strongly encouraged to become very familiar with the regional anatomy and position of the femoral artery before attempting this surgery.

13.4 About the FHO

Prognosis with an FHO is good to excellent [16–18]. Cats are reported to have a good to excellent long-term functional outcome with unilateral or bilateral FHOs [16]. One retrospective study on FHO in 94 dogs and cats found 82.6% of the dogs had excellent results. This same success rate was found when only the large breed dogs were assessed (over 30 kg, mean of 38.5 kg) [17]. Coxofemoral luxations, acetabular fractures, and fractures of the femoral head and neck were the most common reasons for an FHO in that study [17]. Simultaneous bilateral FHOs (patients weighing between 19 and 31 kg) were reported to have good to excellent outcomes in all cases, according to owners [18].

The importance of the postoperative care and rehabilitation should not be underestimated for the success of this procedure. The clients must understand the value of the exercises and participate in their pet's postoperative rehabilitation. A diligent rehabilitation program with regular progress checks and appropriate pain management is essential for success with this surgery as well as an excellent pain management regime. The use of NSAIDs for 3–4 weeks postoperatively, providing there are no contraindications for that patient, will help the patient participate in the rehabilitation program that is essential to a more complete recovery [19]. Each patient should be monitored closely and treated according to his or her needs. Veterinarians dealing with FHO patients are encouraged to become familiar with the basic necessary rehabilitation techniques [20, 21]. The recovery tends to be much faster for patients receiving an FHO for acute problems as compared with those with chronic diseases such as severe OA.

Complications with the FHO include: severe lameness with pain in the hip area that may require a revision surgery, stiffness when first getting up and after strenuous exercise, iatrogenic sciatic nerve deficit, and ongoing lameness due to lack of postoperative rehabilitation.

Many general practitioners are comfortable and competent with this procedure. It is best to learn how to do the surgery by attending workshops or by working with a mentor rather than relying solely on the description from a surgery textbook. At surgery one can expect significant bruising and swelling of the regional tissues as well as malpositioning of the bony landmarks, which can make the approach more challenging. If the fracture is chronic, then fibrosis will also be an added challenge. A review of the regional anatomy and patience at the time of surgery are necessary. Any fragments located within the acetabulum should be removed (capitis).

An FHO in a small to medium-size patient with appropriate postoperative rehabilitation can have a very good to excellent outcome. A total hip replacement (or surgical repair of the problem) may be a better alternative for large to giant breed dogs; although if absolutely not feasible the FHO should not be dismissed, but clients should be forewarned that the recovery might be slower and the outcome not as positive as for a smaller patient.

References

1 DeCamp, C.E., Johnston, S.A., Déjardin, L.M., and Schaefer, S.L. (2016). Fractures of the pelvis. In: *Brinker, Piermattei and Flo's Handbook of Small Animal Orthopaedics and Fracture Repair*, 5e, 437–455. St Louis, MO: Elsevier.

2 Anson, L.W., DeYoung, D.J., Richardson, D.C., and Betts, C.W. (1988). Clinical evaluation of canine acetabular fractures stabilized with an acetabular plate. *Vet. Surg.* 17: 220–225.

3 Boudrieau, R.J. and Kleine, L.J. (1988). Nonsurgically managed caudal acetabular fractures in dogs: 15 cases (1979–1984). *J. Am. Vet. Med. Assoc.* 193: 701–705.

4 Basher, A.W., Walter, M.C., and Newton, C.D. (1986). Coxofemoral luxation in the dog and cat. *Vet. Surg.* 15: 356–362.

5 Kieves, N.R., Lotsikas, P.J., Schulz, K.S., and Canapp, S.O. (2014). Hip toggle stabilization using the TightRope™ System in dogs: Technique and long-term outcome. *Vet. Surg.* 43: 515–522.

6 Martini, F.M., Simonazzi, B., and Del Bue, M. (2001). Extra-articular absorbable suture stabilization of coxofemoral luxations in dogs. *Vet. Surg.* 30: 468–475.

7 Campbell, J.R., Lawson, D.D., and Wyburn, R.S. (1965). Coxofemoral luxation in the dog. *Vet. Rec.* 77: 1173–1177.

8 Bone, D.L., Walker, M., and Cantwell, H.D. (1984). Traumatic coxofemoral luxation in dogs. *Results of repair. Vet. Surg.* 13: 263–270.

9 Sissener, T.R., Whitelock, R.G., and Langley-Hobbs, S.J. (2009). Long term results of transarticular pinning for surgical stabilization of coxofemoral luxation in 20 cats. *J. Small Anim. Pract.* 50: 112–117.

10 Trostel, C.T., Peck, J.N., and deHaan, J.J. (2000). Spontaneous bilateral coxofemoral luxation in four dogs. *J. Am. Anim. Hosp. Assoc.* 36: 268–276.

11 Grayton, J., Allen, P., and Biller, D. (2014). Case report: Proximal femoral physeal dysplasia in a cat and a review of the literature. *Isr. J. Vet. Med.* 69: 40–44.

12 McNicholas, W.T., Wilkens, B.E., Blevins, W.E. et al. (2002). Spontaneous femoral capital physeal fractures in adult cats: 26 cases (1996–2001). *J. Am. Vet. Med. Assoc.* 221: 1731–1736.

13 DeCamp, C.E., Johnston, S.A., Déjardin, L.M., and Schaefer, S.L. (2016). Fractures of the femur and patella. In: *Brinker, Piermattei and Flo's Handbook of Small Animal Orthopaedics and Fracture Repair*, 5e, 518–596. St Louis, MO: Elsevier.

14 Daly, W.R. (1978). Femoral head and neck fractures in the dog and cat: A review of 115 cases. *Vet. Surg.* 7: 29–38.

15 Fischer, H.R., Norton, J., Kobluk, C.N. et al. (2004). Surgical reduction and stabilization for repair of femoral capital physeal fractures in cats: 13 cases (1998–2002). *J. Am. Vet. Med. Assoc.* 224: 1478–1482.

16 Yap, F.W., Dunn, A.L., Garcia-Fernandez, P.M. et al. (2015). Femoral head and neck excision in cats: medium- to long-term functional outcome in 18 cats. *J. Feline Med. Surg.* 17: 704–710.

17 Berzon, J.L., Howard, P.E., Covell, S.J. et al. (1980). A retrospective study of the efficacy of femoral head and neck excisions in 94 dogs and cats. *Vet. Surg.* 9: 88–92.

18 Rawson, E.A., Aronsohn, M.G., and Burk, R.L. (2005). Simultaneous bilateral femoral head and neck ostectomy for the treatment of canine hip dysplasia. *J. Am. Anim. Hosp. Assoc.* 41: 166–170.

19 Grisneaux, E., Dupuis, J., Pibarot, P. et al. (2003). Effects of postoperative administration of ketoprofen or carprofen on short- and long-term results of femoral head and neck excision in dogs. *J. Am. Vet. Med. Assoc.* 223: 1006–1012.

20 Pyke, J. and Sylvestre, A. (2014). Rehabilitation in Small Animal Practice. https://itunes.apple.com/ca/book/rehabilitation-in-small-animal-practice/id928891810?mt=11.

21 Pyke, J. and Sylvestre, A. (2015). iRehab my dog. https://itunes.apple.com/ca/book/i-rehab-my-dog/id1070374203?mt=11.

14

Femur

Thomas W.G. Gibson[1] and Anne M. Sylvestre[2]

[1] *Ontario Veterinary College, University of Guelph, Guelph, Ontario, Canada*
[2] *Focus and Flourish, Cambridge, Ontario, Canada*

Fractures of the shaft of the femur are among the most common fractures presented to a referral hospital (33–44%) [1, 2]. In a large study looking at the prevalence of fracture types in general practice, however, femoral fractures accounted for only 19.3% of all fractures seen in dogs (fractures of the radius and tibia were more frequent) [3]. Cats will more commonly fracture a femur (36.5%) than any other bone [3]. Figure 14.1 identifies the relevant landmarks of the femur.

Femoral fractures can result from a high-velocity trauma such as a vehicular accident or a low-velocity type of trauma such as becoming wrapped up in a leash or caught up in a fence. The large muscles that envelope the femur help to assist with stabilizing the fragments (when compared with a distal tibia or paw) and bring vascularity to the bone. This is good for the healing process but does tend to result in profuse swelling and hematoma formation at the fracture site. The thigh cannot be effectively bandaged or splinted. A Robert Jones, or other padded bandage, applied to a femoral fracture (even a distal one) will *not* stabilize the fracture but will act as a fulcrum and create more instability, pain, and soft tissue trauma (Figure 14.2). It is best to simply confine a patient with a femoral fracture to a small space, to limit movement, and treat the pain rather than bandage.

Nerve damage, although possible, is very uncommon with a femoral fracture. However, the abundant swelling in the thigh as well as narcotic pain medications may prevent a proper response to a toe pinch or patellar reflex test. Although it is important to assess the neurologic status carefully, one must also give the patient the benefit of the doubt regarding peripheral nerve function. If the withdrawal or pain response is poor, the patient should be reassessed once the swelling and opiate effects have diminished.

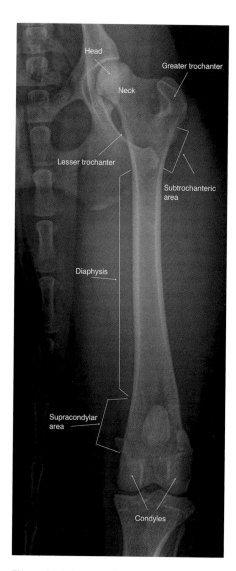

Figure 14.1 A ventrodorsal projection of the femur identifying its relevant bony landmarks.

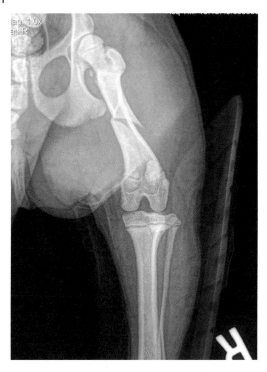

Figure 14.2 A ventrodorsal radiograph of a dog with a femoral fracture that was "stabilized with a splint." It should be noted that the top of the splint is located at the level of the fracture.

14.1 Fractures

14.1.1 Avulsion Fractures of the Greater Trochanter (Figure 14.3)

Avulsion fractures of the greater trochanter can occur in isolation or concurrently with capital physeal and/or femoral neck fractures. As the greater trochanter is the insertion point of the gluteal muscles, there can be considerable traction on this apophysis resulting in separation with trauma. This traction also needs to be considered when contemplating fracture repair methods.

Treatment of choice: Conservative management may be elected for, consisting of strict cage rest for 4–6 weeks if displacement of the greater trochanter is minimal. Recheck radiographs after 2 weeks of rest may be prudent in order to determine if any further displacement has occurred necessitating internal fixation. Internal fixation is accomplished by a craniolateral approach to the hip joint; reduction of the fracture and stabilization are the treatment options of choice. Stabilization is typically achieved using parallel K-wires placed perpendicularly to the fracture line and augmented with a tension band using orthopedic wire. Alternatively a lag screw

combined with an anti-rotational K-wire can be used. Use of a screw should be reserved for larger dogs due to the risk of fracturing the small, avulsed fragment during screw placement.

Postoperative management: Activity restriction is recommended until radiographic signs of healing have occurred. Controlled activity in the form of on-leash walks and formal physical therapy is recommended.

Prognosis: Patients with an avulsion fracture of the greater trochanter tend to have a good outcome. Complications include pin migration or pin and/or wire failure, particularly if the patient is not adequately exercise restricted.

14.1.2 Fractures of the Femoral Shaft

Approximately 50–65% of femoral fractures occur in the diaphysis [1, 2]. The types of fractures of the femoral shaft vary from simple to markedly comminuted. *All femoral fractures* should be considered for surgical repair as this bone cannot be splinted.

14.1.2.1 Fractures of the Proximal Shaft of the Femur (Figure 14.4)

These subtrochanteric fractures are less common. They rarely occur in isolation but rather in conjunction with fractures of the mid-diaphysis.

Treatment of choice: Fractures in the proximal femur tend to be much more challenging to repair. The approach is more difficult because of the vasculature and muscle attachments to this part of the bone. A combination of the craniolateral approach to the hip and a lateral approach to the femur is necessary. Precise contouring of the plate to accurately embrace the metaphysis and greater trochanter is difficult, and the proximity of the hip joint requires careful insertion of the screws or pins; compromise to the vasculature of the femoral neck is also a concern. Fractures in this area of the femur are best left for the experienced surgeon.

Postoperative management: The femur cannot be adequately bandaged and therefore appropriate activity restriction is recommended (Chapter 3).

Prognosis: The prognosis will vary according to the complexity (number of fragments, open vs closed) and location (femoral neck and hip joint affected) of the fracture lines; however, in general, proximal femoral shaft fractures have a good to adequate prognosis with internal fixation. Complicating factors directly related to this type of fracture may include ongoing pain due to the implants irritating the hip joint, coxofemoral osteoarthritis, and/or coxofemoral subluxation (depending on the fracture configuration).

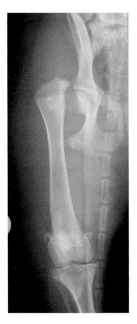
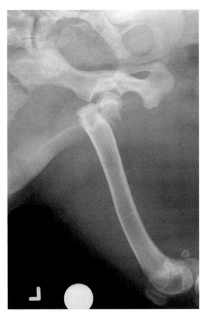
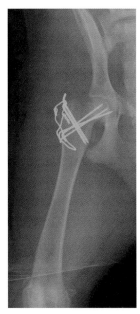
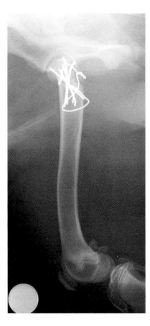

Figure 14.3 Pre- and postoperative radiographs of an immature dog with a capital physeal fracture and concurrent avulsion fracture of the greater trochanter. The capital physeal fracture has been stabilized with diverging K-wires. The trochanter has been stabilized using K-wires and a double twist tension band with orthopedic wire.

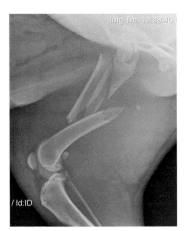
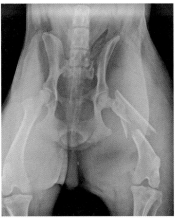
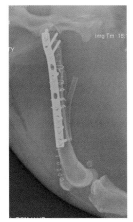
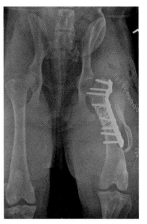

Figure 14.4 Pre- and postoperative projections of a comminuted fracture of the left femur through the proximal shaft, mid-shaft, and femoral neck. It was repaired with cerclage wires, plate, and a femoral head ostectomy. The plate was contoured to fit the shape of the proximal femur.

14.1.2.2 Mid-shaft two-Piece or Two Pieces and a Wedge Fractures

Fractures located in the mid-diaphysis are the most common type of femoral fracture. Typically, they are transverse or long oblique and of a simple configuration (two pieces or two pieces and wedge fragment).

Treatment of choice: Long obliques (length of fracture line is at least twice that of the diameter of the bone) are readily repaired with an intra-medullary pin and cerclage wires (Figure 14.5), which is the least expensive yet a very efficient repair method. A plate or plate and pin can also be used for this fracture configuration. The short oblique and transverse fractures should be repaired with a plate (Figure 14.6), plate and pin, or pin and external fixator. Two-piece mid-diaphyseal fractures are good choices for a general practitioner with the appropriate equipment and training in fracture fixation. The bone, although deep is relatively easy to approach. The large muscles will require retraction with Gelpi, Weitlainer, or handheld retractors and an assistant. Proper implant selection for the patient is the prime concern.

Postoperative management: The femur cannot be adequately bandaged and therefore appropriate activity restriction is recommended (Chapter 3).

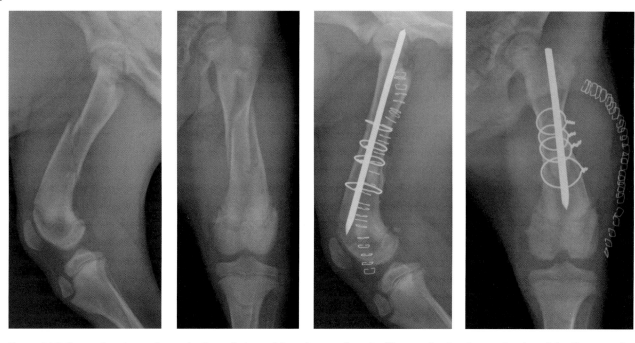

Figure 14.5 Pre- and postoperative projections of a long oblique fracture (length of fracture line is at least twice that of the diameter of the bone) of the left mid-femur that was repaired with a pin and cerclage wires.

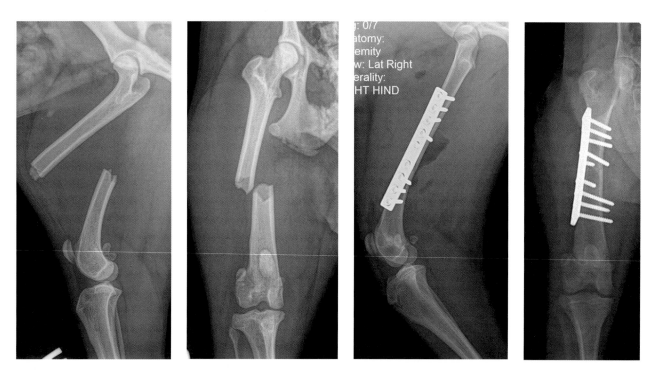

Figure 14.6 Pre- and postoperative projections of a transverse fracture of the left mid-femur that was repaired with a plate.

Prognosis: Prognosis is very good and complications are few providing the repair is technically accurate and of adequate strength. Therefore, clients can be strongly encouraged to proceed with surgical repair of these types of fractures.

14.1.2.3 Mid-shaft Fractures with Segmental or Multiple Pieces (Figure 14.7)

These more complex fractures are technically challenging to repair and are best left for the trained surgeon.

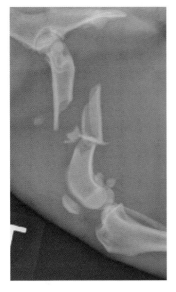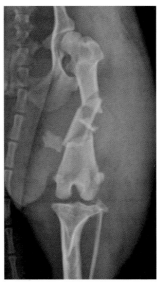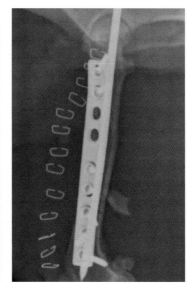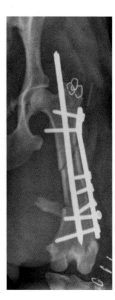

Figure 14.7 Pre- and postoperative projections of a segmental fracture of the left mid-femur that was repaired with a pin and plate.

Treatment of choice: Often a combination of techniques is required, such as plate–pin, plate with interfragmentary screws, pin and Type I external fixator, a long bridging plate, or an interlocking nail [4, 5].

Postoperative management: The femur cannot be adequately bandaged and therefore appropriate activity restriction is recommended (Chapter 3).

Prognosis: Prognosis is very good for the patient with successful osteosynthesis. However, the complication rate with these more complex configurations can be higher. The more common complications include implant failure and infection.

14.1.2.4   Fractures of the Distal Shaft
of the Femur (Figure 14.8)

Fractures in the supracondylar area of the femur account for approximately 11% of all femoral shaft fractures. Fortunately, very few extend to the articular surface [1, 6].

Treatment of choice: These fractures can be repaired with a specialized plate (distal femoral plate, reconstruction plate), a pin–plate combination, or a pin and external fixator (hybrid or ring) [7]. Fractures in this location are much more difficult to repair than mid-shaft fractures. The approach is challenging because of the muscular and capsular attachments and it can be difficult to fit the plate to this section of the bone. These fractures are best left for the trained surgeon.

Postoperative management: The femur cannot be adequately bandaged and therefore appropriate activity restriction is recommended (Chapter 3).

Prognosis: The prognosis will vary according to the complexity (number of fragments, open vs closed) and location (more distal than mid and if the stifle joint is involved) of the fracture; however, in general, femoral shaft fractures have a good prognosis with internal fixation. Complicating factors directly related to this type of fracture may include ongoing pain due to the implants irritating the stifle joint capsule, quadriceps contracture (this is mainly a problem in the immature patient), luxating patella, implant failure, or infection.

14.1.3   Physeal Fractures of the Distal Femur (Figure 14.9)

Fractures of the distal femur that involve the distal physis are a relatively common injury in immature dogs and cats. Due to the strong muscular and ligamentous attachments present, caudal displacement of the distal fragment is frequent.

Treatment of choice: These fractures are usually Salter–Harris I or II fractures. Early reduction and stabilization of these fractures with cross pins is recommended. This will reduce the likelihood of growth impairment or angular limb deformities. Delay in reduction will also result in muscle contraction making reduction more difficult. Closed reduction can be attempted but is challenging and the degree of displacement in the majority of these fractures necessitates an open approach to achieve accurate reduction. Less frequently Salter–Harris III or IV fractures can occur. These fractures

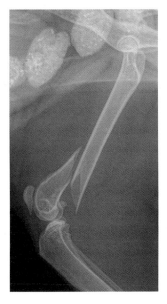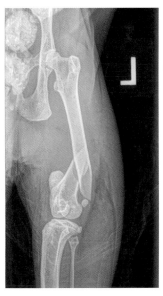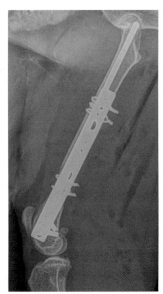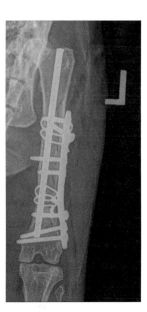

Figure 14.8 Pre- and postoperative projections of a short oblique fracture of the left distal femur of a cat that was repaired with a pin and plate technique.

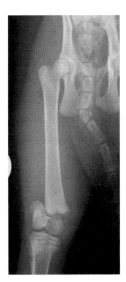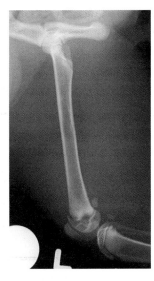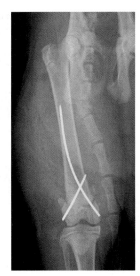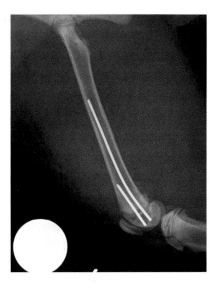

Figure 14.9 Pre- and postoperative craniocaudal and lateral radiographs of a laterally displaced Salter–Harris I fracture of the distal femur in an immature cat. The pin initiated on the medial side is placed in a dynamic fashion, while the lateral pin is placed as a crossed pin. The craniocaudal view shows the pins crossing well above the fracture line. *Source:* Photo courtesy of the Ontario Veterinary College.

involve the articular surface and therefore require accurate anatomic reconstruction. These repairs should be reserved for the experienced surgeon.

Postoperative management: The femur cannot be adequately bandaged and therefore appropriate activity restriction is recommended (Chapter 3).

Prognosis: The prognosis for full return to function is good. Under-reduction of the fracture, varus or valgus reduction, and inadequate pin purchase can all result in fracture failure and poor outcomes. As with all physeal injuries, owners should be warned of the possibility of premature physeal closure and associated limb shortening and/or angular limb deformity as well as pin migration and the need to remove implants. Frequent communication with the client as well as rechecks should occur to ensure the dog or cat is using the limb postoperatively. Failure of adequate limb use combined with callus formation and entrapment of soft tissues may result in "fracture disease" or quadriceps tie-down, usually resulting in the need for limb amputation. Recheck radiographs performed 4–6 weeks post repair will usually confirm fracture healing.

14.2 Managing Expectations with Recommended Treatments

Prognosis for femoral fractures that are surgically repaired is very good, so clients should be strongly encouraged to seek appropriate care and make the financial commitment. Even the complex fracture carries a good prognosis with repair. The femur is a well-muscled bone with an excellent blood supply so it tends to heal well. This bone cannot be bandaged so owners need not be concerned about bandage care. A surgeon may opt to use a non-weight bearing type of sling (Robinson or 90-90) for 10–14 days postoperative if the fracture is very complex and the repair tenuous.

A general practitioner who has the appropriate equipment and has had some training in fracture repair should consider surgically stabilizing two-piece mid-diaphyseal fractures of the femur. The approach to the femur is well described and straightforward. Training is necessary to understand which type of repair to choose based on the fracture configuration, and how to properly apply it. As a rule of thumb, the femur does well with a stronger repair, so selecting a more rigid repair technique such as stack plating, pin–plate, or pin–external fixator may be helpful. Fractures that involve the proximal or distal ends of the femur are much more difficult to repair than the mid-shaft ones and should be left for the more experienced surgeon.

14.3 Alternatives When Treatment of Choice is Not an Option

Appropriately immobilizing the femur with a splint is neither possible nor practical. Non-surgical management of a femoral fracture will very likely result in a malunion given that the natural pull of the thigh muscles will cause the fragments to be displaced.

Fortunately, the large muscles that surround femur tend to help stabilize the fragments of a *two-piece mid-shaft femoral* fracture and maintain a reasonable alignment of the hip and stifle joints. Although *not a desirable treatment option*, a mid-shaft femoral fracture can heal and may result in a reasonably functional limb without surgery (Figure 14.10). Good pain management and confinement to a small area such as a crate are paramount. A Robinson sling to help prevent weight bearing may be useful. This option is better suited to the pediatric patient as they will heal quickly. It is important to monitor these patients closely and to ensure that they are getting adequate care and pain management. Regaining their ability to perform activities of daily living such as standing to eat or comfortably positioning themselves for a bowel movement will take time. Adding a stool softener to help prevent constipation should be considered. Follow-up radiographs can be taken at 2–4 weeks (based on the patient's age) to assess the healing progress. A slow, gradual return to regular exercise can be recommended once a bridging callus is visible on radiographs. Of course, a mid-shaft amputation is also an alternative option.

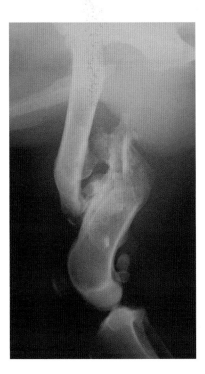 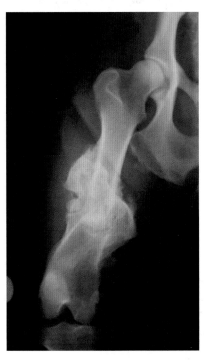

Figure 14.10 Mediolateral and craniocaudal views of the femur of a newly adopted mature dog that was presented to a local hospital for annual vaccines. The mid-shaft femoral fracture had healed without surgery, creating a significant malunion yet the stifle and hip joints are reasonably well aligned despite the malunion. This dog had a palpably thickened thigh but no obvious gait abnormality.

Fractures of the *proximal or distal femur* (including physeal fractures) are more likely to have a pronounced malunion that will likely preclude proper function of the limb without surgical repair (Figure 14.11). A mid- or proximal shaft (based on the location of the fracture) amputation is a better alternative for these patients. If the fracture is only minimally displaced (Figure 14.12), a good outcome may be possible with conservative management.

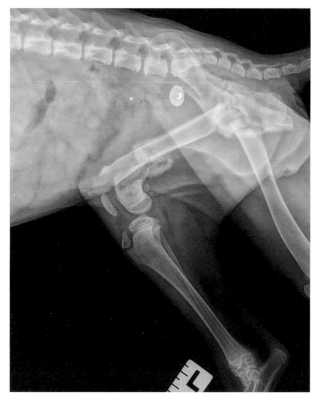

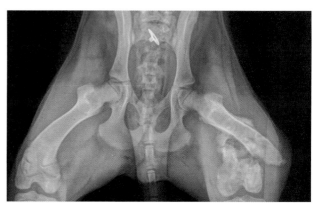

Figure 14.11 A markedly displaced healed fracture of the distal femoral physis in a young border collie presented to the humane society. The limb is not painful and there was no crepitus or instability but the dog would/could not use the limb. A mid-femoral amputation was recommended.

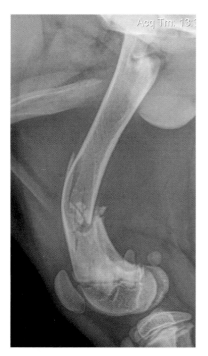

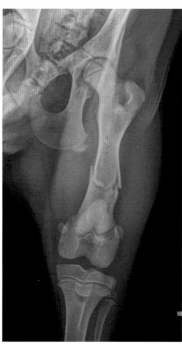

Figure 14.12 An example of a minimally displaced fracture of the left femur of an immature Labrador retriever that was managed conservatively.

References

1 Unger, M., Montavon, P.M., and Heim, U.F.A. (1990). Classification of fractures of the long bones in the dog and cat: Introduction and clinical application. *Vet. Comp. Orthop. Traumatol.* 3: 41–50.

2 Miller, C.W., Sumner-Smith, G., Sheridan, C., and Pennock, P.W. (1998). Using the Unger system to classify 386 long bone fractures in dogs. *J. Small Anim. Pract.* 39: 390–393.

3 Roush, J.K. (2015). Pet health by numbers: Prevalence of bone fractures in dogs and cats. Today's Veterinary Practice. Retrieved from: http://todaysveterinarypractice. navc.com/pet-health-by-the-numbers-prevalence-of-bone-fractures-in-dogs-cats.

4 Johnson, A.L., Smith, C.W., and Schaeffer, D.J. (1998). Fragment reconstruction and bone plate fixation versus bridging plate fixation for treating highly comminuted femoral fractures in dogs: 35 cases. *J. Am. Vet. Med. Assoc.* 213: 1157–1161.

5 Dueland, R.T., Johnson, K.A., Roe, S.C. et al. (1999). Interlocking nail treatment of diaphyseal long-bone fractures in dogs. *J. Am. Vet. Med. Assoc.* 214: 59–66.

6 Braden, T.D., Eicker, S.W., Abdinoor, D., and Prieur, W.D. (1995). Characteristics of 1000 femur fractures in the dog and cat. *Vet. Comp. Orthop. Traumatol.* 8: 203–209.

7 Kirby, K.A., Lewis, D.D., Lafuente, R.M. et al. (2008). Management of humeral and femoral fractures in dogs and cats with linear-circular hybrid external skeletal fixators. *J. Am. Anim. Hosp. Assoc.* 44: 180–197.

15

Stifle Joint

Anne M. Sylvestre

Focus and Flourish, Cambridge, Ontario, Canada

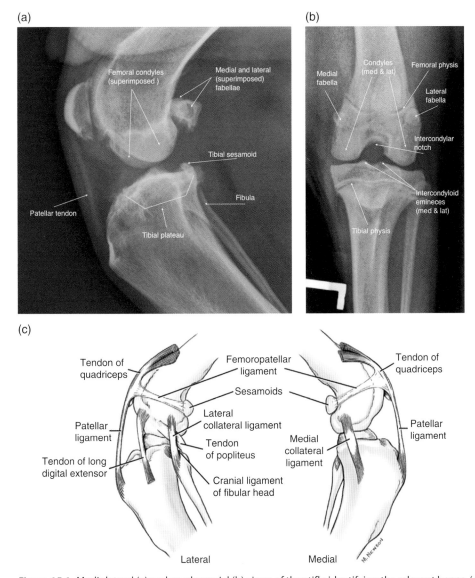

(a)

Femoral condyles (superimposed)
Medial and lateral (superimposed) fabellae
Tibial sesamoid
Fibula
Patellar tendon
Tibial plateau

(b)

Medial fabella
Condyles (med & lat)
Femoral physis
Lateral fabella
Intercondylar notch
Intercondyloid emineces (med & lat)
Tibial physis

(c)

Tendon of quadriceps
Femoropatellar ligament
Sesamoids
Tendon of quadriceps
Patellar ligament
Lateral collateral ligament
Medial collateral ligament
Patellar ligament
Tendon of long digital extensor
Tendon of popliteus
Cranial ligament of fibular head
M. Newton
Lateral
Medial

Figure 15.1 Mediolateral (a) and caudocranial (b) views of the stifle identifying the relevant bones. (c) Ligaments of the left stifle joint. *Source:* From [1].

Fracture Management for the Small Animal Practitioner, First Edition. Edited by Anne M. Sylvestre.

In this chapter, fractures and traumatic luxations of the stifle joint will be discussed. Cranial cruciate ligament tears and non-traumatic patella luxations are not addressed in this book. Trauma to the stifle joint may be associated with extensive soft tissue damage such as collateral ligament, cruciate ligament, or meniscal damage and hemarthrosis. It is important to assess the joint, lavage, debride, and manage the associated soft tissue damage accordingly at surgery. Figure 15.1 shows the relevant bony and ligamentous structures of the stifle joint.

15.1 Fractures and Luxations

15.1.1 Articular Distal Femoral Fractures

Fortunately fractures of the articular surface of the distal femur are very uncommon, accounting for only 3.5% of all femoral fractures [2]. Because these fractures are uncommon, there is very little information on outcomes and complication rates in the literature. However, with accurate reconstruction and rigid internal fixation the prognosis for return to function should be very good. Osteoarthritis will develop in that joint but with appropriate management should not prevent the patient from enjoying regular activity.

15.1.1.1 Unilateral Condylar Fractures
These occur rarely. The lateral or medial condyle can fracture from the femur (Figure 15.2).

Treatment of choice: The articular surface must be reconstructed with accuracy and stability. This is typically achieved with lag screws and Kirschner wires. These repairs are very difficult and best left in the hands of a trained surgeon. Appropriately equipped referral centers can reduce and stabilize some of these fractures closed, using fluoroscopy, a technique known as minimally invasive osteosynthesis.

Postoperative management: It is difficult to adequately bandage the stifle. Restricted activity until the fracture has healed, along with a rehabilitation protocol, are indicated (Chapter 3).

Prognosis: With accurate reconstruction and rigid internal fixation the prognosis for return to function should be very good. Osteoarthritis will develop in that joint but with appropriate management should not prevent the patient from enjoying regular activity.

15.1.1.2 "T" or "Y" Fractures
These occur a little more frequently than unicondylar fractures described above, but are still very uncommon [2]. They are an intercondylar fracture with a supracondylar component (Figure 15.3).

Treatment of choice: For a successful outcome, the articular surface must be accurately reconstructed and stabilized with sufficient strength to prevent motion of the fragments and implants. These are best repaired with lag screws and the addition of a specially created condylar or reconstruction plate. These fractures are very challenging to repair.

Postoperative management: The motion in the stifle can be restricted with a padded bandage, although this can be difficult to maintain; commercially available stifle braces are also a good choice. For large breed dogs, a trans-articular hinged fixator may be necessary to help immobilize the joint. A non-weight bearing sling such as a 90-90 or Robinson may be used as well. Marked activity restriction for 6–8 weeks is indicated followed by a gradual return to regular activity. Close postoperative monitoring of the patient is indicated to help minimize potential complications.

Prognosis: With accurate reconstruction and rigid internal fixation the prognosis for return to function should be very good. Osteoarthritis will develop in that joint but with appropriate management should not prevent the patient from enjoying regular activity.

15.1.2 Patellar Fractures (Figure 15.4)

Patellar fractures are rare in small animals. The patella is a sesamoid located within the quadriceps mechanism and is therefore subject to strong distraction forces. Patellar fractures can occur as a result of trauma or spontaneously. The non-traumatic ones have been reported as a complication of the TPLO (tibial plateau leveling osteotomy) procedure and as a spontaneous occurrence in cats [3–5]. In these non-traumatic cases, the displacement of the fragments is minimal and the patients typically do well with non-surgical management.

Treatment of choice: Traumatic patella fractures are best repaired with a tension band mechanism. The repair is difficult because the fragments are small and can fracture when a pin or drill bit is driven through the fragment and the high tensile force of the quadriceps muscle. These fractures are best left to the trained surgeon.

Postoperative management: Bandages do not tend to adequately counteract distraction forces, especially at the level of the stifle. For large breed dogs, a trans-articular hinged fixator may be necessary. Marked activity restriction for 6–8 weeks is indicated followed by a gradual return to regular activity. Close postoperative monitoring of the patient is indicated to help minimize potential complications.

Prognosis: The prognosis for return to function of the limb can be good providing the fracture heals; however, an athletic dog is not likely to return to competition even after successful healing of the fracture.

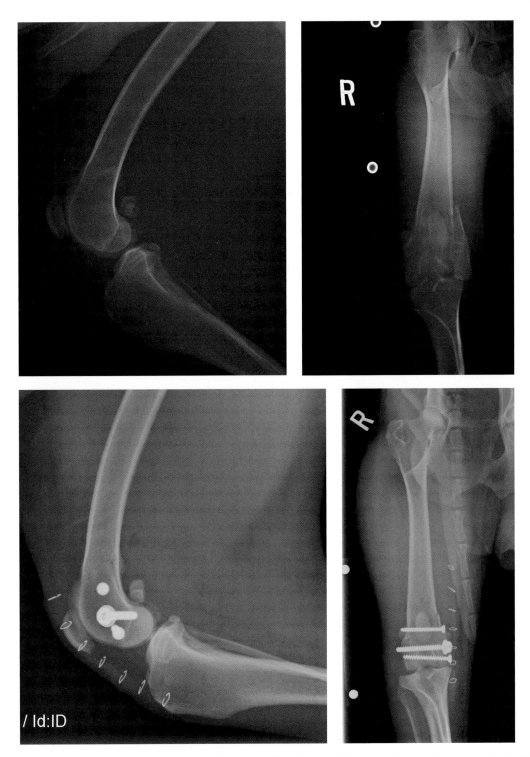

Figure 15.2 Pre- and postoperative views of a canine stifle with a medial condylar fracture that was repaired with screws placed in a lag fashion. *Source:* Photos courtesy of Dr. M. Rochat.

Complications with repair include implant failure and failure of the repair as well as irritation of the soft tissues by the implants requiring their removal. Some authors recommend a complete patellectomy for fractures of the patella. The outcome for this procedure in dogs has not been reported in the literature but the results in people have been found to be suboptimal although variable [6].

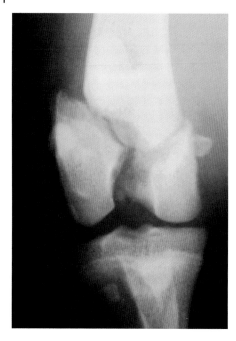

Figure 15.3 Caudocranial view of a canine stifle with a "Y" fracture. *Source:* Photo courtesy of Dr. M. Rochat.

15.1.3 Traumatic Patellar Luxations

These are uncommon. The patient will have a history of an acute trauma, such as running into a post or other solid object. There will be external signs of trauma: marked swelling, effusion, and skin trauma or bruising. The patella will typically luxate medially although it can move both medially and laterally in the very acute phase due to marked swelling and effusion. Radiographs should be taken to ensure that there are no fractures and the integrity of the collateral ligaments should be assessed (see below) as well as that of the cruciate ligaments.

Treatment of choice: It is best to manage these luxations with restricted activity and pain control for 10–14 days following the traumatic event as many will settle back into the groove once the swelling and effusion have subsided. Those that do not do this usually settle medially and will require surgical correction. It is possible that some of these patients have an anatomical predisposition toward patellar luxation. Stabilization involves imbricating the lateral femoropatellar ligament, joint capsule, and the fascia lata with a heavy gauge suture material. Because the luxation is traumatic, these patients typically have an anatomically normal trochlear groove and tibial crest position.

Postoperative management: Activity restriction for 4 weeks followed by a gradual return to regular activity is indicated.

Prognosis: The prognosis for a traumatic patellar luxation managed conservatively or with surgery, is very good to excellent.

For information on *non-traumatic patellar* luxations of small and large breed dogs the reader is directed to *Brinker, Piermattei and Flo's Handbook of Small Animal Orthopedics and Fracture Repair* [7].

15.1.4 Collateral Ligament Damage

Injuries to the medial or lateral collateral ligament are not common and occur as a result of a significant trauma. The integrity of the cranial cruciate ligaments must be assessed as they too may be damaged at the time of the trauma. At presentation, the joint will be swollen and painful.

Diagnosis: Evaluation of the collateral ligaments is done with the stifle *in extension*, and the drawer motion, if present, reduced. If the stifle joint can be angled into a varus position, then the lateral collateral ligament is damaged. If it can be placed in a valgus position, then the medial collateral ligament is damaged (Figure 15.5).
Treatment of choice: Surgical reconstruction of the damaged ligaments is the treatment of choice. There are many different methods of repair described, and the technique chosen will depend on the type of injury. Reconstruction using bone anchors (Everost™) with nylon and crimps works well (Figure 15.6).
Postoperative management: The motion in the stifle can be restricted with a padded bandage although it can be difficult to create a bandage that remains above the stifle especially in certain dog breeds. Commercially available stifle braces are also a good choice. For large breed dogs, a trans-articular hinged fixator may be necessary. Marked activity restriction for 6–8 weeks is indicated followed by a gradual return to regular activity (Chapter 3).
Prognosis: Patients can expect a good return to function with surgical stabilization of the ligaments although the ensuing osteoarthritis will need to be managed.

15.1.5 Luxation of the Stifle Joint (Figure 15.6)

This type of luxation implies damage to multiple ligaments and is also termed "deranged stifle." It is an uncommon occurrence and can be associated with damage to all four ligaments of the stifle joint (both cruciate and both collateral ligaments) as well as the menisci. This type of injury is seen with high-velocity traumas such as automobile

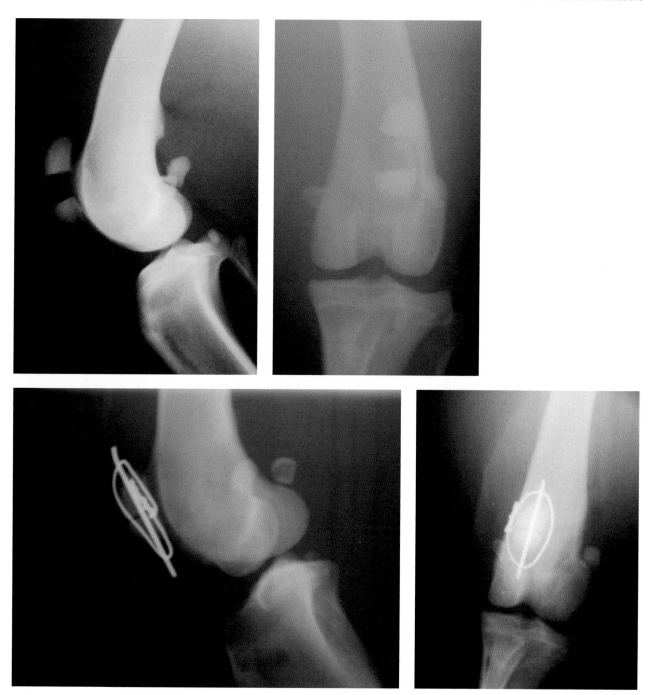

Figure 15.4 Pre- and postoperative views of a canine patella with a mid-body fracture that was repaired with a tension band system. *Source:* Photos courtesy of Dr. M. Rochat.

accidents and, therefore, is often associated with other injuries. The stifle will be markedly swollen, effusive, and unstable. The joint can be supported with a thick soft padded or Robert Jones bandage until such time as the patient can be safely anesthetized for a definitive repair. Hind limb bandages used to immobilize a stifle can be difficult to place, and to maintain in place, especially in dogs with shorter limbs and heavily muscled thighs. Should the bandage slip and not remain well above the stifle, it may accentuate the patient's discomfort and should be removed. This type of injury is very painful and the patient should receive appropriate medications. The extent of the damage to the joint can be thoroughly assessed under general anesthesia.

(a)　　　　　　　　　　　(b)　　　　　　　　　　　(c)

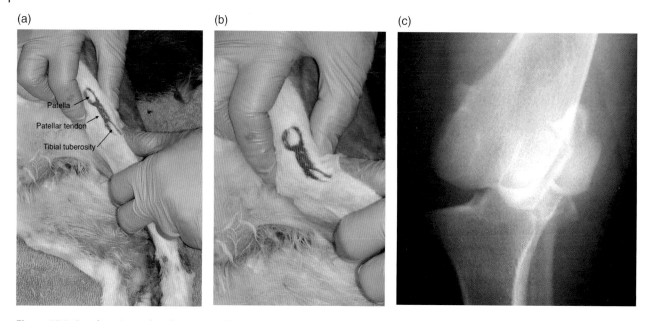

Patella

Patellar tendon

Tibial tuberosity

Figure 15.5 A cadaver is used to demonstrate how to evaluate the medial collateral ligament. The positions of the patella, patellar ligament, and tibial tuberosity have been drawn with a red marker to help with orientation (a). The stifle is placed in extension, and the drawer motion, if present, reduced. The hands are placed on the femur and tibia with the thumbs positioned on the lateral aspect of the stifle (a). Pressure is applied to the lateral and tension on the medial aspects of the stifle in an attempt to "crack it open," if the medial collateral ligament is disrupted, then the joint can be placed into a valgus position (b). (c) A radiograph showing the excess valgus created in the stifle with a damaged medial collateral ligament.

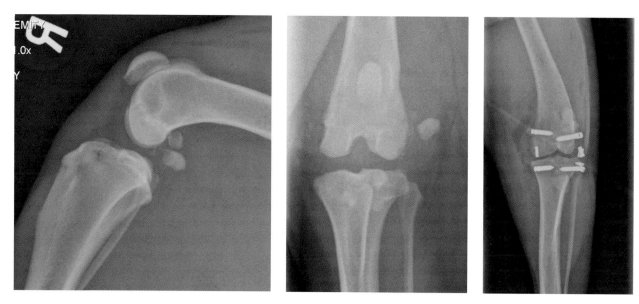

Figure 15.6 Pre- and postoperative views of a canine stifle where the medial and lateral collateral ligaments were reconstructed using bone anchors and nylon with crimps. The increased space between the femur and the tibia is evident on the pre-operative views. *Source:* Photos courtesy of the VCA Canada Mississauga Oakville veterinary emergency Hospital and referral group.

Treatment of choice: At surgery, the joint is explored and, if necessary, meniscal damage is addressed. The collateral ligaments are repaired (as described in Section 15.1.4) next to help realign the joint and then finally, if necessary, the cranial cruciate ligament can be repaired with an extra-capsular technique. Imbrication of the damaged joint capsule and periar-ticular tissues is often sufficient to further stabilize the joint. Small dogs and cats with multiple ligamentous damage can be stabilized with a trans-articular pin immobilizing the stifle in the neutral standing position. Once sufficient fibrosis has occurred, the pin is removed. These surgeries are best left in the hands of a trained surgeon.

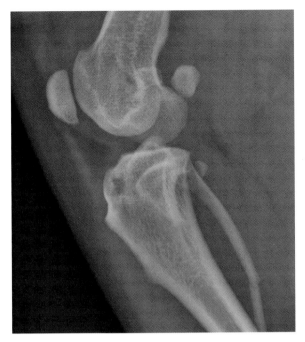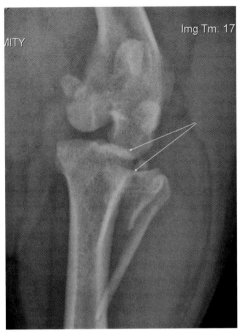

Figure 15.7 Pre-operative views of a canine stifle with an articular fracture of the proximal tibia. The arrows delineate the step between the intact articular surface and the fragment. *Source:* Photos courtesy of the VCA Canada Mississauga Oakville veterinary emergency Hospital and referral group.

Postoperative management: A reconstructed deranged stifle requires restricted activity with gentle passive range of motion (PROM) exercises for approximately 6–8 weeks, until sufficient fibrosis has occurred. If a trans-articular pin has been used to stabilize the joint, PROM exercises should be started once the pin has been removed.

Prognosis: The outcome for these patients is surprisingly very good with surgery given the amount of damage sustained [8]. The small patients with a trans-articular pin tend to have a good outcome with this surgery despite the resulting decrease in range of motion [9].

Cats can present with what appears to be a deranged stifle, as described above, with the femur being positioned caudal to the tibia; however, at surgery, only the cranial cruciate ligament is found to be severed while the other three ligaments remain functionally intact. The author has found this to be a more common occurrence than multiple ligament damage. At surgery, it is important to first reduce the drawer: placing the stifle into the proper anatomical position allows for evaluation of the integrity of the collateral ligaments. In these cases, an extra-capsular cranial cruciate ligament repair with appropriate postoperative care will restore function to the joint with a very good outcome.

15.1.6 Articular Proximal Tibial Fractures (Figure 15.7)

Fractures of the articular surface of the proximal tibia are exceedingly rare.

Treatment of choice: As with all joint fractures, accurate reduction and rigid internal fixation are necessary to maximize a positive outcome. Repair with a lag screw and Kirschner wire as well as a plate or with a ring fixator is indicated. These repairs are very challenging and are best left in the hands of a trained surgeon.

Postoperative management: The motion in the stifle can be restricted with a padded bandage, although this can be difficult to maintain; commercially available stifle braces are also a good choice. A non-weight bearing sling such as a 90-90 or Robinson may be used as well. Marked activity restriction for 6–8 weeks is indicated followed by a gradual return to regular activity. Close postoperative monitoring of the patient is indicated to help minimize potential complications.

Prognosis: It is difficult to get accurate information on the prognosis for fractures of the tibial articular surface as they are so rare. With accurate reconstruction and rigid internal fixation the prognosis should be good. Osteoarthritis will be present in that joint but with appropriate management should not prevent the patient from enjoying regular activity.

15.2 Managing Expectations with Recommended Treatments

Although there is not a lot of information on prognosis and complication rates for dogs and cats with these traumatic stifle injuries, because they are so uncommon, the few reports that do exist indicate that the outcomes are quite positive. This is the type of information that many owners need to hear to give them the encouragement to seek out the appropriate care for their pet. There is no doubt that the traumas to the stifle joint described in this chapter are significant and that osteoarthritis will ensue; despite that, the pet should be able to enjoy a reasonably active lifestyle with an osteoarthritis management regime (Chapter 3).

The surgeries describe in this chapter are challenging and best left in the hands of an experienced surgeon. Postoperatively, a non-weight bearing sling may be recommended (Robinson sling) for the first 2 weeks after a difficult fracture repair; for large dogs with a complex condition, a trans-articular external fixator may be used to protect the reconstructed stifle joint. Support with a pelvic or abdominal sling may also be helpful and should be considered, especially if the pet has other mobility challenges. The traumatic patellar fractures are likely the more difficult ones to manage postoperatively because of the strong tensile forces placed on the repair and the difficulty with immobilizing the area with external coaptation.

15.3 Alternatives Treatment When Surgery is Not an Option

Joint fractures do better with surgical repair. There are no good alternatives for fractures of the articular surface of the stifle joint. As discussed earlier, non-traumatic, minimally displaced fractures of the patella can do well without surgery. However conservative management of all other articular stifle fractures will result in a residual lameness and/or poor limb use. An amputation may be a better choice. Also, there are no non-surgical treatment alternatives for a stifle luxation that will result in an adequate outcome. However, clients can be reassured that their pet can have a good outcome with surgery and be encouraged to seek the appropriate care.

References

1 Evans, H.E. and de Lahunta, A. (2013). *Miller's Anatomy of the Dog*, 4e. St Louis, MO: Saunders/Elsevier.

2 Unger, M., Montavon, P.M., and Heim, U.F.A. (1990). Classification of fractures of the long bones in the dog and cat: introduction and clinical application. *Vet. Comp. Orthop. Traumatol.* 3: 41–50.

3 Rutherford, S., Bell, J.C., and Ness, M.G. (2012). Fractures of the patella after TPLO in 6 dogs. *Vet. Surg.* 41: 869–875.

4 Salas, N. and Popovitch, C. (2011). Surgical versus conservative management of patella fractures in cats: a retrospective study. *Can. Vet. J.* 52: 1319–1322.

5 Langley-Hobbs, S.J. (2009). Survey of 52 fractures of the patella in 34 cats. *Vet. Rec.* 164: 80–86.

6 Stougard, J. (1970). Patellectomy. *Acta Orthop. Scand.* 41: 110–121.

7 DeCamp, C.E., Johnston, S.A., Déjardin, L.M., and Schaefer, S.L. (2016). *Brinker, Piermattei and Flo's Handbook of Small Animal Orthopaedics and Fracture Repair*, 5e. St Louis, MO: Elsevier.

8 Aron, D. (1988). Traumatic dislocation of the stifle joint: treatment of 12 dogs and 1 cat. *J. Am. Anim. Hosp. Assoc.* 24: 333–340.

9 DeCamp, C.E., Johnston, S.A., Déjardin, L.M., and Schaefer, S.L. (2016). The stifle joint. In: *Brinker, Piermattei and Flo's Handbook of Small Animal Orthopaedics and Fracture Repair*, 5e, 597–669. St Louis, MO: Elsevier.

16

Tibia and Fibula

Thomas W.G. Gibson[1] and Anne M. Sylvestre[2]

[1] Ontario Veterinary College, University of Guelph, Guelph, Ontario, Canada
[2] Focus and Flourish, Cambridge, Ontario, Canada

(a)

(b)

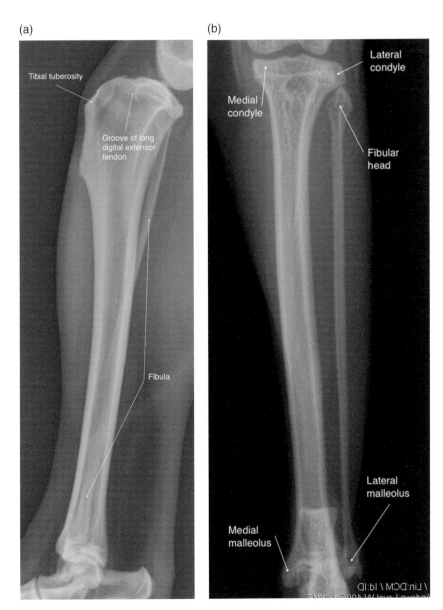

Figure 16.1 Mediolateral (a) and caudocranial (b) projections of the canine tibia identifying its relevant landmarks.

Fracture Management for the Small Animal Practitioner, First Edition. Edited by Anne M. Sylvestre.
© 2019 John Wiley & Sons, Inc. Published 2019 by John Wiley & Sons, Inc.

Fractures of the tibia and fibula are common in dogs and cats, accounting for approximately 20–25% of long bone fractures [1–4]. Fractures of the diaphysis account for 51–81% of all tibial fractures [1, 2, 4].

There are more open tibial fractures than seen with other bones. This is due to the lack of musculature and soft tissues covering this bone. The patient must be examined carefully for skin wounds located close to the fracture site. In many open fractures the bone will protrude through the skin at the time of the impact but then recede back under the skin as the limb settles into its post-impact position. Open fractures must be treated accordingly to decrease the potential for osteomyelitis (see Chapter 2). Figure 16.1 shows the relevant bony landmarks of the tibia and fibula.

16.1 Fractures

16.1.1 Tibial Tuberosity Avulsion Fractures (Figure 16.2)

The tibial tuberosity is an apophysis that acts as the insertion of the quadriceps mechanism due to the attachment of the patellar tendon. As a result, this apophysis can be subjected to large muscular forces when the stifle is flexed, resulting in avulsion of this tuberosity. Displacement can be minimal or severe, resulting in detachment of the tuberosity and proximal displacement of the patella. Lateral radiographs of the contralateral tibia can be helpful to confirm the diagnosis and determine the degree of displacement on the affected side, as this growth plate can appear wide in the normal immature tibia.

Treatment of choice: Conservative management using external coaptation with a lateral splint or cast may be elected for in cases where there is minimal displacement and mild lameness. Coaptation may also be elected for in cases that are more chronic due to a delayed diagnosis as open reduction may be challenging if surgery is delayed. In small patients with minimal displacement, two K-wires may be sufficient to stabilize the fragment. In most cases a pin and tension band is recommended.

Postoperative management: Strict exercise restriction should be recommended until the first radiographic recheck at 3–4 weeks. In animals with potential for further growth, implants should be removed once radiographic healing is evident, typically at 3–6 weeks.

Prognosis: Prognosis for full return to function is good. Complications include pin migration, pin or wire failure, and pin- and wire-induced injury of the overlying soft tissues.

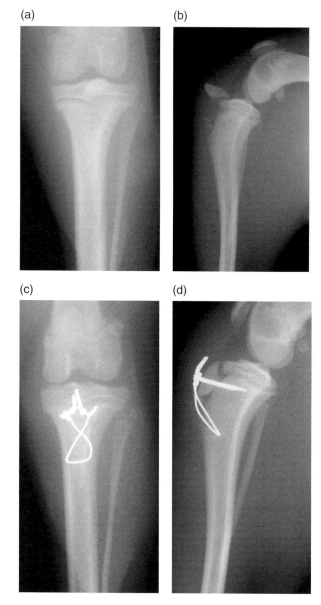

(a) (b) (c) (d)

Figure 16.2 Preoperative caudocranial (a) and mediolateral (b) radiographs of a displaced tibial tuberosity avulsion fracture in an immature dog; and the postoperative caudocranial (c) and mediolateral (d) views. Note the side-by-side pin placement in the fragment and augmentation with a double twist figure-8 wire tension band. *Source:* Photo courtesy of the Ontario Veterinary College.

16.1.2 Tibial Plateau Physeal Fractures (Figure 16.3)

Salter–Harris I or II fractures involving the physis of the tibial plateau occur in immature animals and often involve the growth plate of the tibial tuberosity. In this case the plateau often "slips" caudally and medially.

Treatment of choice: Proper reduction and stabilization with crossed pins, plus or minus a tension band wire are recommended. If diagnosed early, the fracture fragment can be manipulated back into place

(a)
(b)
(c)

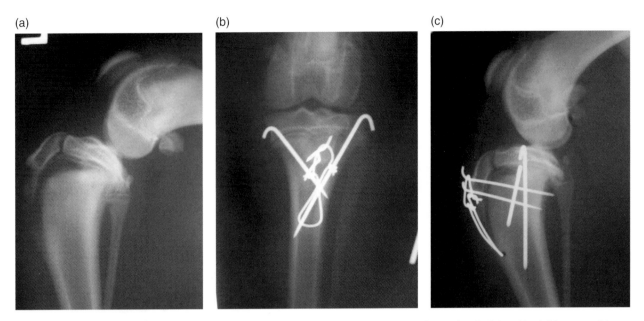

Figure 16.3 Lateral pre-operative (a) and caudocranial (b) and lateral (c) postoperative radiographs of a Salter–Harris I fracture of the tibial plateau in an immature dog. The involvement of the physis of the tibial tuberosity and the addition of pins and a tension band to the tuberosity to add additional stability should be noted. *Source:* Photo courtesy of the Ontario Veterinary College.

with closed reduction by extending the stifle and applying caudal and lateral traction to the metaphysis of the tibia. This will allow placement of the crossed pins in a closed fashion through medial and lateral stab incisions at the level of the tibial plateau. This approach usually requires fluoroscopic guidance to confirm proper reduction and pin placement and is usually reserved for trained surgeons. Otherwise the fracture is reduced via an open reduction and stabilized with cross pins and potentially a tension band wire.

Postoperative management: Strict exercise restriction should be recommended until the first radiographic recheck at 3–4 weeks. In animals with potential for further growth, the pins and tension band apparatus should be removed once radiographic healing is evident, typically at 3–6 weeks.

Prognosis: The prognosis for a full return to function is good. In cases where surgical intervention is not an option or diagnosis has been delayed making adequate reduction of the fragment unlikely, a lateral splint may be placed for 3–4 weeks to prevent any further displacement of the tibial plateau. Conservative management is usually not recommended as poor reduction can result in an abnormal tibial plateau angle and/or the possibility of an angular limb deformity. Serious alteration to stifle biomechanics may occur. These complications can be exacerbated in animals with further growth potential. Owners need to be counseled on the possibility of future angular or rotational growth deformities.

16.1.3 Proximal Tibial Shaft Fractures (Figure 16.4)

Fractures of the proximal shaft of the tibia are not common.

Treatment of choice: They are best repaired with a plate, plate–pin combination, or an external fixator. The configuration of the proximal tibia make it difficult to effectively place cerclage wires; therefore, a pin and cerclage wiring technique is not a method of choice.

Postoperative management: Activity restriction and postsurgical care, as detailed in Chapter 3, should be followed.

Prognosis: The prognosis for this type of fracture is very good providing no other structures (joint, tibial tuberosity) are affected.

16.1.4 Fractures of the Mid- and Mid-to-Distal Portions of the Tibial Shaft

These are the most common fractures of the tibia [1, 3, 5]. A mid-shaft fracture may extend into the distal part of the bone or vice versa making it difficult to accurately classify them according to location alone. Those that extend into the distal fifth of the bone are more difficult to repair because of the configuration of the bone and proximity to the joint.

The medial approach to the tibia is straightforward and a two-piece mid-diaphyseal fracture configuration is one that a general practitioner with the appropriate equipment and training in fracture fixation can readily

(a)   (b)   (c)   (d)

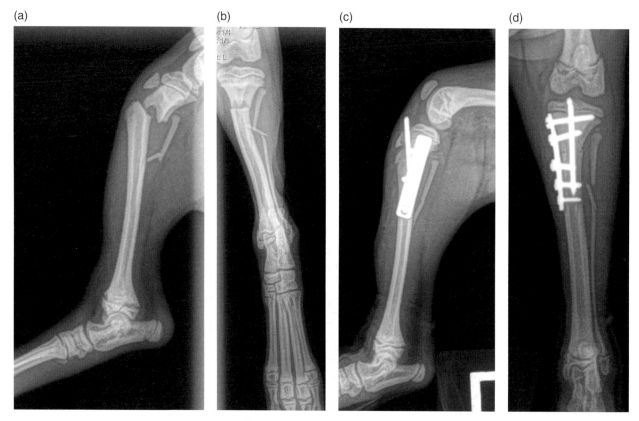

Figure 16.4 Pre mediolateral (a) and caudocranial (b) projections of a fractured proximal tibial shaft; and the postoperative mediolateral (c) and caudocranial (d) views. This fracture was repaired with a pin and plate.

handle. It is important to start with good quality pre-operative mediolateral and caudocranial radiographs of the entire tibia to accurately identify the extent of the fracture and fissure lines. Fractures that extend close to the tibiotarsal joint and those that have significant fissure lines are best left to the trained surgeon.

Overall prognosis: Tibial shaft fractures that are surgically repaired carry a very good to excellent prognosis [3, 5–7]. Some of the more distal fractures or those with fissure lines are technically much more challenging. Accurate implant selection and placement as well as owner and patient compliance will contribute to a lower complication rate. Studies and case series of tibial shaft fractures that are surgically stabilized report successful outcomes without complications in 87.5–91% of cases [3, 7]. Complications seen with diaphyseal fractures of the tibia are not frequent but include: implant failure (breakage/loosening of screws, plates, external fixator pins); intra-medullary pins causing irritation of the subcutaneous soft tissues; pins or rods backing out of the medullary canal; osteomyelitis; and delayed healing. Some of these complications are easily addressed with a minor procedure (pin removal), extra time, or perhaps with a minor second

surgery such as for plate/screw removal. Catastrophic failures where a major second and maybe third procedure are necessary do occur but are very infrequent.

16.1.4.1 Fractures of the Mid- and Mid-to-Distal Portions of the Tibia That are Incomplete or/and With the Fibula Intact (Figure 16.5)

Fractures of the tibial shaft with an intact fibula occur in approximately 16% of tibial fractures [5]. This type of fracture usually occurs owing to a low-impact trauma. The resultant fracture is typically a simple two-fragment configuration with minimal displacement.

Treatment of choice: These fractures can be treated with external coaptation.
Patient management: A custom-made or lateral splint is applied and managed (Chapter 4) until radiographic evidence of bony healing is evident. Appropriate activity restriction and patient care should be followed (Chapter 3).
Prognosis: Very good to excellent results can be expected [8] with theses fractures. Complications are usually associated with bandage/splint management (bandage sores, loss of range of motion in the tarsus). As with many splinted fractures, a malunion may be apparent

(a)

(b)

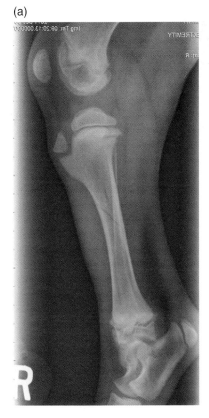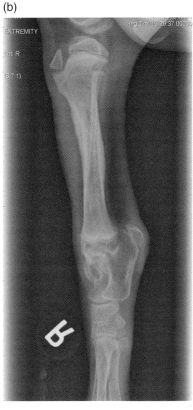

Figure 16.5 Mediolateral projections of an acute (a) and healed (b) minimally displaced fracture of the right tibia of a young dog that was treated with a splint. The fibula was intact.

on the radiographs of the healed bone. These malunions are often not clinically significant. The bone will remodel according to Wolff's law, which states that the bones of a healthy individual will adapt to the loads under which it is placed. To avoid dealing with the frequent bandage changes and potential complications with splints, a unilateral/uniplanar (simple configuration) external fixator can be applied with minimal hassle and good owner satisfaction [9].

16.1.4.2 Simple Fractures (Two Pieces or Two Main Pieces with Few Small Fragments) of the Tibia and Fibula

Tibial fractures that are complete (fibula included) are best addressed with surgery as they are inherently unstable and the tibia is a difficult bone to properly immobilize with external coaptation.

Treatment of choice: Transverse and short oblique fractures, where the fracture length is less than twice the width of the bone (Figure 16.6), are best repaired with a plate, a pin–plate combination, or an external fixator. Long oblique and spiral fractures (Figure 16.7) are the most common type of diaphyseal tibial fractures [5]. These fractures are best repaired with: pin and cerclage wires; pin–plate combination; pin–external fixator; plate and inter-fragmentary screws; or interlocking nail. Caution should be exercised when

examining these configurations as there may be fissures and the fracture lines can extend into or very close to the tibiotarsal joint. Good quality pre-operative radiographs of the entire tibia are important to accurately identify the extent of these fractures.

Postoperative management: The limb may be bandaged for a few days after surgery to help manage the swelling. Otherwise activity restriction and post-surgical care, as detailed in Chapter 3, should be followed.

Prognosis: The prognosis with surgical repair is very good to excellent.

16.1.4.3 Comminuted Fractures of the Mid-Shaft of the Tibia (Figure 16.8)

Treatment of choice: These are more challenging to repair and best left in the hands of a trained surgeon. The repair technique employed will be based on the specific fracture configuration and the surgeon's preference. Commonly used techniques include: plate with cerclage wires and inter-fragmentary screws; pin–plate–cerclage wire combination; external fixator; locking plates; intramedullary nails; and extension plates.

Postoperative management: The surgeon may opt to place the limb in a splint for a few weeks postoperatively based on the stability of the repair and the dog's personality. Chapter 3 has further details on postoperative care.

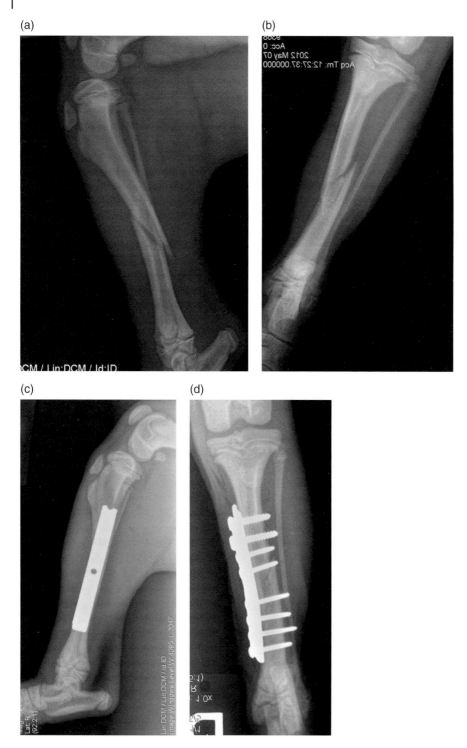

Figure 16.6 Pre mediolateral (a) and caudocranial (b) projections of a short oblique tibial fracture and its postoperative mediolateral (c) and caudocranial (d) views. The length of the oblique fracture line is less than 2× that of the width of the bone. This fracture was repaired with stacked cuttable plates.

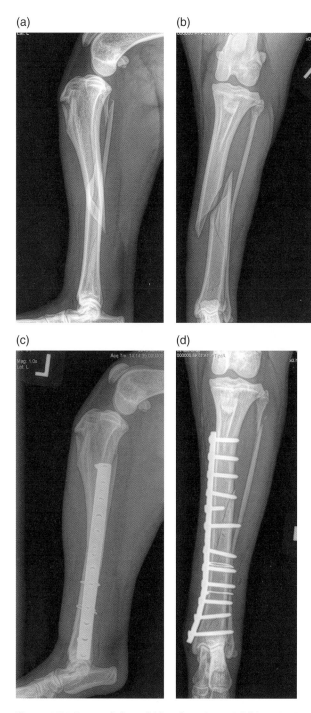

Figure 16.7 Pre mediolateral (a) and caudocranial (b) projections of a long oblique tibial fracture and it post-operative mediolateral (c) and caudocranial (d) views. The length of the oblique fracture line is more than 2× the width of the bone. There are prominent fissure lines on the caudocranial view. These are not uncommon with long oblique fractures of the tibia. This fracture was repaired with a plate and cerclage wires.

Prognosis: The prognosis for these fractures is very good to excellent once the fracture has healed but the potential for complications to occur during the healing process is higher than with a two-piece fracture configuration [6].

16.1.5 Fractures of the Distal Tibial Shaft (Figure 16.9)

Whether simple or comminuted, these are very challenging fractures to deal with because of the necessity to accurately configure and position the implants, the proximity of the tibiotarsal joint, soft tissue attachments, and the typically small size of the bone fragments in this location.

Treatment of choice: Repair techniques of choice are: pin and cerclage wires; plate; pin–plate; or external fixators (hybrid or ring). These fractures are best left in the hands of the trained surgeon.

Postoperative management: The surgeon may opt to place the limb in a splint for a few weeks postoperatively based on the stability of the repair and the dog's personality. Activity restriction, husbandry and rehabilitation as detailed in Chapter 3 are also indicated.

Prognosis: The prognosis for return to activity is very good once the fracture has healed but the potential for complications to occur during the healing process is higher than with two-piece fracture configurations.

16.1.6 Physeal Fractures of the Distal Tibia/Fibula (Figure 16.10)

Physeal fractures of the distal tibia and fibula are a relatively common occurrence in immature animals experiencing trauma. These fractures need to be distinguished from other injuries of the tarsus such as tarsal fractures and luxations. In most cases both these fractures are Salter–Harris I or II fractures involving both physes of the distal tibia and fibula resulting in caudal displacement of the tarsus.

Treatment of choice: In rare cases where the fracture can be reduced closed using traction and manipulation of the tarsus with some intrinsic stability present, casting or external coaptation with a lateral splint can be attempted. The vast majority of these fractures require open reduction and stabilization, usually with crossed pins.

Postoperative management: Strict exercise restriction should be recommended until the first radiographic recheck at 3–4 weeks. A lateral splint or a bivalve cast may provide additional support until evidence of radiographic healing is present.

Prognosis: The prognosis for full return to function is good. Pins may be removed if problems arise related to the thin soft tissue coverage in this area.

16.1.7 Fractures of the Fibular Shaft Alone (Figure 16.11)

These are uncommon in dogs and cats. They usually are a result of a blunt trauma.

Treatment of choice: These fractures are readily managed with restricted activity and pain medication. A splint

(a) (b) (c) (d)

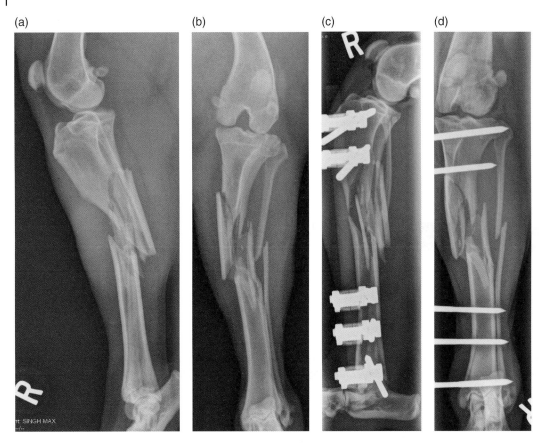

Figure 16.8 Pre mediolateral (a) and caudocranial (b) projections of a comminuted mid-shaft fracture of the tibia and its postoperative mediolateral (c) and caudocranial (d) views. This fracture was stabilized with an external fixator.

is not necessary for these as the intact tibia serves as an internal stabilizer for the fracture.

Prognosis: The prognosis is excellent.

When the *very distal* fibula is fractured (a lateral malleolar fracture), an instability of the tibiotarsal joint is often the result as this is where the lateral collateral ligament originates. This specific type of fracture is discussed in Chapter 17 on fractures of the tarsal joint.

16.2 Managing Expectations with Recommended Treatments

The prognosis for tibial fractures that are surgically repaired is very good to excellent and, overall, complications are few; therefore, the client should be strongly encouraged to seek the appropriate care despite the potential financial concerns. If the fracture configuration is complex, then the patient may have a splint or bandage postoperatively. The owner should be aware that regular bandage changes may be necessary (Chapter 4).

A general practitioner who has the appropriate equipment and has had some training in fracture repair should consider surgically stabilizing mid-diaphyseal fractures

of the tibia. The approach is very straightforward. Training is necessary to understand which type of repair to choose based on the fracture configuration. Fractures that involve the distal end of the tibia are much more difficult to repair than the mid-shaft ones and should be left for the more experienced surgeon.

The tibia can be managed with a splint but it is one of the more difficult bones to properly manage this way because of the configuration of the hind limb. Although many owners like the idea of avoiding surgery because of the cost and the emotional implications, it is important that they are made to understand that splint management can be frustrating and difficult. Splinted tibial fractures are prone to longer healing times, bandage slippage, and the formation of decubital sores. Client education is important.

16.3 Alternatives When Treatment of Choice is Not an Option

If surgical repair is not an option for a patient with a fracture of the mid- or mid-to-distal tibial diaphysis, then external coaptation using a lateral or custom-made

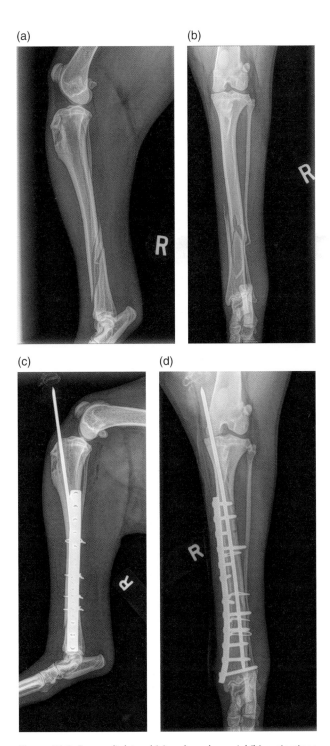

(a)   (b)

(c)   (d)

Figure 16.9 Pre mediolateral (a) and caudocranial (b) projections of a distal tibial shaft fracture and it post-operative mediolateral (c) and caudocranial (d) views. This fracture was repaired with a pin–plate combination. The pin was cut short subsequent to the radiograph being taken.

splint can be applied. Ideally, the bandage/splint should immobilize the stifle as well as the tarsus; this can be difficult to accomplish because of the shape of the hind limb, especially in the chondrodystrophic breeds. More

distally located fractures can be adequately immobilized with a bandage/splint that does not include the stifle. Proximally located fractures that are splinted must include the stifle, and be replaced if they slip below the stifle, to function properly.

There are only a few reports that include outcomes of patients with conservatively managed tibial fractures. One had nine dogs with two-piece diaphyseal tibial and fibular fractures managed with external coaptation alone; eight out of nine dogs had a good to excellent outcome [3]. The ages of the dogs were not reported. Another report had approximately half of their immature patients with complete tibial shaft fractures treated successfully with external coaptation [5]. Another study reported on conservatively managed tibial fractures *with the fibula intact*; dogs less than 1 year of age had an excellent outcome and healed within an expected time period, while mature dogs (>24 months) had delayed healing times (approximately 4 months), although all had a good outcome [8]. The fractures in this study were simple (two-piece) or two-piece with a wedge fragment, transverse or oblique configurations. From these studies we can reason that simple tibial diaphyseal fractures can heal with external coaptation; however, mature patients are likely to take longer to achieve bony union. Therefore, owners and veterinarians should be prepared to deal with splint changes for a longer period of time. There are no data on comminuted fractures treated with splints alone but one can speculate that an increased number of delayed and non-unions as well as malunions could be anticipated. The malunion, in most cases, may not be clinically significant [8].

In summary, a tibial diaphyseal fracture addressed conservatively can heal well and with a good outcome, especially if the patient is young and the fracture is simple in configuration. However, it is important to appreciate the potential frustrations and difficulties associated with long-term splinting of the tibia. Given the high success rate and positive outcomes with surgically repaired tibial shaft fractures, it is worth taking the time to properly educate the pet owner so that they can make an informed decision rather than an emotional one.

Fractures that are located in the proximal and distal-most portions of the bone tend to have a less optimal outcome with conservative management than the ones located in the mid- and mid-distal sections because of the proximity to the joints and the small size of the fragments making closed reduction difficult. Encouraging owners to pursue surgical repair, if at all possible, is best for these fractures.

The alternative to splinting would be a mid-femoral amputation. The cost of this procedure would be less than that of a fracture repair but still requires a substantial outlay of funds. Again, given the high success and low complication rates of surgically repaired tibial fractures, it would be worth having the owners reconsider the value of their pet's well-being over that of the financial savings.

(a)   (b)   (c)   (d)

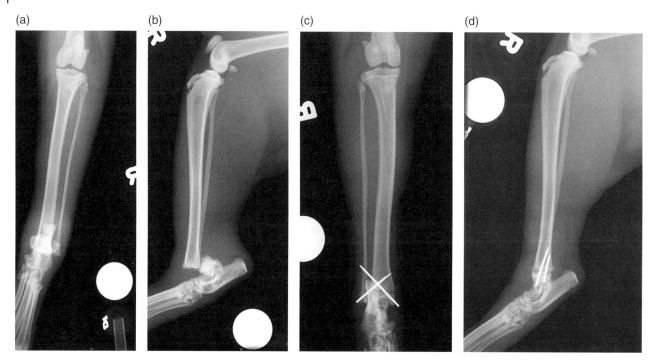

Figure 16.10 Preopreative craniocaudal (a) and mediolateral (b) and postoperative craniocaudal (c) and mediolateral (d) radiographs of a Salter–Harris I fracture of the distal tibia and fibula in an immature cat that was repaired with crossed K-wires. The caudal displacement of the tarsus in the pre-operative lateral view is evident. *Source:* Photo courtesy of the Ontario Veterinary College.

(a)   (b)

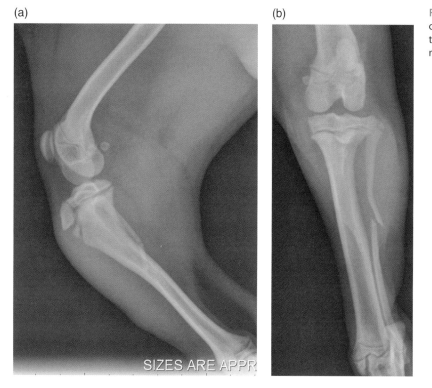

Figure 16.11 Mediolateral (a) and caudocranial (b) projections of a fracture of the fibula. This fracture was managed with restricted activity and pain medication.

References

1 Unger, M., Montavon, P.M., and Heim, U.F.A. (1990). Classification of fractures of the long bones in the dog and cat: introduction and clinical application. *Vet. Comp. Orthop. Traumatol.* 3: 41–50.

2 Roush, J.K. (2015). Pet health by numbers: Prevalence of bone fractures in dogs and cats. Today's Veterinary Practice. Retrieved from: http://todaysveterinarypractice. navc.com/pet-health-by-the-numbers-prevalence-of-bone-fractures-in-dogs-cats.

3 Miller, C.W., Sumner-Smith, G., Sheridan, C., and Pennock, P.W. (1998). Using the Unger system to classify 386 long bone fractures in dogs. *J. Small Anim. Pract.* 39: 390–393.

4 Bennour, E.M., Abushhiwa, M.A., Ben Ali, L. et al. (2014). A retrospective study on appendicular fractures in dogs and cats in Tripoli—Libya. *J. Vet. Adv.* 4: 425–431.

5 Boone, E.G., Johnson, A.L., Montavon, P.M. et al. (1986). Fractures of the tibial diaphysis in dogs and cats. *J. Am. Vet. Med. Assoc.* 188: 41–45.

6 Dudley, M., Johnson, A.L., Olmstead, M. et al. (1997). Open reduction and bone plate stabilization, compared with closed reduction and external fixation, for treatment of comminuted tibial fractures: 47 cases (1980–1995) in dogs. *J. Am. Vet. Med. Assoc.* 21: 1008–1012.

7 Baroncelli, A.B., Peirone, B., Winter, M.D. et al. (2012). Retrospective comparison between minimally invasive plate osteosynthesis and open plating for tibial fractures in dogs. *Vet. Comp. Orthop. Traumatol.* 5: 410–417.

8 Zaal, M.D. and Hazewinkel, H.A. (1997). Treatment of isolated tibial fractures in cats and dogs. *Vet. Q.* 4: 191–194.

9 Aronsohn, M.G. and Burk, R.L. (2009). Unilateral uniplanar external skeletal fixation for isolated diaphysial tibial fractures in skeletally immature dogs. *Vet. Surg.* 38: 654–658.

17

Tarsal Joint

Anne M. Sylvestre

Focus and Flourish, Cambridge, Ontario, Canada

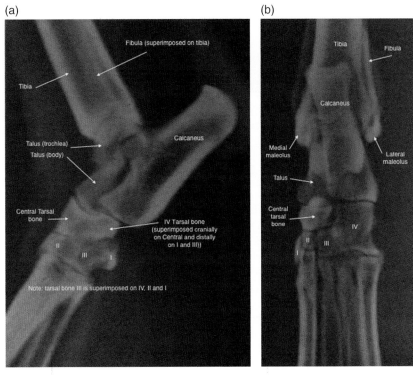

(a)

(b)

Figure 17.1 Mediolateral (a) and craniocaudal (b) views of the tarsus identifying the relevant bones. (c) Ligaments of the left tarsus. C, calcaneus; I–V, metatarsals; T, talus; TII, TIII, TIV, second, third, fourth tarsals; TC, central tarsal. *Source:* From [1].

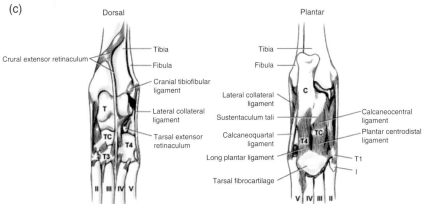

(c)

Fracture Management for the Small Animal Practitioner, First Edition. Edited by Anne M. Sylvestre.
© 2019 John Wiley & Sons, Inc. Published 2019 by John Wiley & Sons, Inc.

The tarsus is a complex joint. It is composed of seven bones, all of which articulate with one another and stabilized in position by numerous ligaments (Figure 17.1). The joints of the tarsus include: (1) the tarsocrural (or tibiotarsal) joint, which is the articulation between the tibia, talus, and fibula (the human term "talocrural" is also used to refer to this joint); (2) the talocalcaneal joint, which is the articulation between the calcaneus and talus; (3) the proximal intertarsal joint, which refers to the articulation between the talus, calcaneus, central, and fourth tarsal bones; (4) the distal intertarsal joint, which is the articulation between the small numbered bones and central and fourth tarsal bones; and (5) the tarsometatarsal joint, which is the distal-most articulation between the numbered bones and the metatarsal bones. Diagnoses of injuries to this area can be made using radiographs but computerized tomography (CT) scans may also be necessary in some cases to show lesions that may be missed on radiographs. Radiographic interpretation can be challenging because of the complexity of this joint. Fortunately the widespread use of digital radiography has made it easy to engage the expertise of a board-certified radiologist to help with these cases. Stress views should be considered for patients with an injury to this joint to assess for ligamentous instabilities.

17.1 Fractures and Ligamentous Injuries

17.1.1 Articular Distal Tibial Fractures

These fractures, whether simple or complex, are rare.

Treatment of choice: A "chip" fracture, where a small articular fragment separates from the tibia (Figure 17.2), is best treated by removing the fragment as they are usually too small for a screw. More complex fractures (which are very rare) should have reconstruction of the articular surface if possible with a ring fixator or several lag screws and a trans-articular external fixator to stabilize the fragments. These surgeries are best left for the trained surgeon. An arthrodesis may be the better choice in many of these cases as reconstruction may not be possible. Arthrodesis is discussed below.

Postoperative management: The tarsus should be immobilized post-operatively for 4–6 weeks. This can be accomplished with a lateral of custom splint; a custom-made brace or a trans-articular external fixator. This latter technique may be preferred in larger dogs.

Prognosis: The prognosis with reconstruction will depend on how precisely the articular surface can be realigned and joint stability reestablished.

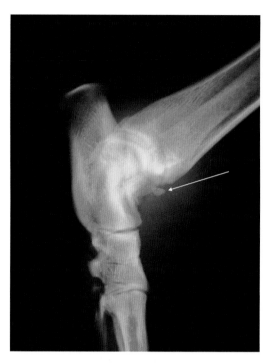

Figure 17.2 A mediolateral projection of a "chip" fracture of the craniodistal tibial articular surface (arrow).

17.1.2 Fractures of the Medial Malleolus or the Lateral Malleolus (Figure 17.3)

The medial malleolus is located on the distal-most aspect of the medial tibia and the lateral malleolus is the distal-most component of the fibula. Fractures of either of these structures will cause a significant instability in the tarsus as the collateral ligaments originate from these points. The section on collateral ligament injuries below has more information on how to assess the tarsus for collateral instabilities (Section 17.1.3).

Treatment of choice: Surgical repair is necessary to reestablish stability, and therefore, proper function of the joint. The fragment can be secured back in place with a lag screw, Kirschner wires, or a tension band system. The fragment is often small and therefore difficult to work with. This surgery is best left in the hands of a trained surgeon.

Postoperative management: The surgeon may choose to support the joint with a splint for 3–4 weeks post-operatively. Activity restriction for another 2–4 weeks followed by a gradual return to regular activity is indicated (Chapter 3).

Prognosis: The prognosis with surgery is very good; irritation of the soft tissues by the pins or pin migration can occur and is managed by removing the pins once the bone has healed (approximately 8 weeks).

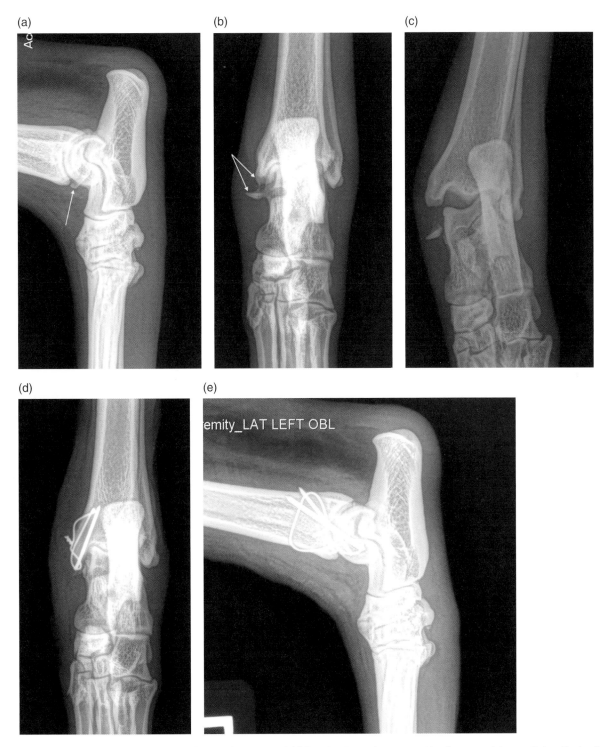

Figure 17.3 Preoperative mediolateral (a) and craniocaudal (b) projections of a tarsus with a fracture of the medial malleolus (arrow). (c) A stress view showing the increased joint space medially associated with the instability caused by the malleolar fracture. Postoperative craniocaudal (d) and mediolateral (e) projections of the repair with a tension band wire system. *Source:* Photos courtesy of the VCA Canada Mississauga Oakville veterinary emergency Hospital and referral group.

Removing these pins is a minor procedure and should not be a deterrent to proceeding with the initial repair.

17.1.3 Medial or Lateral Collateral Ligament Injuries

Collateral ligament injury, whether medial or lateral, will result in an instability to the tarsus. The instability is the same as that for a malleolar fracture (Section 17.1.2) but without an associated fracture. The patient will present with a marked lameness and swelling around the tarsus but no fractures are visible on radiographs.

Diagnosis: Diagnosis is made by palpation and stress radiography (Figure 17.4). To palpate the instability, one hand is placed on the distal tibia, the other on the metatarsals, and the hock is placed in extension. To assess the medial collateral ligament, pressure is applied to the lateral aspect of the joint in order to "crack it open medially." To assess the lateral collateral ligament, pressure is applied to the medial surface of the tarsus in an attempt to "crack the joint open laterally." Both the medial and lateral collateral ligaments have a short and a long branch. Diagnosis can be difficult when only one of the branches is torn because the laxity will not be as obvious [2]. It is useful to compare the degree of laxity to the contralateral tarsus (Figure 17.5).

Treatment of choice: Reconstruction of the torn ligament is the treatment of choice. This can be accomplished by reattaching the avulsed ligament using a screw and spiked washer; suturing the damaged ligament using the locking loop, or continuous cruciate suture pattern if there is sufficient ligamentous material to work with; or by reconstructing the ligament using bone tunnels or bone anchors and prosthetic suture material. The purpose of the prosthetic suture is to stabilize the joint until sufficient strength has been regained through fibrosis of the healing tissues. These surgeries are best left in the hands of the trained surgeon.

Postoperative management: Postoperatively, the limb is placed in a lateral or custom-made splint for approximately 4 weeks followed by a soft padded bandage for 2 weeks and continued restricted activity for a total of 8 weeks. Commercially available braces may also be helpful for these cases. Activity restriction and appropriate patient care, as described in Chapter 3, are indicated.

Prognosis: The prognosis with repair is very good [3]. Potential complications include irritation of the soft tissues by the implants, infection, and loss of range of motion. Without surgery, closed injuries to collateral ligaments rarely have an acceptable outcome for return to an active lifestyle.

17.1.4 Luxations of the Tarsocrural Joint (Figure 17.6)

A tarsocrural luxation implies that there is marked damage to the collateral ligaments (often both medial and lateral). Surgical correction of the problem is necessary for a functional limb.

Treatment of choice: There are several repair options: (1) An open reduction is performed and the damaged ligaments are reconstructed as described in Section 17.1.3. (2) A pantarsal arthrodesis is another option (see Section 17.4 for details). Postoperatively the joint is supported with external coaptation for 6 weeks. (3) An open reduction is performed and a temporary trans-articular pin is inserted from the caudal aspect of the talus into the tibia (Figure 17.6). This technique is best for smaller patients. Care must be taken to position the joint at a functional angle (dogs 130–135°; cats 110–120°).

Postoperative management: With surgical reconstruction of the ligaments, the joint is supported with external coaptation or an external fixator for 6–8 weeks until sufficient fibrosis has occurred. If a temporary trans-articular pin has been placed, the joint is supported with a splinted bandage for 2–4 weeks. The pin can be removed once the healing process is complete (8–10 weeks) and the joint will regain some mobility.

Prognosis: The prognosis for return to function of the limb is good for any of the described techniques. Osteoarthritis will ensue (except with a pancarpal arthrodesis).

17.1.5 Shearing Injuries

These injuries typically occur as a result of automobile accidents. The skin, ligaments, joint capsule, and bone are ground off as the result of the trauma (Figure 17.7). Wound management, including debridement of the exposed joint surface, is the primary concern with this injury.

Treatment of choice: The initial treatment is to manage the wound by debriding the exposed tissues, and stabilizing the joint with a lateral or custom-made splint. Surgical stabilization of the joint is often delayed until the wound bed is clean and showing healthy granulation tissue. The joint can be surgically stabilized by reconstructing the collateral ligaments (as described in Section 17.1.3) or with a pantarsal arthrodesis. The choice may depend on the extent of the injury. Non-surgical management can work well for these cases [4]. The joint is stabilized with external coaptation (or an external fixator or temporary trans-articular pin) while the wound is appropriately managed. The abundance of fibrosis that will be necessary for the wound to close by second intention is often sufficient to stabilize the joint.

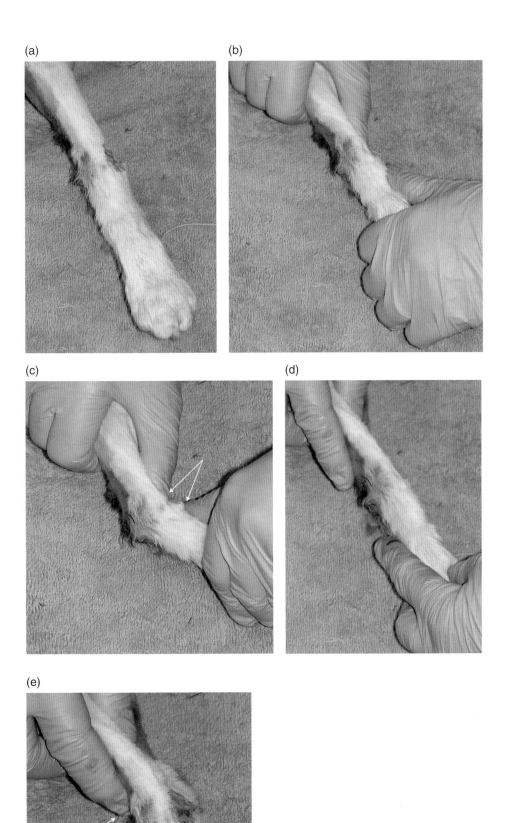

Figure 17.4 A cadaver is used to demonstrate how to assess integrity of the tarsal collateral ligaments. To assess the tarsus for medial instability due to collateral ligament or medial malleolar damage, the patient should be heavily sedated or anesthetized. The tarsus is placed in extension (a). The clinician's hands are placed on either side of the tarsus with the thumbs on the lateral aspect (b). Pressure is applied (arrows c), via the thumbs, to the lateral aspect of the tarsus to "crack" the medial side "open." In subtle cases, it is best to compare the injured side with the contralateral, normal, limb. To test for a lateral instability, pressure is applied to the medial aspect of the tarsus while maintaining it in extension (d and e). Craniocaudal radiographs are taken of the limb in the "normal" and "stressed" position.

(a)　　　　　　　　　(b)　　　　　　　　　(c)

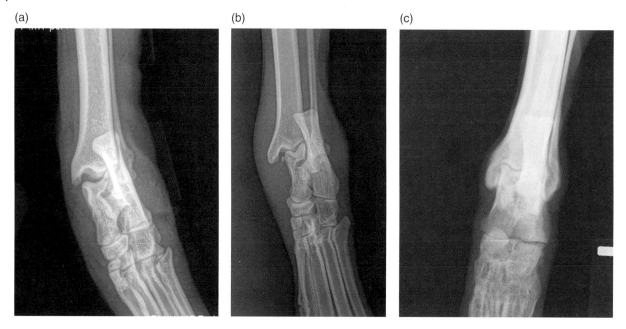

Figure 17.5 Stress views of two patients with medial collateral ligament injuries. (a) This patient has a complete tear of both branches of the medial collateral ligament as evidenced by the greater space in the medial compartment of the tarsocrural joint. (b) This shows a partial tear, there is marked soft tissue swelling but the instability is significantly less than that of patient (a) yet greater than normal (c).

(a)　　　　　　　(b)　　　　　　　(c)　　　　　　　(d)

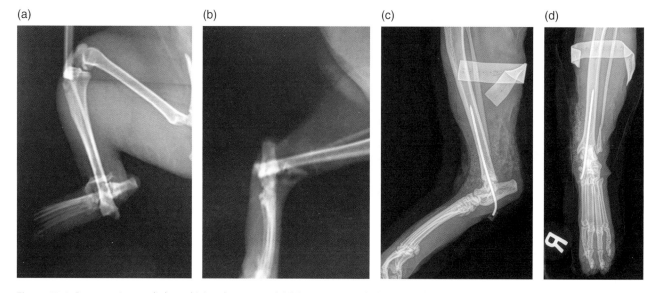

Figure 17.6 Preoperative mediolateral (a) and craniocaudal (b) projections of a luxation of the tarsocrural joint in a cat. The luxation was stabilized with a trans-articular pin (c, d). *Source:* Photos courtesy of the VCA Canada Mississauga Oakville veterinary emergency Hospital and referral group.

Postoperative management: Wound management is the primary focus in these patients. Numerous bandage changes and hospital visits are typically required. The total duration of the healing process can last close to 2 months. Activity restriction and appropriate patient care, as described in Chapter 3, are indicated.

Prognosis: The prognosis for patients with shearing injuries to the tarsus is dependent on the amount of damage that occurs at the time of injury and success in

achieving joint stability; most patients will have a good limb function with treatment [5, 6].

17.1.6 Fractures of the Calcaneus (Figure 17.8)

These fractures can result in severe ambulatory issues because the tendon of the gastrocnemius muscle inserts on this bone. These are common fractures in the *racing greyhound*. The fractures in the racing dog are considered

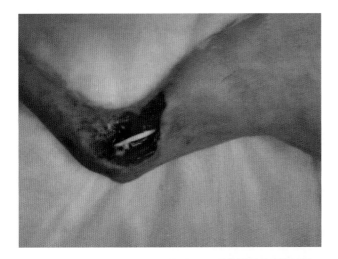

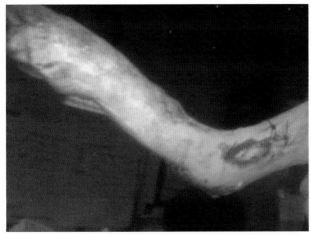

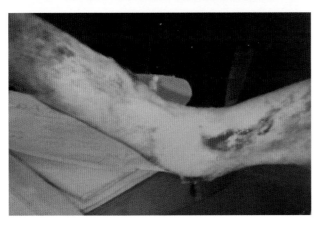

Figure 17.7 Serial pictures of a cat with a shearing injury to the medial aspect of the tarsocrural joint. The joint was stabilized with a trans-articular pin and the wound allowed to heal via second intention. This is the same patient as is depicted in Figure 17.6. *Source:* Photos courtesy of the VCA Canada Mississauga Oakville veterinary emergency Hospital and referral group.

to be stress induced; they have specific patterns and a very good prognosis with surgical repair [7]. In the *non-racing dogs*, these fractures are a result of trauma. They may be articular or extra-articular, and of varying configurations.

Treatment of choice: Surgical repair is necessary to re-establish proper function because the strong distraction forces of the Achilles mechanism on the calcaneus cannot be neutralized with a cast or splint. The repair can be accomplished using a tension band wire system, small plate, or lag screw. Some minimally displaced, extra-articular fractures can be successfully treated conservatively with a lateral or custom-made splint for 6–8 weeks [7].

Postoperative management: A splint, or other more effective immobilization technique (external fixator, internal trans-calcaneal screw), will be applied to the limb for 6–8 weeks postoperatively.

Prognosis: The complication rate with this type of fracture, in the *non-racing dog,* is considered high (52%) and is often associated with a second surgery and poorer outcomes [7]. These patients require close monitoring postoperatively to help minimize complications. Once the fracture is healed, these patients tend to have a good outcome with full use of the limb. These cases are best left in the hands of the experienced surgeon.

17.1.6.1 Injuries of the Achilles Tendon Mechanism

Although not technically an injury of the tarsal joint, this section is included here as the patient will often present with a plantigrade stance giving the impression of a tarsal injury. The Achilles mechanism, also known as the common calcanean tendon, is composed of three tendons: the gastrocnemius, the superficial digital flexor, and the common tendon of insertion of the biceps femoris, semitendinosus, and gracilis muscles. The gastrocnemius tendon is the largest and most powerful. It inserts on the tuber calcaneus. The superficial digital flexor tendon is the most superficial. It crosses over the tuber calcaneus to continue distally and split into each digital branch. It is anchored onto the tuber calcaneus by medial and lateral retinacular insertions.

Lacerations or rupture of the Achilles tendon are not always associated with a skin wound. The patient will have a plantigrade stance and palpation of the area will reveal a lack of a continuous "cordlike" tendon attaching to the tuber calcaneus and often the swollen nodular end of the severed tendon can be palpated.

Treatment of choice: Primary repair is the treatment of choice. The severed ends of the tendon are debrided. The ends are sutured together using a heavy gauge strong suture (PDS™ or Nylon) in a continuous cruciate (Figure 17.9) or locking loop fashion (Figure 17.10). Placing the hock joint in slight extension will help relax the tension at the suture line.

Postoperative management: In acute cases (repaired within hours of the injury) a simple heavy padded bandage for 10–14 days postoperative to decrease

(a)

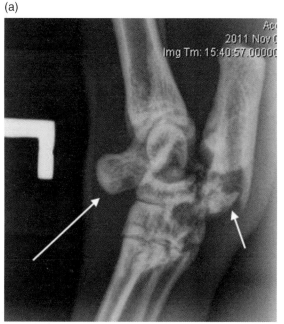

(b)

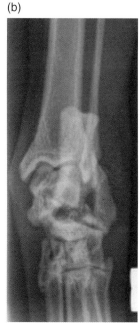

Figure 17.8 Preoperative mediolateral (a) and craniocaudal (b) projections of a traumatic complex articular fracture of the base of the calcaneus (short arrow) as well as a luxation of the base of the talus (long arrow). The injuries were stabilized with pins and a tension band system (c,d). *Source:* Photos courtesy of the VCA Canada Mississauga Oakville veterinary emergency Hospital and referral group.

(c)

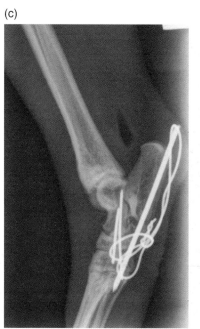

(d)

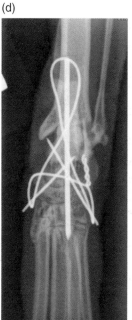

swelling and offer some resistance to range of motion in the hock is indicated, along with significant restriction in activity. If the injury is more chronic, the tension at the suture line will be greater and the hock may need to be held in mild extension for a longer period of time. The motion in the hock joint can be restricted using an external fixator, a splint, or a custom-made brace for 8 weeks postoperatively.

Prognosis: The prognosis is very good to excellent in acute cases. The more chronic ones can be difficult to re-attach and properly immobilize. They are best left in the hands of the trained surgeon.

Avulsion of the gastrocnemius tendon from its attachment on the tuber calcaneus tends to occur in larger dogs. Avulsion can occur as a result of normal activity, allowing for speculation about a potential degenerative process, as seen in humans.

Treatment of choice: Repair is aimed at reattaching the avulsed tendon to the calcaneus bone. This is accomplished by drilling anchor holes into the calcaneus

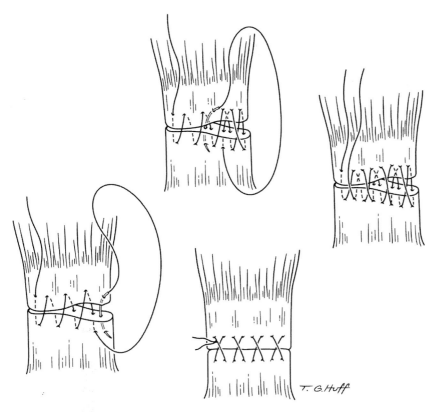

Figure 17.9 An example of the continuous cruciate pattern for suturing tendons. *Source:* From [8].

T. G. Huff

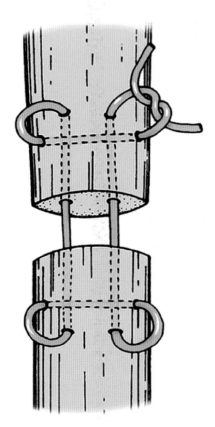

Figure 17.10 An example of the locking loop pattern for suturing tendons. *Source:* [9].

through which the heavy gauge suture material is threaded. The tendon is reattached using one of the suture patterns described above.

Postoperative management: Postoperatively the joint is immobilized with external coaptation or a fixator for 6–8 weeks (Figure 17.11). This surgery is best left in the hands of a trained surgeon.

Prognosis: The prognosis is guarded. Complications include failure of the repair, necessitating a revision, and fracture of the calcaneus.

Luxations of the superficial digital flexor tendon can occur during vigorous activity. This issue has been reported to be most prevalent in the collie breeds [10]. The patient may present with mild to moderate lameness; swelling at the level of the tuber calcaneus may be present and a popping sensation is palpable when the hock is flexed and extended. The tendon tends to luxate medially.

Treatment of choice: Surgical repair is aimed at reconstructing the retinacular attachment of the tendon with a heavy gauge suture material. Although the repair per se is not difficult, it can be challenging to identify the appropriate structures that require suturing.

Postoperative management: The patient is placed in a short lateral or custom splint for 2–4 weeks with activity restriction for a total of 4–6 weeks.

(a)

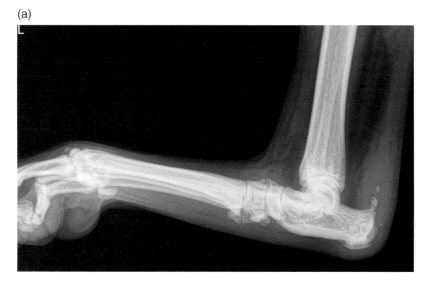

Figure 17.11 Pre- (a) and postoperative (b,c) radiographs of a dog with a chronic avulsion of the gastrocnemius tendon. The repair was protected by immobilizing the tarsus with a ring fixator.

(b) (c)

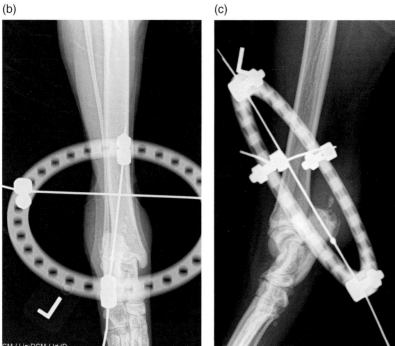

Prognosis: The prognosis is excellent, especially if repaired during the acute phase, rather than in the chronic phase once significant fibrosis has developed.

17.1.7 Fractures/Luxations of the Talus

There are three components to the talus: the trochlear ridges, the neck (which is the junction of the body and the ridges), and the body (Figure 17.1). The trochlear ridges are covered with cartilage and articulate directly with the distal tibia.

17.1.7.1 Fractures of the Trochlear Ridges

These can be very difficult to see on radiographs and often require specific views or a CT scan.

Treatment of choice: Reconstruction of the articular surface can be difficult with a variable prognosis. Therefore, a pantarsal arthrodesis may be the preferred treatment (Section 17.4 has details on pantarsal arthrodesis).

17.1.7.2 Fractures of the Body or Neck

A fracture through the body (lower part) or the neck (upper part) of the talus is uncommon.

Treatment of choice: These fractures are best managed with an open reduction and screw or wire fixation. The neck fractures can be associated with a luxation of the body. Repair of the fracture is often sufficient to maintain the body in reduction.

(a)

(b)

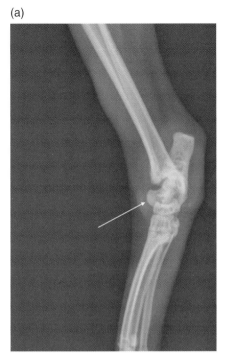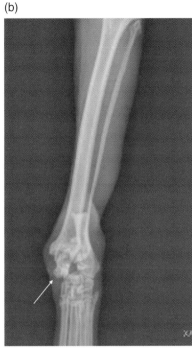

Figure 17.12 Mediolateral (a) and craniocaudal (b) projections of tarsus of a cat with a luxation of the base of the talus (arrow). Unfortunately, the owners declined repair despite the good prognosis and a mid-femoral amputation was performed.

Postoperative management: A splint is applied postoperatively for 4 weeks. In a small dog or cat where there is minimal displacement at the fracture line, conservative management with a splint may be adequate.

Prognosis: The prognosis with repair is very good.

17.1.7.3 Luxation of the Base of the Talus (Figure 17.12)

This is not a common injury. Careful radiographic detail is necessary for diagnosis.

Treatment of choice: The best treatment option is to surgically reduce and stabilize the body of the talus by securing it to the calcaneus with a small screw. Small dogs and cats may have a satisfactory outcome with a closed reduction and splinting [10].

Postoperative management: After surgery, or a closed reduction, the joint is supported with a splint for 4–6 weeks. Activity is restricted for 6–8 weeks followed by a gradual return to regular exercise (Chapter 3).

Prognosis: The prognosis with this repair is excellent.

17.1.8 Fractures/Luxations of the Central Tarsal Bone (Figure 17.13)

These are most commonly seen in the *racing greyhound*. They vary in configuration from simple non-displaced to comminuted fractures [10]. Surgical repair is the best approach for all types in order to return the dog to racing condition. With the exception of comminuted fractures, the prognosis for return to racing is very good. Comminuted fractures carry a poor

prognosis for return to racing but a good outcome *for non-racing activities* [10].

A fracture or fracture/luxation of the central tarsal bone occurs infrequently in the *non-racing dog*.

Treatment of choice: Surgical repair with a positional screw is necessary to re-establish proper function.

Postoperative management: A lateral or custom-made splint is often applied for 4 weeks postoperatively. Activity is restricted for 6–8 weeks followed by a gradual return to regular exercise (Chapter 3).

Prognosis: The prognosis with repair is very good to excellent [12, 13]. A fracture/luxation of the central tarsal bone has been reported to occur during free exercise in border collies [13].

17.1.9 Fractures of the Numbered Tarsal Bones

These fractures are not common. They are more frequently seen in the *racing greyhound* and require surgical repair. More detailed information on this injury in racing greyhounds is available elsewhere [10]. In *non-racing dogs*, the fourth tarsal bone is the one that is typically injured.

Treatment of choice: This fracture is usually not significantly displaced and can be successfully treated with external coaptation [10].

Patient management: The tarsus is immobilized with a lateral or custom-made splint that extends to mid-tibia for 6–8 weeks. Activity is restricted for 6–8 weeks followed by a gradual return to regular exercise (Chapter 3).

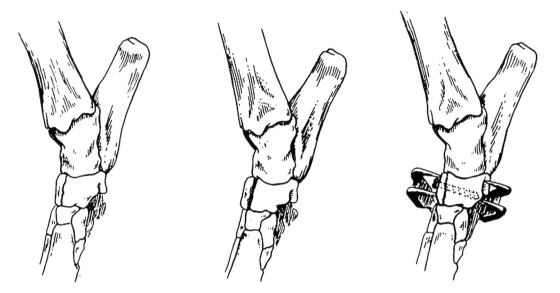

Figure 17.13 An example of a slab fracture with mild displacement of the central tarsal bone. These are uncommon fractures. *Source:* From [17].

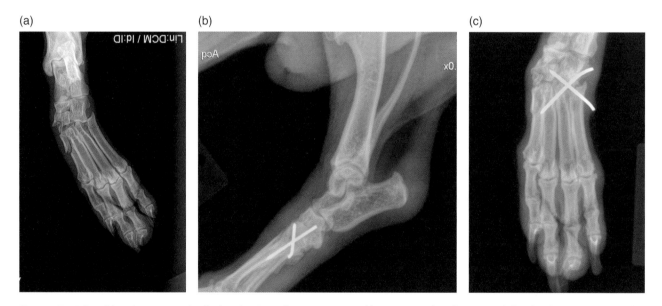

(a)   (b)   (c)

Figure 17.14 Pre- (a) and postoperative (b,c) projections of a tarsometatarsal luxation in a dog that was stabilized with cross pins. *Source:* Photos courtesy of the VCA Canada Mississauga Oakville veterinary emergency Hospital and referral group.

Prognosis: The prognosis for return to function is good although there may be lameness noted after strenuous activity.

17.1.10 Luxation of the Intertarsal and/or Tarsometatarsal Joints (Figure 17.14)

Luxation of the intertarsal and tarsometatarsal joints will result in varying degrees of plantigrade stance and, potentially, medial or lateral instabilities. Injuries in this portion of the hock joint are best treated with partial tarsal arthrodesis (the details are in Section 17.5). The prognosis with surgery is good.

17.2 Managing Expectations with Recommended Treatments

Injuries to the tarsus in general will result in a significant lameness. The prognosis with repair by an experienced surgeon, however, is very good in most cases. Owners should be encouraged to seek the appropriate care.

The financial and time commitments are usually rewarded with a positive outcome. Owners can expect that their pet will have some sort of external coaptation to help immobilize the joint during the healing process. Therefore, regular splint changes or monitoring of the external fixator will be necessary as morbidity (decubital sores) associated with splinting can be significant in this area.

As with any joint injury, OA will develop. The pet can enjoy a good lifestyle with a proper OA management regime (Chapter 3).

Partial tarsal arthrodesis has a good prognosis and low complication rate. The overall function of the tarsus will be only slightly altered. Pantarsal arthrodesis is a much more difficult procedure and the function of the tarsus will be completely altered; having said that, the outcome for the patient is good. Both these surgeries should be performed by a trained surgeon; owners should be encouraged to seek the appropriate care.

17.3 Alternatives When Treatment of Choice is Not an Option

Surgery is definitely the treatment of choice for most injuries to the tarsus. Should surgery not be a possibility, then management with a splint for approximately 8 weeks may be considered however the outcome will likely be less than desirable.

Non-surgical management of *fractures* to the bones of the tarsus will result in varying degrees of ongoing lameness depending on the fracture location, degree of displacement, and the size of the dog. A possible exception to this outcome is fractures of the fourth tarsal bone in non-racing dogs (see Section 17.1.8). Fractures involving an articular surface or resulting in an instability (e.g. malleolar fractures) are likely to result in an ongoing, continuous weight bearing lameness. Articular "chip" fractures can perhaps be treated conservatively by immobilizing with a splint for 6–8 weeks but an intermittent lameness may ensue, especially with exercise. Non-articular fractures without instability that are managed with external coaptation (e.g. fracture of the body of the talus) are likely to show a lameness with activity. The client should be made to understand that the outcome with surgery for many of the tarsal injuries can be very good and encouraged to seek the services of a trained surgeon, especially since the alternatives to surgery are not likely to give the desired outcome.

Non-surgical management of *luxations* located in the tarsus will result in varying degrees of ongoing lameness and/or plantigrade stance, depending on the location of the luxation. The joint can be splinted for 8–10 weeks in the hopes of achieving sufficient fibrosis, but the result will likely be disappointing. A custom-made brace can be used to help the pet ambulate if a repair is not possible, but the dog's ability to exercise freely may be significantly diminished. The brace should be worn at least when the animal goes out for exercise, but for those patients with severe ligamentous damage it should be worn most of the day.

If the surgical treatment of choice is not a possibility for a patient it may be worthwhile trying conservative management before considering amputating the limb.

17.4 About Pantarsal Arthrodesis (Figure 17.15)

The goal of this procedure is to fuse all the joints of the hock so that motion is no longer possible. To achieve this, the articular cartilage of all the bones in the tarsus is removed using a high-speed burr. The joint is then stabilized using an external fixator, a specially constructed plate applied to the lateral or medial aspect of the joint, or an appropriately contoured bone plate placed on the cranial aspect of the joint. The fixation method spans from the distal third of the tibia to the distal third of the metatarsals, approximately. This surgery is best left in the hands of the trained surgeon. If a plating technique is utilized, then the joint is supported with external coaptation (a lateral or custom-made splint) until there is radiographic evidence of bony fusion. If an external fixator is used, then it should remain on until there is bony fusion visible on radiographs (10–12 weeks). The prognosis for return to function of the limb is good [5, 6, 14]. Very active patients need to alter their lifestyle somewhat after an arthrodesis. However, given the complexity of many of the injuries that require a pantarsal arthrodesis, this type of outcome is usually very acceptable to most owners and their pets. OA of the hock joint is no longer a concern in these patients since the joint is now fused. Complication rates can be high and include: necrosis of skin, plate breakage, pin or screw loosening, incomplete fusion, and infection [5, 15].

17.5 About Partial Tarsal Arthrodesis (Figure 17.16)

Most of the motion in the hock stems from the large tarsocrural joint. The intertarsal and tarsometatarsal joints offer only a small amount of movement; however, an instability to these smaller joints will cause a significant lameness. A partial tarsal arthrodesis involves fusing only a portion of the tarsus and leaving the remainder of the tarsal joints intact.

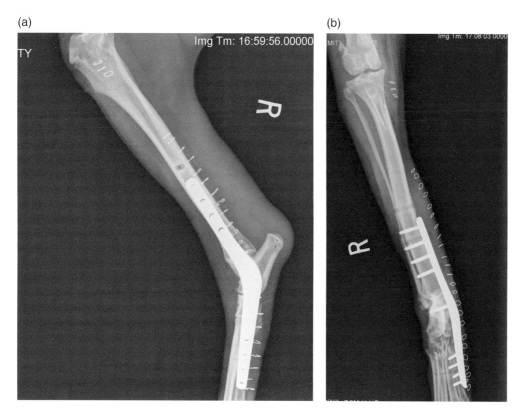

Figure 17.15 Pantarsal arthrodesis performed using a specialized plate that was applied to the lateral side of the limb (a,b). The skin staples over the proximal tibia indicate the location where bone graft was obtained. *Source:* Photos courtesy of Dr. M. Rochat.

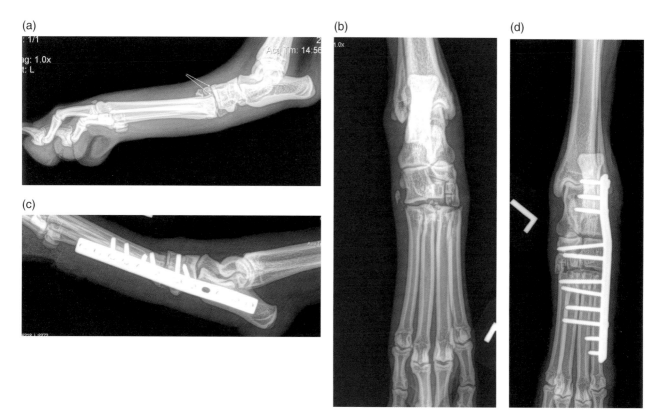

Figure 17.16 Preoperative mediolateral (a) and craniocaudal (b) radiographs of a dog with a tarsometatarsal luxation. The arrows point to the step between the row of numbered tarsal bones and the metatarsal bones. The postoperative mediolateral (c) and craniocaudal (d) views show that the luxation was repaired with a partial arthrodesis using a lateral plate. *Source:* Photos courtesy of the VCA Canada Mississauga Oakville veterinary emergency Hospital and referral group.

Fusion of the tarsocrural joint (tibia–talus) alone is not advised as these patients tend to have a poorer outcome than those with a pantarsal arthrodesis (Section 17.4) [10].

The smaller intertarsal and/or tarsometatarsal joints can be fused while sparing the larger, more mobile tarsocrural joint. The technique involves removing the articular cartilage of the affected joints using a high-speed burr and stabilizing with a plate, external fixator, cross pins, or a tension band system. The prognosis with a partial tarsal arthrodesis is very good to excellent and the complications are much less than with the pantarsal arthrodesis [11, 16–18].

References

1 Evans, H.E. and de Lahunta, A. (2013). *Miller's Anatomy of the Dog*, 4e. St Louis, MO: Saunders/Elsevier.

2 Aron, D.N. and Purinton, P.T. (1985). Collateral ligaments of the tarsocrural joint. An anatomic and functional study. *Vet. Surg.* 14: 173–177.

3 Fox, S.M., Guerin, S.R., Burbidge, H.M., and Lindsay, R.G. (1997). Reconstruction of the medial collateral ligament for tarsocrural luxation in the dog: a preliminary study. *J. Am. Anim. Hosp. Assoc.* 33: 268–274.

4 Beardsley, S.L. and Schrader, S.C. (1995). Treatment of dogs with wounds on the limbs caused be shearing forces: 98 cases (1975–1993). *J. Am. Vet. Med. Assoc.* 207: 1071–1075.

5 Benson, J.A. and Boudrieau, R.J. (2002). Severe carpal and tarsal shearing injuries treated with an immediate arthrodesis in seven dogs. *J. Am. Anim. Hosp. Assoc.* 38: 370–380.

6 Diamond, D.W., Besso, J., and Boudrieau, R.J. (1999). Evaluation of joint stabilization for treatment of shearing injuries of the tarsus in 20 dogs. *J. Am. Anim. Hosp. Assoc.* 35: 147–153.

7 Perry, K.L., Adams, R.J., Woods, S., and Bruce, M. (2017). Calcaneal fractures in non-racing dogs and cats: complications, outcome, and associated risk factors. *Vet. Surg.* 46: 39–51.

8 DeCamp, C.E., Johnston, S.A., Déjardin, L.M., and Schaefer, S.L. (2016). *Brinker, Piermattei and Flo's Handbook of Small Animal Orthopedics and Fracture Repair*, 5e. St Louis, MO: Elsevier.

9 Tobias, K.M. and Johnston, S.A. (2012). *Veterinary Surgery Small Animal*. St Louis, MO: Elsevier/Saunders.

10 DeCamp, C.E., Johnston, S.A., Déjardin, L.M., and Schaefer, S.L. (2016). Fractures and other orthopedic injuries of the tarsus, metatarsus and phalanges. In: *Brinker, Piermattei and Flo's Handbook of Small Animal Orthopaedics and Fracture Repair*, 5e, 707–785. St Louis, MO: Elsevier.

11 Fettig, A.A., McCarthy, R.J., and Kowaleski, M.P. (2002). Intertarsal and tarsometatarsal arthrodesis using 2.0/2.7-mm or 3.7–3.5-mm hybrid dynamic compression plates. *J. Am. Anim. Hosp. Assoc.* 38: 364–369.

12 Cinti, F., Pisani, G., Penazzi, C. et al. (2016). Central tarsal bone fracture in a cat. *Vet. Comp. Orthop. Traumatol.* 29: 170–173.

13 Guillard, M. (2007). Central tarsal bone fracture in the border collie. *J. Sm. Anim. Pract.* 48: 414–417.

14 Fitzpatrick, N. and Farrell, S.D. (2013). Feline pantarsal arthrodesis using precontoured dorsal plates applied according to the principles of percutaneous plate arthrodesis. *Vet. Comp. Orthop. Traumatol.* 26: 399–407.

15 Roch, S.P., Clements, D.N., Mitchell, R.A. et al. (2008). Complications following tarsal arthrodesis using bone plate fixation in dogs. *J. Sm. Anim. Pract.* 49: 117–126.

16 Scrimgeour, A.B., Bruce, W.J., Bridges, J.P. et al. (2012). Long-term outcomes after partial tarsal arthrodesis in working farm dogs in New Zealand. *N. Z. Vet. J.* 60: 50–55.

17 Dyce, J., Whitelock, R.G., Robinson, K.V. et al. (1998). Arthrodesis of the tarsometatarsal joint using a laterally applied plate in 10 dogs. *J. Sm. Anim. Pract.* 39: 19–22.

18 Allen, M.J., Dyce, J., and Houlton, J.E.F. (1993). Calcaneoquartal arthrodesis in the dog. *J. Sm. Anim. Pract.* 34: 205–210.

18

Paw (Manus and Pes)

Anne M. Sylvestre

Focus and Flourish, Cambridge, Ontario, Canada

Fractures of the metacarpals (MC), metatarsals (MT), and phalanges as seen in the pet population are discussed in this chapter. Racing greyhounds are prone to injuries of this region. Treatment of greyhound fractures, if the intent is for return to racing, is best left in the hands of the trained surgeon, and will not be discussed further here.

Fractures of the manus (forepaw) or pes (hind paw) can often occur as a result of a low-velocity trauma (stepped on by a person, wrapped in a leash). Fortunately in these cases the associated soft tissue trauma is often minimal. When there has been considerably more trauma such as caused by a vehicular or roadside accident, then there may be substantial damage to the skin, which may affect the decision making process.

The bones of the paw are mostly dependent on the endosteal blood supply. The periosteal blood supply is not as extensive in these bones as compared with the more proximal, larger bones. This poorer blood supply translates into *slower healing times* and *increased complications* with surgery. The first digit (dewclaw) may or may not be present in dogs. The third and fourth digits are the main weight bearing bones of the paw.

18.1 Fractures and Luxations

18.1.1 MC/MT Fractures

The MC and MT bones are composed of the base (proximal end), the shaft, and the head (distal end). The MC/MT articulate proximally with the numbered bones of the carpus/tarsus, respectively, and distally with the first phalanx of each digit.

18.1.1.1 One, or More, MC/MT Remain(s) Intact (Figure 18.1)

When one or some of the MC/MT remain(s) intact then it (they) can act as an internal splint, creating a good situation for external coaptation.

Treatment of choice: A commercial metasplint or "spoon splint" can be used or one can be custom-made using moldable fiberglass material. The entire paw must comfortably fit within the splint.

For fractures of the *forepaw* the splint should be on the palmar surface of the bandaged paw and it should not be too wide or too tight. The splint should extend just proximal to the carpus. Consideration should be given to placing a donut over the accessory carpal bone and carpal pad to prevent the formation of wounds over these protuberances.

For fractures of the *hind paw* the splint should be placed on the plantar aspect of the bandaged foot and it should comfortably cradle the entire paw. The splinted bandage should extend to the proximal aspect of the calcaneus bone, but does not need to incorporate the tarsocrural joint.

Patient management: Follow-up radiographs should be taken every 4 weeks and the splint can be replaced by a soft padded bandage for 1–2 weeks once bony callus formation is evident on radiographs. Healing times can be as long as 10–12 weeks. Proper splint care is imperative (Chapter 4 has more detail on this topic).

Prognosis: These patients have an excellent prognosis for full return to activity. The biggest challenges with managing these fractures are preventing and/or addressing splint-induced problems.

Fracture Management for the Small Animal Practitioner, First Edition. Edited by Anne M. Sylvestre.
© 2019 John Wiley & Sons, Inc. Published 2019 by John Wiley & Sons, Inc.

(a)

(b)

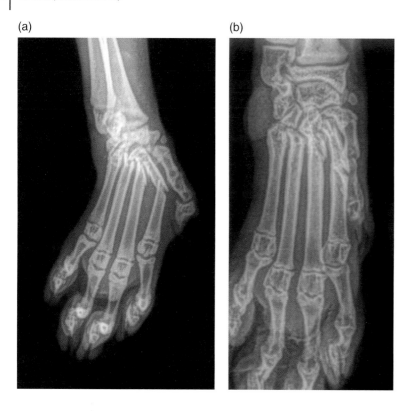

Figure 18.1 Dorsopalmar projections of fractures of the shaft of the second and the base third metacarpal in a cat treated conservatively. Acute (a) and 8 weeks later (b).

18.1.1.2 Fractures of all four MC/MT (Figure 18.2)

When all four MC/MT are fractured, there is no inherent stability to the paw.

Treatment of choice: External coaptation with a splint as described in the previous section is a good treatment option. Surgical repair is also a good treatment choice. Placing an intra-medullary Kirschner wire within the MC/MT is the recommended internal fixation technique [1]; mini bone plates can be used on the large to giant breed dogs. The goal of surgery is to stabilize the paw as a whole rather than each individual bone. Therefore a minimum of two of the MC/MT should be repaired but there is no need to repair all four. It is preferable to repair the third and fourth MC/MT as they are the major weight bearing bones. However, the location and configuration of the fractures often dictate which bones will be repaired. It is best to repair the bones with the fracture configuration/location that are easiest to stabilize (mid-shaft, two pieces) and therefore offer the best chance of success. Surgical repair of the MC/MT fractures can be difficult and have many complications; it is best left in the hands of a trained surgeon. External coaptation is often necessary after internal fixation of the bones of the paw as the small implants may break before the bones can heal.

Patient management: The patient is placed in a splint for approximately 6–8 weeks following surgery

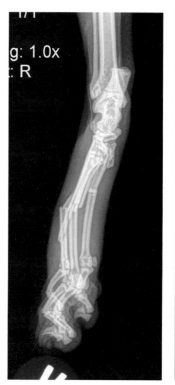
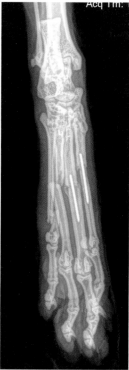

Figure 18.2 Pre- and 6 weeks postoperative views of the pes of a cat with all four metatarsals fractured. Two of the four fractures were stabilized with an intra-medullary pin. Bony calluses are evident on the pinned metatarsals.

before being placed in a soft padded bandage for 1–2 weeks. Follow-up radiographs should be taken every 4 weeks to assess healing. If external coaptation is the only treatment method used, then the splint can be replaced by a soft padded bandage for 1–2 weeks once bony callus formation is evident on radiographs. Healing times can be as long as 12–16 weeks. Proper splint care is imperative (Chapter 4 has more detail on this topic). Implants may need to be removed if they are irritating the surrounding tissues. One report indicated that 25% of patients required a second surgery to remove the implants [2].

Prognosis: Overall, the prognosis for MC/MT fractures of the paw is very good. Studies have found that there is no significant difference in the outcomes between surgically vs conservatively managed patients [2, 3]. The majority of patients have an excellent outcome (no lameness) while those without an excellent outcome were found to have minor gait abnormalities or discomfort. Healing times with surgery were considerably longer than with conservative management. Some surgeons strongly recommend surgical repair when all four MC/MT are fractured, stating a high incidence of non-union and malunion without surgery. However,

surgery does have a high complication rate and prolonged healing times [2, 3].

18.1.1.3 Fractures of the Base of the MC/MT (Proximal End) (Figure 18.3)

These typically involve the second or fifth MC/MT bones. An instability of the carpo-metacarpal or tarso-metatarsal joint may be present as collateral ligaments attach at these sites.

Treatment of choice: Surgical repair with a tension band wire mechanism is recommended. These fractures can also be managed conservatively with a palmar/plantar splint.

Postoperative management: The patient is placed in a palmar/plantar splint postoperatively, for 4–6 weeks, followed by a soft padded bandage for 1–2 weeks. If external coaptation is the only treatment method, then follow-up radiographs should be taken every 4 weeks and the splint can be replaced by a soft padded bandage for 1–2 weeks once bony callus formation is evident on radiographs. Proper splint care is imperative (Chapter 4 has more detail on this topic).

Prognosis: The outcomes with surgical repair is excellent; with a splint alone, a slight varus or valgus angulation may ensue.

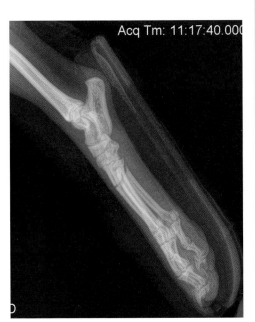
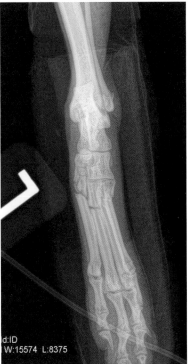

Figure 18.3 Mediolateral and craniocaudal projections of the hind paw of a dog with fractures of the proximal metatarsals. There was no significant instability at the tarso-metatarsal joint. This patient was treated with external coaptation.

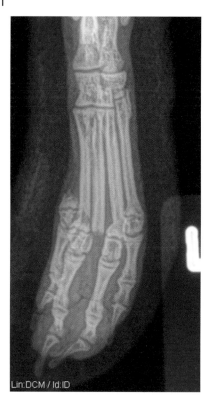

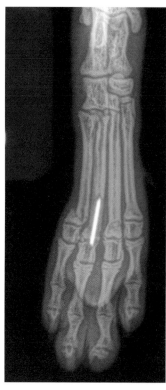

Lin:DCM / Id:ID

Figure 18.4 Dorsoplantar view of very distal metatarsal fractures of the pes. Only the fourth metatarsal was repaired as it had a larger distal fragment to work with; the repair served to help realign the digits. The second metatarsal was intact acting as a second stabilizer.

18.1.1.4 Fractures of the Head of the MC/MT (Distal End) (Figure 18.4)

These may result in an instability of the joint because the collateral ligaments of the MC/MT-phalangeal joint originates from this part of the bone.

Treatment of choice: Surgery to restore stability to the joint may be the better option. This surgery can be quite challenging because of the small size of the fragments. It is best left in the hands of a trained surgeon.
Amputation of the digit through the affected MC/MT is an alternative treatment choice if only one digit is affected.
Postoperative management: The patient is placed in a palmar/plantar splint postoperatively, until the fracture has healed. Proper splint care is imperative (Chapter 4 has more detail on this topic).
Prognosis: Most patients will have a good outcome; however, a mild to moderate lameness after exercise can occur as osteoarthritis can develop in the adjacent joint.

18.1.2 Phalangeal Fractures (Figure 18.5)

These are not common fractures. They can occur as a result of a low-velocity trauma such as getting entangled in a leash or caught in a fence.

Treatment of choice: These are typically managed with external coaptation consisting of a short palmar or

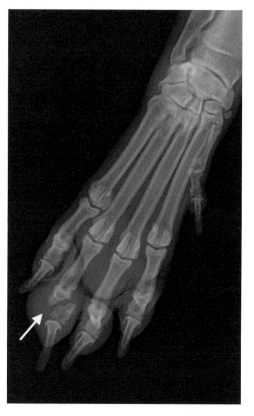

Figure 18.5 Dorsoplantar view of a bulldog presented to the humane society with a fractured second phalanx of a fourth digit (arrow). The fracture was treated conservatively and the lameness resolved.

plantar splint that encases the toes. They can also be surgically repaired with an intra-medullary Kirschner wire but their small size makes the procedure very difficult. Amputation of the digit with the fractured bone is also a good option when only one digit is involved, especially if it's the second or fifth digit. Removal of the digit is simpler than internal fixation and less fraught with complications.

Patient management: If the fracture is treated with external coaptation alone, the splint should be replaced by a soft padded bandage for 1–2 weeks once a bony or fibrous union develops. Proper splint care is imperative (Chapter 4 has more detail on this topic). Healing of a phalangeal fracture in an adult dog can take approximately 8–10 weeks. However, a bony callus does not always develop, leaving only a fibrous union between the fragments. The digit should not be painful on palpation and the patient should be able to ambulate comfortably.

Prognosis: The prognosis for return to function with a phalangeal fracture managed conservatively is very good.

18.1.3 Luxations of the Inter-Phalangeal or MC/MT-Phalangeal Joints

These are not very common in cats or pet dogs.

Treatment of choice: These luxations can be managed conservatively with a short palmar or plantar splint that incorporates the paw. Surgical reconstruction is difficult because of the small size of the bones but may be a better choice for the competing athlete. Amputation of the digit is also a viable treatment choice.

Patient management: Proper splint care is imperative (Chapter 4 has more detail on this topic). The paw should be splinted until sufficient fibrosis develops to ankylose the joint. This may take between 6 and 8 weeks. Once ankylosed, the digit should not be painful on palpation.

Prognosis: The outcome is likely to be acceptable in the non-athletic patient. A very active dog may show a lameness with rigorous activity because of the osteoarthritis. Osteoarthritis will develop.

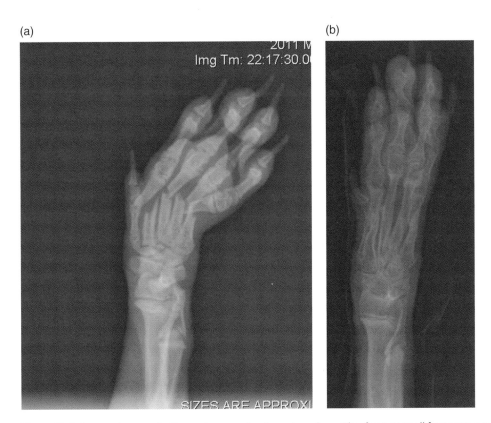

(a)

(b)

2011 M
Img Tm: 22:17:30.0

SIZES ARE APPROXI

Figure 18.6 Dorsopalmar projections of manus of an immature dog with a fracture to all four metacarpals that were treated conservatively. Acute (a) and 4 weeks later (b).

18.2 Managing Expectation with Recommended Treatments

Overall outcomes with fractures of the digits are very good but the management of these injuries can sometimes be frustrating. Longer healing time for fractures of the paw can be expected (8–12 weeks rather than 6–8 weeks) as these bones have a poorer blood supply. The potential issues with prolonged splinting and the frequent bandage changes necessary can be a source of frustration for the owners, the patient, and the medical team. Surgery does not preclude the need for a splint and it can also slow down the healing process. Owners may require some encouragement and positive reinforcement throughout this process.

18.3 Alternatives When Treatment of Choice is Not an Option

External coaptation is a good choice for managing fractures of the paw, even when all four MC/MT bones are affected. Immature patients will heal more quickly (Figure 18.6). If a single digit is affected, then an amputation of that digit is a reasonable treatment option if splint care is an issue.

References

1 Degasperi, B., Gradner, G., and Dupre, G. (2007). Intramedullary pinning of metacarpal and metatarsal fractures in cats using a simple distraction technique. *Vet. Surg.* 36: 382–388.

2 Kapatkin, A., Howe-Smith, R., and Shofer, F. (2000). Conservative versus surgical treatment of metacarpal and metatarsal fractures in dogs. *Vet. Comp. Orthop. Traumatol.* 13: 123–127.

3 Kornmayer, M., Failing, K., and Matis, U. (2014). Long-term prognosis of metacarpal and metatarsal fractures in dogs. A retrospective analysis of medical histories in 100 re-evaluated patients. *Vet. Comp. Orthop. Traumatol.* 27: 45–53.

Section 4

Fracture Repair Techniques

19

Essential Information on Fracture Repair
Anne M. Sylvestre

Focus and Flourish, Cambridge, Ontario, Canada

A veterinary student is taught the principles of fracture management in school but does not graduate with the skills to surgically repair a fracture. Fracture repair requires postgraduate training. There are a multitude of practical workshops available to learn the basic skills necessary. One cannot adequately learn how to repair a bone by reading a book, no matter how detailed the information may be: one learns how to repair a fracture by experiencing it. The reader is encouraged to attend at least one workshop [1, 2, 3] (preferably several) where cadavers are used for practice, and/or to work with a seasoned veterinarian with surgical skills before attempting to do one of these procedures on his or her own. The information on surgical repair of fractures in this book is basic: it is meant to help focus the reader on some of the key technical points, to refresh one's memory, and hopefully help a less experienced surgeon successfully accomplish the task of repairing a bone while minimizing stress. The simple, basic goal of fracture fixation is to place and maintain the bone in an anatomical and stable manner so that it can heal. Anatomical reduction does not equate "perfect" reduction: it means to keep the bone reasonably aligned in every plane (frontal, sagittal, and rotational).

There are three main ways to stabilize a diaphyseal fracture, each requiring a different set of skills and instrumentation.

1) Intramedullary (IM) fixation, where the implant is placed within the IM canal. IM pins, rods, and nails are examples of this type of fixation.
2) Bone plating, where the bone is stabilized by attaching a rigid plate across the fracture line using screws. There are a variety of plating techniques, the most common being the technique where the plate is screwed directly onto the reconstructed bone—a variety of plate types are used to accomplish this. The locking plate technique is where the screws are locked into the plate before being placed into the bone,

allowing for a much more rigid repair. Elastic osteosynthesis is ideal in the young patient; the plate is secured to the distal and proximal ends of the bone with screws, but not along the fractured portion of the diaphysis, allowing for a less rigid fixation and more dynamic repair at the fracture site. Plates can also be placed using minimally invasive methods.
3) External fixation is where the fracture is stabilized by implants that are mostly external to the skin. External fixators have evolved tremendously over the years. They can be linear, circular, hinged, or hybrids.

Physeal fractures are also common. Unfortunately, these fractures are very difficult to recreate in a workshop setting for teaching purposes; therefore, the best way to learn how to repair these is by working with a seasoned surgeon. The same is true for articular fractures.

Each category of repair has its advantages, disadvantages, and ideal applications. A board-certified surgeon is well versed in a variety of techniques and can pick the most appropriate one for a particular patient. It may not be practical for a general practitioner to be well versed in all the different fracture fixation methods but in order to be able to repair a wide variety of fractures, one should learn how to use pins and cerclage wires as well as one other technique (plating or external fixators). It is best to learn how to use *one* system (e.g. standard plating system or linear external fixators) and to become proficient at that system by taking more courses on that same topic rather than trying to learn several systems, and becoming proficient in none. Taking courses and becoming equipped in several different systems (e.g. standard plating systems, locking plating systems, specialty plating systems) will result in the accumulation of inventory but not in the improvement of skills.

The most common fracture seen in an urban setting is the radius ulna distal third fracture of toy breed dogs. These fractures are best repaired with a plate. In a rural practice, higher velocity traumas resulting in more

Fracture Management for the Small Animal Practitioner, First Edition. Edited by Anne M. Sylvestre.
© 2019 John Wiley & Sons, Inc. Published 2019 by John Wiley & Sons, Inc.

complex femoral and tibial fractures may be more common. Repairs with pins and plates or external fixators are indicated. General practitioners should opt to take courses on repair techniques based on their demographics.

19.1 Forces Applied to a Bone

In order to repair a fractured bone, one must understand the forces applied to the bone and how the various repair methods can counteract those forces. This understanding is what allows a surgeon to select the appropriate repair method. The terms "forces" and "stresses" are often used interchangeably, although they have different meanings. Forces are applied to the bone, whereas stresses occur within the bone structure. Suffice it to say that when the forces applied to the bone exceed the strength of the bone, and therefore the stress that the bone structure can handle, a fracture will occur. The goal when stabilizing a fracture is to select a repair method that will adequately counteract the forces that are now affecting the fracture line(s). The forces to consider are: compression, tension, torsional, shear, and bending (Figure 19.1).

- Compression forces occur as a result of a load applied parallel to the long axis of the bone (therefore sometimes called an axial load).

- Tension, or distractive, forces occur when two forces pull on an area in opposite directions. For example, the pull of the quadriceps muscle group, via the patellar tendon, on the tibial tuberosity; this distractive force can result in an avulsion fracture.
- Torsional, also known as rotational, forces cause the bone to twist along its long axis resulting in a rotational deformation and ultimately displacement of the fragments.
- Bending occurs as a result of axial forces that are eccentrically loaded on a bone (such as the femur). The net effect is compression of the loaded side of the bone and tension on the opposite side.
- Shear stress results from two forces acting parallel to one in another but in opposite directions, causing the two fragments to slide along one another.

19.2 Techniques for Reducing a Fracture

When a bone breaks, the contractile force of the muscle will cause the ends to override. Ensuring that the muscles are relaxed and/or stretched can greatly assist the surgeon in reducing the fracture. Hanging the limb under general anesthesia while the patient is being prepared for

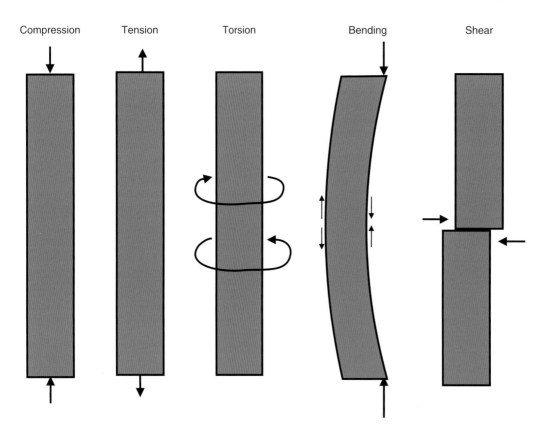

Figure 19.1 The diagrams depict the forces acting upon a bone. See text for details.

surgery is helpful, as well as having a very good analgesia regime on board.

Reducing a fracture can be the hardest part of the surgery. There is no single move or maneuver that will reduce all fractures, easily and quickly. Manipulations of the fragments, patience, and trying out some of the techniques below will get the job done: holding the fragments in a distracted position while the muscles relax a bit more, then attempting again to reduce. Each time the muscles are held under a bit more tension will help to allow the fragments to come closer to being reduced. The key is to have patience and to allow the muscles to relax. Therefore, repetition of the maneuvers is as important as doing the maneuver itself.

19.2.1 Distraction

The (main) fragments are grasped with an instrument and gently but forcibly distracted until the ends are apposable.

Kern bone holding forceps work well here for grasping the bone fragments in medium to large dogs. Thumb forceps often suffice on the very small bones (Figure 19.2).

19.2.2 Lever

A periosteal elevator is positioned between the fragments. A gentle distractive force is applied by using the instrument to lever the pieces apart and then allowing them to fall back into place (Figure 19.3).

19.2.3 Toggle

The fractured edges are toggled together and then digital pressure is slowly and gently applied to push them back down into place. Several attempts may be necessary to allow the muscle to sufficiently relax to allow the fracture to become safely reduced. This maneuver is especially useful with a transverse fracture (Figure 19.4).

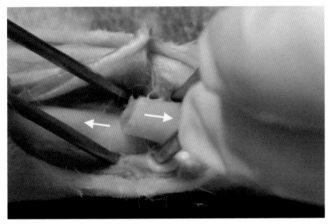
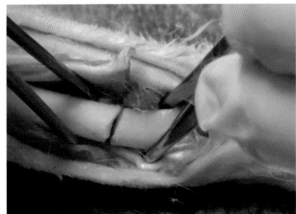

Figure 19.2 A fracture can be reduced by distracting the two main fragments until the muscles have relaxed enough so that the pieces can be apposed.

(a)

(b)

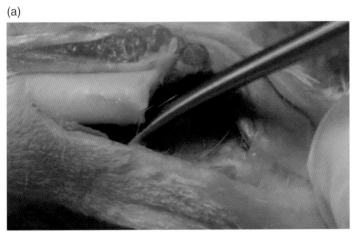
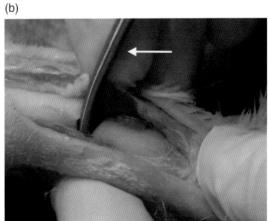

Figure 19.3 In this cadaver demonstration of levering a fracture into reduction, a periosteal elevator is positioned between the fragments (a). Pressure is applied onto the elevator in the direction of the arrow to ease the fragments into reduction (b).

(a)

(b)

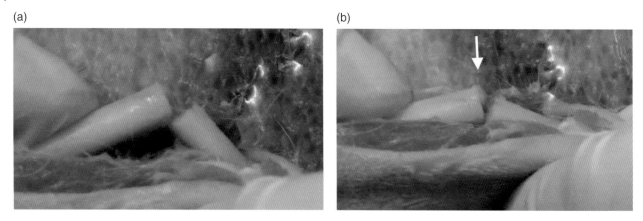

Figure 19.4 In this cadaver demonstration of the toggle technique for reducing a fracture, the fragments are positioned so that their far cortices are apposed (a). Pressure is applied onto the fragment ends (arrow) in order to ease the fragments into reduction (b).

(a)

(b)

(c)

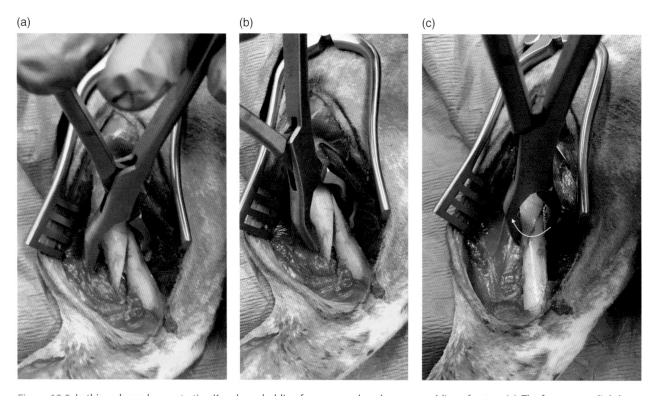

Figure 19.5 In this cadaver demonstration Kern bone holding forceps are placed across an oblique fracture (a). The forceps are slightly angled to align with the fragment edges (b), and then gently closed while being slightly rotated to cause the fragment ends to further distract (c).

19.2.4 Oblique Fractures

Bone holding forceps can be used to align an oblique fracture (easiest if it is a long oblique) into reduction. The distraction technique is used to roughly align the fracture but the musculature will tend to keep the edges overriding. Bone holding forceps (Kerns) are held across the fracture line so that the jaws are slightly angled to roughly align with the fragment edges. The forceps are gently closed (by digital pressure, not with the locking mechanism) while being slightly rotated in the direction that causes the fracture ends to further distract. The fracture configuration and the applied pressures will cause the overriding ends to slide back into place (Figure 19.5).

(a)

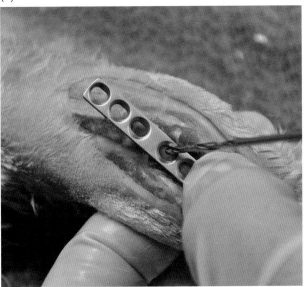

(b)

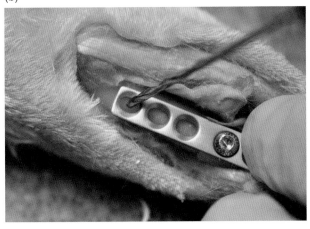

Figure 19.6 In this cadaver demonstration, the plate is secured to the distal fragment with one screw, while the fracture is not reduced (a). The plate can be used to help toggle, align, and hold the fracture in reduction (b).

19.2.5 Using the Plate

A plate is secured on one of the fragments (usually the smaller one) and is used to help lever, position, and hold the fracture reduced. This method is especially useful with a short oblique fracture in the distal radius (Figure 19.6).

19.3 Instrumentation

19.3.1 Drills

There are a variety of types of drill that will work well for orthopedic surgery. The key is to have a drill that has

sufficient power and can be used in a sterile manner (Figure 19.7).

19.3.1.1 Orthopedic Drills

Orthopedic drills can be pneumatic, electric, or battery-powered. The battery-operated ones are probably the easiest to work with because there is no need to have compressed air or nitrogen tanks or an electrical connection. The drills are autoclavable and the batteries have a long duration when fully charged. Various attachments are usually available to make this instrument more versatile. They are typically lightweight with ergonomic designs so they are comfortable and will not tire the surgeon's hand during long procedures. These drills will cost between $15 000 and $30 000 depending on the brand and number of attachments. These drills are well worth their price tag in a high-volume referral practice and often the pneumatic (compressed air version) is preferred because of its even lighter weight. Some of the popular brands are: Synthes™, Aesculap™, and Stryker™. Everost™ has a less ergonomic autoclavable battery-powered drill available. It can be purchased with a choice of attachments and the battery has a long duration. It is a heavier drill but with a leaner price tag ($5000–$7000) [4]. The author refers to it as the Mercedes ML350 as it is big and bulky but very smooth and reliable.

19.3.1.2 Hardware Store Battery-Powered Drills

Hardware store battery-powered drills can be used in orthopedics but must somehow be made sterile. The key factors to consider when purchasing a hardware store battery-powered drill are: weight, wobble, and voltage. Selecting a high-quality drill tends to help keep the wobble to a minimum. The drill must be greater than 10 V in order to have enough power to drill through some of the harder cortical bones. However, higher voltage means a heavier (and more awkward) drill. The 12 V drill tends to be powerful enough yet the battery is still compact and lightweight. These drills *cannot* be autoclaved but can be made sterile in the following ways:

i) Sterilizing with ethylene oxide (EO) gas is possible. Some small animal practices do have gas sterilizers. The battery should *not* be sterilized but it can easily be shrouded with a sterile surgical glove and/or cohesive bandage material (Vet Wrap).

ii) Arbutus™ is a Canadian company that has created a sterilizable chuck and shroud that can be attached to a hardware store battery-powered driver. A driver is slightly different than a drill; its normal use is with quick coupling drill bits and screwdriver attachments. Arbutus Medical™ recommends the DeWalt 12 V driver. Although the chuck and shroud could be used with a regular hardware drill, the friction

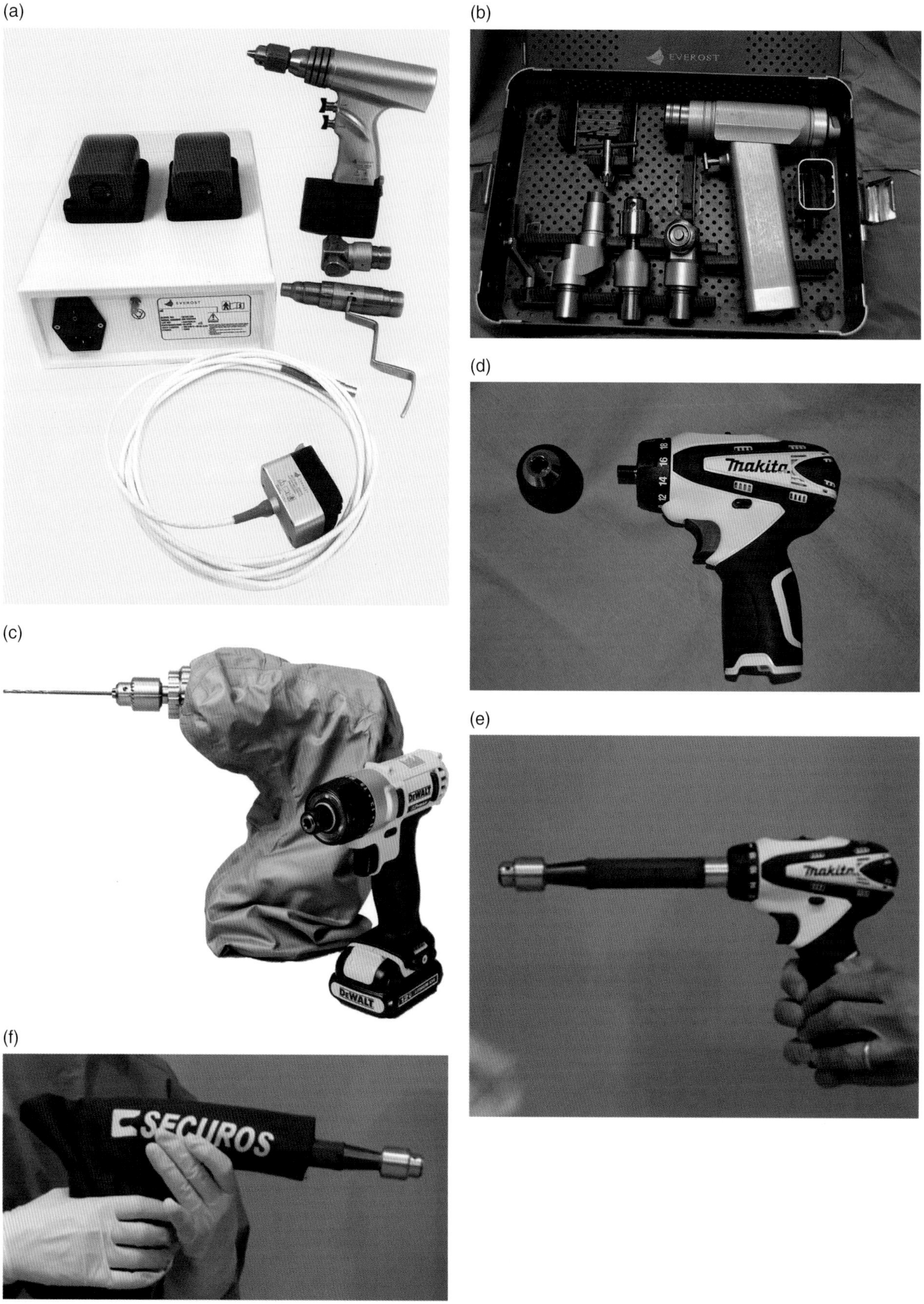

(a)

(b)

(d)

(c)

(e)

(f)

Figure 19.7 Various types of drills that can be used in surgery. An autoclavable, lightweight, compact, high-end, battery-powered drill (a). An Everost autoclavable battery-powered drill that is heavier and much less compact than that of a (b). Autoclavable commercially available (Arbutus medical) secure chuck and shroud that are used with a common battery-powered driver. (c) A common battery-powered drill that is adapted to fit a surgical chuck and fitted shroud. The chuck portion of the drill is removed (d) and a surgical chuck is sterilely attached in its place (e) and then the drill can be covered with a sterile shroud (f). A video demonstration on how to sterilely shroud the drill is available at www.focusandflourish.com.

between the drill chuck and the shroud will rapidly cause the shroud to deteriorate. More information on this drill attachment can be obtained from the Arbutus website [5].

iii) A shroud and regular Jacobs chuck can be used with a hardware store battery-powered drill. The chuck component of the drill needs to be removed so that a sterile Jacob's chuck can be attached in its place. For a video on how to sterilely use a Jacobs chuck and hardware drill combination, visit www.focusandflourish.com.

19.3.2 Fracture Repair General Instruments

The general fracture repair instruments necessary will vary slightly based on the size of the patient and implants being used.

- Periosteal elevators come in various shapes and sizes. The Freer elevator (Figure 19.8) is popular, inexpensive, and readily available. It may be a bit too small for some of the larger patients, in which case a more robust elevator may be preferred.
- Bone holding forceps (Figure 19.9) come in a variety of styles and sizes. There is not one single type of bone holding forceps that will function in every circumstance and all are too heavy for the very small patient. It is best if they are self-retaining, such as ratchet or speed-lock types. The 5.5″ size is versatile so a good

starting place when getting equipped. Larger sizes will be necessary for the large breeds of dogs.

- Retractors are useful when dealing with most fractures. Gelpi and Weitlaners (Figure 19.10) are popular self-retaining retractors. The 5.5″ size is versatile so a good starting place when getting equipped. Larger sizes will be necessary for the large breeds of dogs.
- Suction, although very helpful, is not necessary in the small patients where sponges will suffice. Suction is particularly useful with joint fractures and fractures of bones that are surrounded with heavy musculature such as the humerus, femur, and pelvis.

(a)

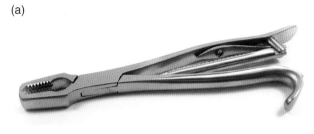

(b)

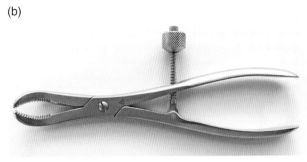

(c)

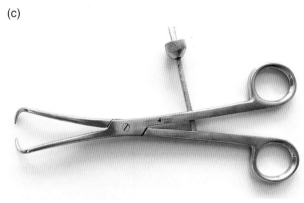

Figure 19.9 Commonly used bone holding forceps: Kern (a); clamshell style forceps with speed-lock mechanism (b), and point-to-point forceps (c).

(a)

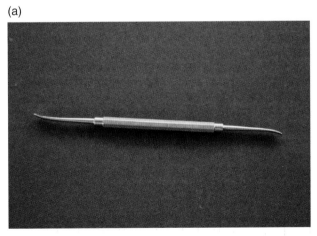

(b)

Figure 19.8 Periosteal elevators: Freer (a) and a larger wooden-handled Synthes/AO elevator (b).

(a)

(b)

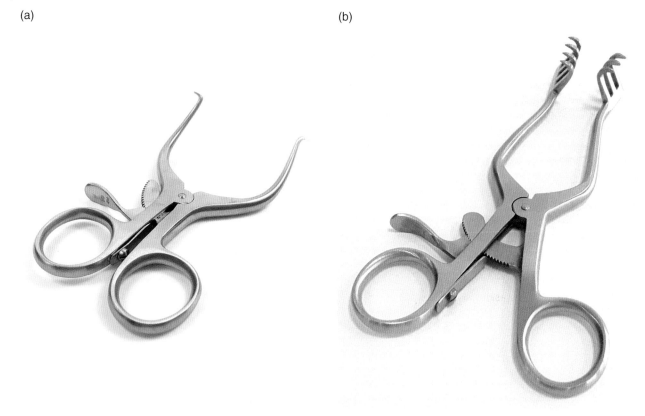

Figure 19.10 Commonly used retractors are the Gelpi (a) and the Weitlaner (b). *Source:* Photos courtesy of Scil Animal Care Company, Canada.

References

1 Focus and Flourish (n.d.) Focus and Flourish homepage. Retrieved from https://focusandflourish.com (accessed November 5, 2018).

2 Everost (n.d.) Everost homepage. Retrieved from http://everost.com/educational-program.html

3 AOVET (n.d.) AOVET homepage. Retrieved from https://aovet.aofoundation.org (accessed November 5, 2018).

4 Everost (n.d.) Everost power systems. Retrieved from http://www.everost.com/products-power-systems.html (accessed November 5, 2018).

5 Arbutus Medical (n.d.) Arbutus Medical veterinary homepage. Retrieved from http://arbutusmedical.ca/vet/drillcover-vet (accessed November 5, 2018).

20

Pins and Wires
Catherine Popovitch

Veterinary Specialty and Emergency Center, Levittown, Pennsylvania, USA

This section discusses the basic principles of fracture repair using intra-medullary pins and cerclage wires. This repair technique is reserved for long oblique and spiral diaphyseal fractures.

20.1 Case Selection

Younger patients and smaller dogs and cats are often ideal candidate for fracture repair using pin and wire. Stable fracture configurations such as long obliques (length of the fracture line is at least twice the diameter of the bone) and spirals are the best fractures for pin fixation. Transverse fractures are not rotationally stable with a single pin and require the addition of a plate or external fixator. Cerclage wires cannot be applied to a transverse fracture as hemicerclage wires cannot adequately counteract rotational forces.

20.2 Instrumentation (Figure 20.1)

Pins are placed by hand with a Jacobs chuck. Hand placement allows better control and feel of the direction of the pin. In cases where the bone is very hard, such as the calcaneous or olecranon, power can be used. Bone clamps such as speed-locks, Kerns, or point-to-points are necessary to help manipulate the bone fragments and maintain reduction. Selection of pins should include from 0.045″ up to 1/4″, preferably smooth, trocar-tipped pins. It is recommended to have several pins of each diameter and at least a second pin of the same length to evaluate the positioning of the inserted intra-medullary pin.

A range of cerclage wires should include 22, 20, 18, and 16 gauge. Large, inexpensive needle holders can be used to twist the wire; wire specific twisters have a sturdier and wider box shape that makes properly twisting the

wire easier. As an alternative, eyelet wire and a tensioner can also be used.

A pin cutter that can be sterilized and can cut up to a 1/8 in. pin is ideal and a smaller pair of cutters is needed for the cerclage wires. A pin punch (and mallet) is optional but can be very helpful.

Non-surgical cutters can be used but they may not be sterilizable, which increases the risk of infection.

20.3 Fundamentals of Application

20.3.1 Cerclage Wires

The cerclage wires function to hold the bone in reduction. Bone clamps such as speed-locks, Kerns, or point-to-points are used to place and hold the bone fragments in reduction while the wires are placed.

The wire is passed as close to the bone as possible. It is important to avoid entrapping the soft tissues between the wire and the bone. A wire passer can be helpful for this. Wires are placed at least 5 mm from the fracture ends, and 1–1.5 cm apart (Figure 20.2). A minimum of two wires should be used. If the conical shape of the bone causes the wire to slip, a bone rasp can be used to notch the bone, giving the wire a place to seat. The twisting of the wire is started by crossing the wires ends over one another and grabbing in the center of the cross with a needle driver or wire twister. Gentle upward tension is applied to the needle driver as it is slowly turned to evenly intertwine the wire ends along one another and to prevent one wire from wrapping itself around the other (Figure 20.3). Proper twisting prevents loosening of the wire.

The wire "knot" should be cut leaving three twists on the wire. The cut wire ends should be bent in areas where the soft tissue coverage is minimal, such as the medial aspect of the tibia. When using an eyelet wire and accompanying tensioner the wire is bent over while making the

Fracture Management for the Small Animal Practitioner, First Edition. Edited by Anne M. Sylvestre.
© 2019 John Wiley & Sons, Inc. Published 2019 by John Wiley & Sons, Inc.

final twist; this reduces the loss of tension. It is better to use a wire that is too large rather than one that is too small. Cerclage wires are never to be used as the sole fixation method of any diaphyseal fracture.

20.3.2 Pins

If one is uncertain as to which is the correct pin size for the bone, it is best to start with a smaller pin. Switching from a larger pin to a smaller one will result in it not seating well in the bone. A pin of the same length is also needed to measure how far the pin has been advanced in the bone. The pin selection size is estimated by measuring the width of the medullary canal on the radiographs. A singular pin should take upto 60–75% of the medullary canal at its narrowest part. Ultimately, the correct pin size is determined by inserting it into the fracture end and evaluating the fill of the medullary cavity.

Multiple pins (stack pinning) are not recommended. It was thought that stack pinning provided better rotational stability, but clinically this has not been shown to be the case. They also have a higher complication rate [1].

Pins can be placed in a normograde fashion, by inserting the pin from one end of the bone (usually proximal end) into the medullary canal; or retrograde, by inserting it at the fracture site, driving it out of one end of the bone (usually proximal) and then redirecting it back into the opposite fragment. Normograde pinning is recommended when possible as it allows for better control of where the pin exits the bone. Pins placed retrograde may exit too close to tendons (patellar tendon in the tibia), nerves (sciatic in the femur), or the articular surface (humerus).

Lowering the surgery table can be helpful to allow for a better angle when directing the pin. Having only a few centimeters of pin protruding from the chuck when starting placement prevents bending of smaller pins and gives a mechanical advantage with larger pins. Bone clamps are helpful to stabilize the bone while driving the pin into the fragment. The fracture is reduced and the pin is seated into the other (usually the distal) fragment of the bone, avoiding penetration into the joint. Specific landmarks will vary depending on the bone.

The pin should be cut as short and close to the bone as possible: approximately 5 mm. To accomplish this, the incision can be extended to where the pin enters the bone. This allows better visualization and allows the pin cutter to be placed closer to the bone. Another method is to back the pin out 2–3 cm after it has been seated, cut the pin, and then reinsert it using a punch (or bone tamp) and mallet. It is important to stabilize the bone and watch the fracture site while cutting the pin as it can shift. Pins left too long very often result in complications including: pain, seroma formation, or nerve impingement.

(a)

(b)

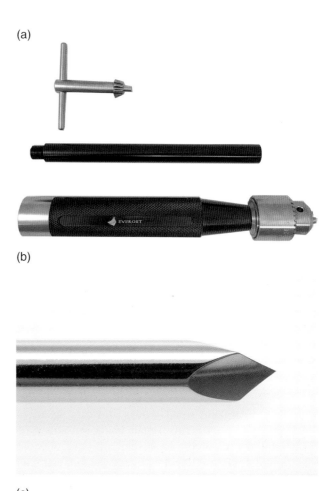

(c)

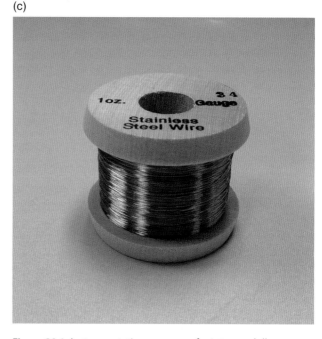

Figure 20.1 Instrumentation necessary for intra-medullary pinning. (a) Hand chuck with protective sleeve and key; (b) trocar-tipped smooth intra-medullary pin; (c) a spool of cerclage wire; (d) a wire twister; (e) cerclage wire with eyelet and tensioner; (f) pin cutter large enough to cut a 1/8″ diameter pin; (g) smaller cutters for the cerclage wires; (h) a pin punch (and mallet, not shown) are used to bury the end of the pin within the bone.

(d)

(e)

(f)

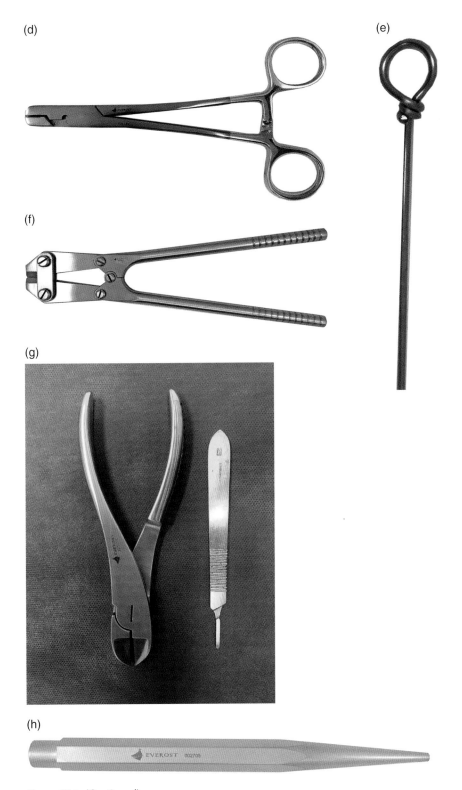

(g)

(h)

Figure 20.1 (Continued)

The pin should be cut in surgery so it is done in a sterile environment. However, if there are concerns regarding the pin placement, it can be cut after the radiographs are taken. Measures should be taken to keep the exposed end of the pin sterile and prevent it from injuring the patient and personnel during transportation. Placing sterile gauze over the exposed pin end and wrapping it with sterile bandaging material (Coflex™) will help with keeping the end of the pin sterile. After proper placement of the pin is confirmed on radiographs, the patient

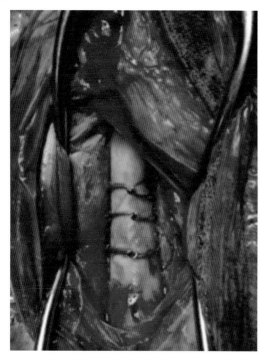

Figure 20.2 Intra-operative photo showing the spacing of 1–1.5 cm between each cerclage wire.

is taken back to the operating room where the pin can be cut using sterile technique and the skin over the pin sutured closed.

20.4 Pinning Techniques for Various Long Bones

20.4.1 Humerus

Many simple fractures of the humerus are amenable to repair using an intra-medullary pin and cerclage wires.

Pins may be placed normograde or retrograde. Normograde is the technique of choice. The selection of pin size depends on the location of the fracture. In fractures of the proximal to middle diaphysis, a larger pin can be used and inserted to the level of the supratrochlear foramen. Normograde pins are inserted on the lateral ridge of the greater tubercle (Figure 20.4). The pin is started perpendicular to the bone. When the point is seated, it is redirected distally down the shaft. The pin is inserted and seated just proximal to the supracondylar notch. In cases of more distal humeral shaft fractures a smaller pin can be used and directed into the medial condyle to provide increased stability. It is technically more challenging to direct the pins into the medial condyle either normograde or retrograde [2].

If placing a pin retrograde it is started at the fracture and driven proximally aiming to exit out of the lateral edge of the greater tubercle.

Postoperatively, fractures of the humerus may be supported with a spica bandage. A bandage that ends mid-humerus should be avoided as it may act as a fulcrum and place more stress on the fracture repair. If the repair is not supported with a bandage or a splint, restriction of activity is very important until the fracture has healed.

Radiographs are recommended every 4 weeks until healing has occurred. It is not necessary to remove the pin or wires unless they are causing a problem.

20.4.2 Radius

An intra-medullary pin *should never be used* for fractures of the radius. The radius is covered at either end by articular cartilage. It is not possible to place an intra-medullary pin without damaging the articular cartilage and impinging on the joint. Also the medullary canal of the radius is very small and does not accommodate a pin well.

20.4.3 Femur

Many simple fractures, long oblique and spiral, of the femur are amenable to repair using a pin and wires. Also more complex fractures in small dogs and cats and younger patients can be reconstructed and repaired with a pin and cerclage wires.

Normograde is the preferred method of insertion. The pin is inserted at or just medial to the greater trochanter (Figure 20.5).

Care needs to be taken to protect the sciatic nerve, which sits medial and caudal to the greater trochanter. One of the reasons retrograde insertion of the pin is not recommended in the femur is the possibility it can exit close to the sciatic. The pin is driven into the distal fragment of the femur up to but not penetrating the intercondylar fossa. Another pin of the same length is used to measure the depth of placement. The stifle is flexed and extended to ensure there is no impingement. Pins should be cut as short as possible. Pins left too long result in the development of seromas and can be painful if they cause irritation to the sciatic nerve. Postoperatively, restriction of activity is very important until the fracture has healed. The femur is not amenable to bandaging, as a bandage may act as a fulcrum and place more stress on the fracture repair. Radiographs are recommended every 4 weeks until healing has occurred. It is not necessary to remove the pin or wires unless they are causing a problem.

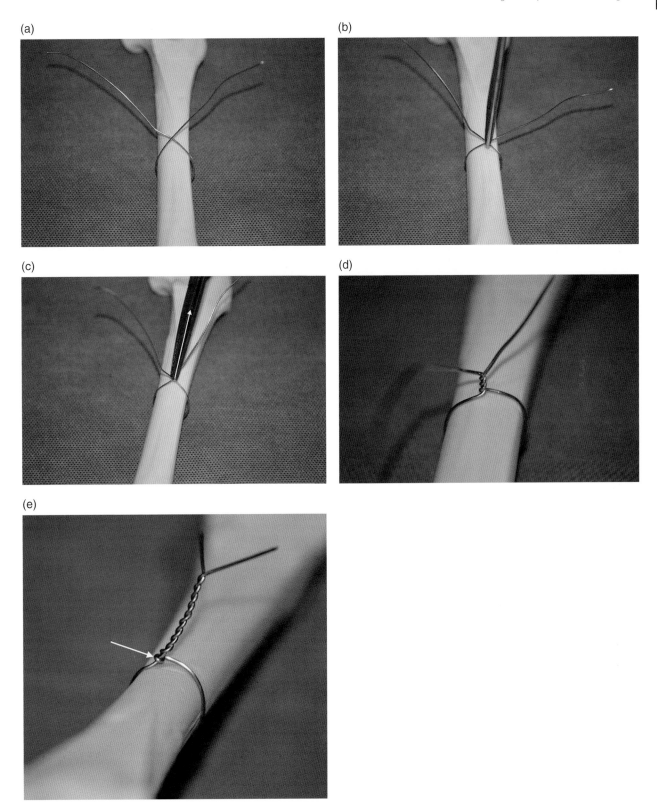

Figure 20.3 This series of photographs illustrates how to twist a cerclage wire. (a) The wire ends are crossed over one another. (b) The needle driver (or a wire twister) is placed in the center of the "cross." (c) The needle driver is slowly twisted in the direction of the "crossover" while applying a steady, gentle upward pull on the instrument. (d) The result should be an even intertwining of the two wires as opposed to one wire "wrapping itself around the other" (e).

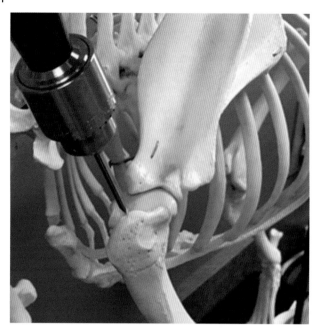

Figure 20.4 Positioning of the pin for normograde placement in the humerus. The pin is inserted on the lateral ridge of the greater tubercle.

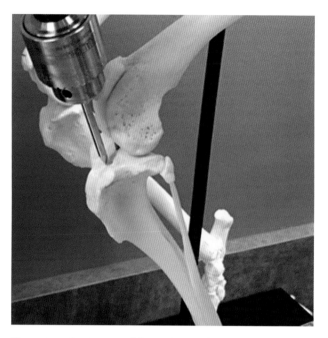

Figure 20.6 Positioning of the pin for normograde placement in the tibia. The pin is inserted just medial to the patellar tendon along the cranial aspect of the articular surface of the proximal tibia.

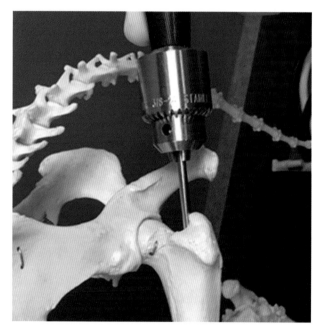

Figure 20.5 Positioning of the pin for normograde placement in the femur. The pin is inserted just medial to the greater trochanter.

20.4.4 Tibia

Fractures of the tibia are a common long bone fractures. Similar to the radius there is not much soft tissue between the skin and bone and this results in a high rate of open fractures. Oblique, spiral, and minimally fragmented fractures are amenable to repair using pin and cerclage wire. Small dogs, cats, and skeletally immature dogs are the best candidates for this type of repair.

Only normograde pinning should be used in the tibia. Pins placed retrograde may exit in an area on the tibial plateau and can damage the insertion of the cranial cruciate ligament or interfere with the femoral condyles [3].

Pin placement is started by flexing the stifle to a 90° angle. The pin should enter the proximal end of the tibia along its cranial aspect and just medial to the patellar ligament (Figure 20.6). Placing the pin too caudal in the tibia will result in limitation of full extension of the stifle. A slightly smaller pin can be used to allow slight bending, which accommodates the curvature of the tibia. The pin is seated into the distal metaphysis, ensuring the tarsal joint is not entered. The medial malleolus is a landmark used to measure the depth of pin placement. Wires are cut short or twisted down to avoid complications such as wires protruding through the skin, given that there is so little soft tissue coverage over the medial tibia. This is especially high risk in thin-skinned dogs such as greyhounds and also in cats. Postoperatively, the limb is placed in a splint or padded bandage for 2–4 weeks. This supports and increases the success of the repair.

Radiographs are taken every 4 weeks until the fracture has healed. The pin and wires are only removed if they are causing problems. More often the wires alone may need to be removed if they are causing irritation to the overlying skin.

References

1 Gibson, K.L. and vanEe, R.T. (1991). Stack pining of long bone fractures: a retrospective study. *Vet. Clin. Orthop. Trauma.* 4: 48–53.

2 Milgram, J. and Hod, N. (2012). Normograde and retrograde pinning of the distal fragment in humeral fractures of the dog. *Vet. Surg.* 41: 671–675.

3 Dixon, B.C. and Tomlinson, J.L. (1994). Effects of three pinning techniques on proximal pin location and articular damage in the canine tibia. *Vet. Surg.* 23: 448–445.

21

Plating

Anne M. Sylvestre

Focus and Flourish, Cambridge, Ontario, Canada

The information in this chapter is meant to help focus the reader on some of the key points about plating; to refresh one's memory and hopefully help a less experienced surgeon successfully accomplish the task of plating a bone while minimizing stress. Learning to use plates and screws comes from experiencing it, not from reading a book. The veterinarian wishing to start repairing fractures is strongly urged to take at least one, but preferably several, practical workshops on the topic. In order to have success and to avoid frustration and defeat, one should choose carefully which cases are appropriate based on the surgeon's level of experience. The more complicated fractures are best left in the hands of the trained surgeon; if one is not available then an alternative treatment option may be a better choice than attempting a repair that is far beyond one's skill level. A complex fracture has a higher risk of major complications and failure. If the owners are ready to deal (financially and emotionally) with the potential complications then it may be best to refer them as too often a patient is seen in a referral practice with a failed fracture repair and a frustrated and emotionally spent owner. At the initial presentation to the referring veterinarian, the owners expressed their unwillingness to spend the money or travel the distance to see a specialist and yet here they are now. This is about educating and motivating the client to make an appropriate choice. The importance of patient selection and practical training are crucial to achieving success with fracture repair.

21.1 Case Selection

Bone plating is a versatile technique for repairing fractures; it allows for an early return to function because it can restore rigid stability to the fractured bone. Bone plates can be utilized in simple and complex fractures, young or old patients, on all long bones, in very large to very small patients. The basic goal of fracture fixation is to place and maintain the bone in a functional and stable manner so that the fracture can heal. It is not about having perfect postoperative radiographs; it is about reducing the fracture and ensuring that the basic principles of plating have been respected.

21.2 Instrumentation

21.2.1 Bone Screws

The different types of bone screws are: the cortical screw and the cancellous screw. The cancellous screw has fewer threads per unit of length and the threads are quite deep, making it valuable for use in bone that is not very dense, such as in humans with osteoporosis [1] but not as useful in the much denser canine and feline cortical bones [1]. The cortical screw is the most versatile and universally used in small animal orthopedics. A cortical screw can be either self-tapping (the screw cuts the threads within the bone as it is inserted) or not self-tapping, where a bone tap is required to cut the threads within the bone prior to inserting a screw. Implants can be stainless steel or titanium. Stainless steel is less expensive and more ubiquitous, at this time, in veterinary surgery. Self-tapping, stainless steel, cortical screws with a hexagonal head are the most commonly used (Figure 21.1).

A screw is composed of a head, shaft or core, and threads. A screw is identified according to its outer diameter (i.e. core and thread). For instance a 2.7-mm screw has a core of 1.9 mm; the threads are 0.8 mm wide so the total width of the screw is 2.7 mm; hence it is referred to as the "2.7 screw."

In order to use this screw, one would choose a drill bit that is approximately equal in diameter to its core. A 2.0 mm drill bit would be used in this particular example. A complete guide to drill bit and screw sizes is found in Table 21.1.

Fracture Management for the Small Animal Practitioner, First Edition. Edited by Anne M. Sylvestre.

(a) (b) (c)

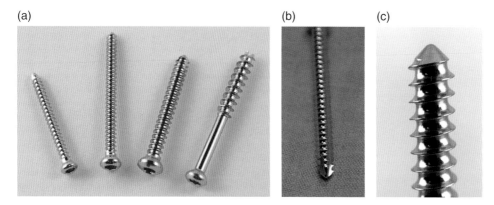

Figure 21.1 (a) Four different types of orthopedic screws. (left to right) Self-tapping cortical; non-self-tapping cortical; fully threaded cancellous; and partially threaded cancellous. The threads of the cancellous screws are wider and spaced further apart. The fluting of a self-tapping screw is visible in (b) as compared with the non-self-tapping screw (c). *Source:* Photos courtesy of Everost.

Table 21.1 This chart indicates which screws, drill bits, and plates sizes are used together.

Screw size	1.5	2.0	2.4	2.7	3.5
Drill bit	1.1	1.5	1.8	2.0	2.5
DCP Plates	1.5	2.0	2.4	2.7	3.5
VCP Plates	VCP 1.5/2.0				
		VCP 2.0/2.7			

VCP, veterinary cuttable plate.

21.2.2 Bone Plates

The following size plates are the more commonly used ones: 1.5 mm, 2.0 mm, 2.7 mm, 3.5 mm and 3.5 mm broad. The plate size refers to the size of screw that should be used with the plate. The commonly used types of plates are (Figure 21.2):

- Dynamic compression plate (DCP): The elliptical holes allow for compression of the fracture site.
- Limited contact dynamic compression plate (LC-DCP): This plate has a scalloped surface on the bone

(a) (b)

(c) (d)

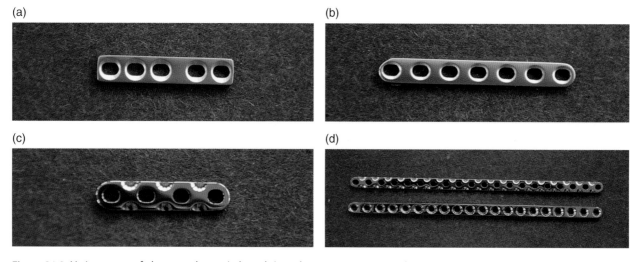

Figure 21.2 Various types of plates are shown. (a, b, and c) are dynamic compression plates (DCPs) as per their elliptical holes. (a) A square edge DCP with spacer, which should be positioned over the fracture line. (b) A round edge DCP without a spacer. (c) A limited contact plate (LC-DCP) identified by the scalloping on the bone side of the plate. (d) A veterinary cuttable plate (VCP), its holes are round, so not a DCP, but its bone side has the scalloping so this is a LCP-VCP. The VCPs are practical as they can be cut to an appropriate length as necessary. *Source:* Photos courtesy of Everost.

side. The intention of the design is to minimize contact between the bone and the plate, thereby maintaining or improving periosteal blood flow. It is important to place the "scalloped" side of the plate on the bone.

- Veterinary cuttable plate (VCP): This plate is very versatile and practical. It is purchased as a long, thin plate (containing 20–50 round holes) that can be cut down to the required length. The screw holes are round and evenly spaced; the plates can be cut to appropriate length with a 9/25″ pin cutter. VCPs come in 1.5/2.0 and 2.0/2.7 sizes. They are useful for animals weighing less than 10 kg. They are not very strong plates on their own, but if more strength is needed (e.g. on a femur or tibia) they can be "stacked."

There are many other types of plates and plating systems available (locking compression plates, reconstruction plates, string-of-pearls, etc.). They have different characteristics that make them useful in various situations. A veterinarian who is looking to become equipped and trained in bone plating should pick a system and learn to become proficient at it. The standard (non-locking) system is likely the simplest, most versatile, and cost-effective system available at this time, especially for an urban practice.

21.2.3 Plating-specific Instruments

The instruments that are necessary in order to be able to use plates and screws are listed below (Figure 21.3):

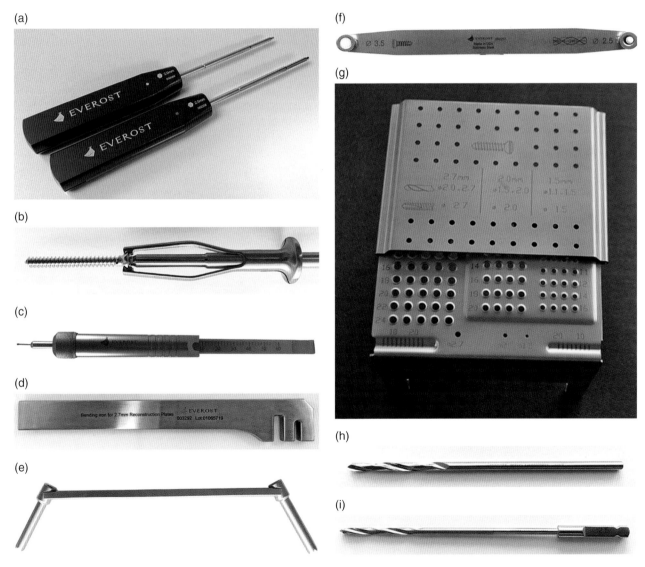

Figure 21.3 The plating-specific instruments necessary in order to be able to use plates and screws are shown here. (a) Hexagonal screwdrivers to be used with 1.5 and 2.0 mm screw and with 2.7 mm and 3.5 mm screws. (b) The screwdriver sleeve holds the screw in place for easy maneuvering. (c) A depth gauge. (d) A bending iron—a pair of these must be purchased. (e) Side view of a drill guide. (f) Top view of a drill guide. (g) Screw rack. (h) Jacobs chuck (JC) drill bit. (i) Quick coupling (QC) drill bit. *Source:* Photos courtesy of Everost.

- Screwdriver: The screwdriver can be purchased as a two-piece item consisting of the shaft and handle, or as a single unit. It is important to purchase the screwdriver sleeve as this will greatly assist in picking up the screws from the screw rack. The screwdriver must fit the type of screw head (most are hexagonal) and the size of screw. The 1.5/2.0 and the 2.7/3.5 screwdrivers must be purchased in order to place the respective size screws.
- Depth gauge: Depth gauges are also size-specific—the 1.5/2.0 for the small screws and the 2.7/3.5 for the larger screws. The larger depth gauge is too big to comfortably fit through the smaller screw hole diameter and the smaller one does not readily "catch" the edge of the far cortex of the 3.5 screw holes. It is best to purchase one of each size.
- Bending irons: Bending irons can be individual hand-held tools or one can purchase a bending press to contour the larger plates. The small (1.5/2.0) plate benders are not adequate for bending the larger plates and the larger ones are too bulky for bending the smaller 2.0 plates.
- Drill guide: A drill guide is a useful instrument to have but not absolutely necessary. It will help hold the drill bit in the center of the plate screw hole ensuring accurate positioning of the screw. It will keep the drill bit from slipping on the surface of the bone.
- Screw rack: A screw rack allows for the storage of the screws according to their size and length. It keeps them readily identifiable and accessible in surgery. A screw rack is a must-have.
- Instrument box: An instrument box is an inexpensive tool that will help keep all the instruments organized, easy to find, and in one place.
- Drill bits: Drill bits are considered a consumable item. Table 21.1 describes the sizes necessary. Drill bits do get dull and can break. It is best to always have a spare, sterilized drill bit of appropriate size available when plating a fracture. Drill bits can have a smooth end to fit in a Jacobs chuck (JC) or have a quick coupling mechanism (QC) for fasting loading into a specialized drill attachment.

21.3 Fundamentals of Application

There are many different techniques that can be employed when applying bone plates and screws. Each one has its merits. The scope of this discussion will deal with the plate and screw construct applied in compression or neutralization manner only. The bridging and buttressing plating techniques are used in fracture locations and configurations that are less common and more complex. Plates can also be applied in a minimally invasive manner; specialized equipment and training are required to accomplish this. These techniques (and many others) are better left for the trained surgeon and are beyond the scope of this book.

A compression plate, not to be confused with placing a fracture line under compression or using a DCP, is named that way because it is placed on the tension side of the bone, thereby effectively maintaining that side under compression. Because bones are eccentrically loaded, they have a side under compression and one under tension. The compression plate and screw construct is strongest when applied to the tension side of the bone. Compression plates are used for simple transverse and short oblique fractures.

A neutralizing plate is also placed on the tension side of a bone in more complex fractures. Once a fracture has been reconstructed with cerclage wire and/or interfragmentary compression screws, the neutralizing plate is then applied to the bone to nullify the bending, distraction, compression, or torsional forces that are acting on the fracture line(s).

21.3.1 Selecting a Plate

The size of the plate is mostly dependent on the weight of the patient but also on the relative size of the bone; therefore, one must consider the body condition score (BCS) of the patient. There are tables that are very good guides to help select the appropriate size plate (Tables 21.2–21.5).

The plate should be long enough to offer a stable and secure fixation. If the fracture is centrally located on the bone, then the plate should cover most of the length of the

Table 21.2 Choosing a plate for the humerus. This chart is to be considered a guideline only.

0 kg	10 kg	20 kg	30 kg	40 kg	50 kg
2.0 DCP or VCP					
	2.7 DCP or VCP				
		3.5 DCP			
			3.5 Broad		

DCP, dynamic compression plate; VCP, veterinary cuttable plate.

Table 21.3 Choosing a plate for the radius. This chart is to be considered a guideline only.

<2kg	>2 kg	10 kg	20 kg	30 kg	40 kg	50 kg
1.5 DCP or VCP						
	2.0 DCP or VCP					
		2.7 DCP or VCP				
			3.5 DCP			
				3.5 Broad		

DCP, dynamic compression plate; VCP, veterinary cuttable plate.

Table 21.4 Choosing a plate for the femur. This chart is to be considered a guideline only.

0 kg	10 kg	20 kg	30 kg	40 kg	50 kg
2.0 DCP or VCP					
	2.7 DCP or VCP				
		3.5 DCP			
			3.5 Broad		

DCP, dynamic compression plate; VCP, veterinary cuttable plate.

Table 21.5 Choosing a plate for the tibia. This chart is to be considered a guideline only.

0 kg	10 kg	20 kg	30 kg	40 kg	50 kg
2.0 DCP or VCP					
	2.7 DCP or VCP				
		3.5 DCP			
			3.5 Broad		

DCP, dynamic compression plate; VCP, veterinary cuttable plate.

diaphysis of the bone. If the fracture is closer to an extremity, as with the commonly seen fracture of the distal third of the radius in toy breed dogs, the plate is selected to fit the maximum number of screws in the smaller (distal in the example) fragment and to have an equal or only slightly larger number of screws in the proximal fragment. For example, if only three screws can be placed on the small distal fragment, then a six- or seven-hole plate should be selected. The *absolute minimum* number of screws necessary to prevent rotation of a fragment is two; however, three screws (at least five cortices) on either side of the fracture is preferred in order to have sufficient stability of the repair. If one of the main fragments is too small to accommodate two screws, then a different repair technique should be selected for that fracture. In general, the hind limb fracture repairs do better with a stronger construct when compared with the radius and ulna fractures.

Once a plate size has been chosen, it can be compared with the size of the bone on the radiograph to help further assess its fit (width and length) to the bone (Figure 21.4). Ultimately, the final decision is made at surgery.

21.3.2 At Surgery

The fracture is reduced and the selected plate is laid on the bone to make a final determination as to whether it is a proper fit (size, length, and number of screw holes per fragment). The plate may require to be contoured to the bone. For most fractures of the diaphysis of the radius, tibia, and femur, very little to no contouring is necessary. Humeral fractures, on the other hand, can require significant plate contouring. A poorly contoured plate will result in loss of reduction of the fracture site once the screws are tightened.

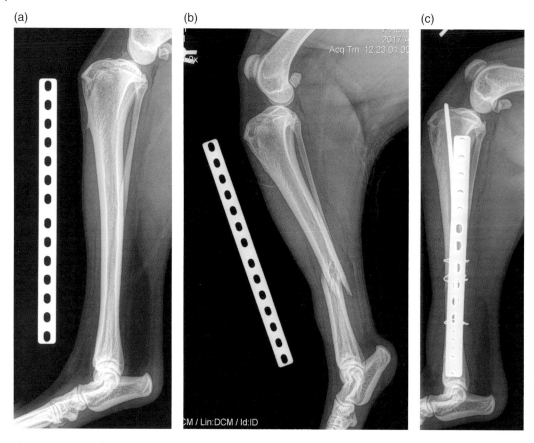

(a)   (b)   (c)

Figure 21.4 Lateral projections of both tibiae of a patient along with a 14-hole dynamic compression plate (DCP) (a, b) in order to assess its fit on the bone. (c) The lateral postoperative view. The 14-hole DCP was used along with an intra-medullary pin to stabilize the fracture. *Source:* Photos courtesy of the VCA Canada Mississauga Oakville veterinary emergency Hospital and referral group.

The minimal distance between a fracture line and a screw is "one screw diameter." It is best to place the most difficult screw first. This will often be the screw adjacent to the fracture on the shortest fragment. A hole is drilled in the center of the plate hole using the appropriate size drill bit (as per the Table 21.1). A depth gauge is then used to determine the length of the screw that will be used. The screw selected should be 2–4 mm longer than the measured depth of the hole so that the far cortex will be fully engaged. The screw is secured into the hole. The second screw is placed into the opposite fragment in the same manner (drill, measure, insert screw). It is important to ensure that the plate is properly aligned with the long axis of the bone and that the fracture is adequately reduced before drilling for the second screw (Figure 21.5). A plate can easily become positioned askew to the long axis of the bone, resulting in the last screw hole being positioned off the bone (Figure 21.6). It is best to place the screws in an alternating fashion between the fragments in order to prevent plate malpositioning and minimize loss of reduction. A screw hole can be drilled on a slight angle to avoid it being too close to a fracture line. All the screws should be tightened before closing. It is easy to

strip a screw, especially the smaller sizes (1.5 and 2.0) and in pediatric patients, so caution must be exercised so as not to overtighten.

21.3.3 Pin–Plate Combination

The pin–plate combination is a useful tool for repairing bones. The pin protects the plate from the bending forces applied to it, while the plate counteracts the rotational forces that the pin does not. This construct provides more strength than with a plate alone [2]. It is a good combination to use for femoral and tibial fractures, especially in the smaller patients, because the 2.0 plates are not very rigid.

The same basic principles are applied as discussed for pinning and plating; however, a pin that fills approximately 35–40% of the diameter of the bone at the narrowest part is chosen. This will allow for the passage of bicortical screws (Figure 21.7).

The pin should be inserted first and tamped into its final position. Positioning the pin first will assist in aligning the major fragments of the bone and maintain the reduction; also it is next to impossible to place a pin once the screws are in place. The plate is then applied to the bone and bicortical screws are placed wherever possible.

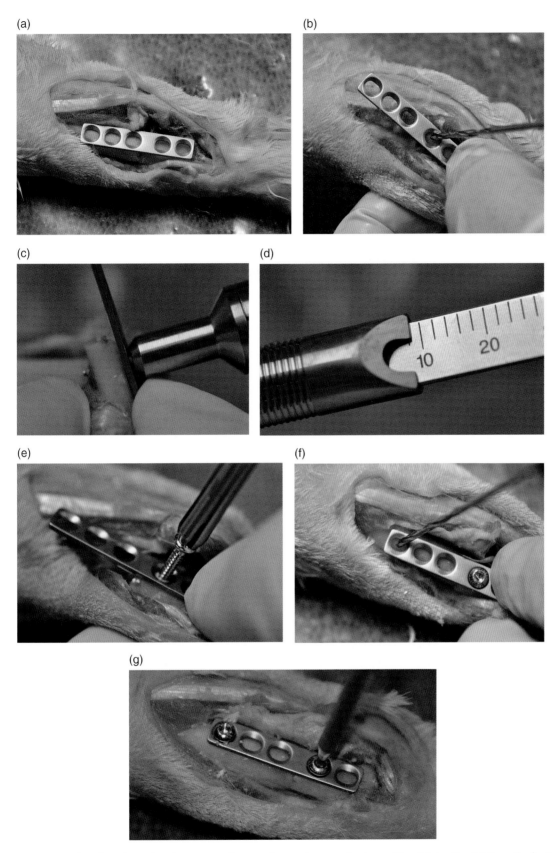

Figure 21.5 A cadaver is used to demonstrate how to place a plate on a fracture of the distal radius. (a) Once the fracture has been reduced, the plate is placed on the bone for a final evaluation of its fit. (b) The most difficult screw hole should be drilled first. In these toy breed radius fractures that is usually the hole next to the fracture line on the distal fragment. (c) Once the hole is drilled, the depth gauge is inserted in the hole and the tip of the instrument is allowed to catch the far cortex; the sleeve is slid down into the screw hole. (d) The resulting depth of the screw hole is read on the graduated portion of the gauge. (e) A screw 2 mm longer than the measured length is selected and placed in the pre-drilled screw hole. (f) The plate is secured to the proximal fragment with a second screw. (g) Once the second screw has been inserted, the first one can be tightened to help keep the fracture stable while the remainder of the screws are placed.

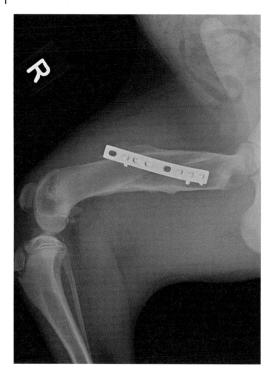

Figure 21.6 A lateral radiograph of a young dog with a femoral fracture that was stabilized with a dynamic compression plate. The plate was positioned on an angle, thereby causing the distal-most screw hole to "miss" the bone.

21.3.4 Stack Plating

VCPs can be stacked, meaning two plates of equal or near equal length can be placed on top of one another and secured to the bone with screws (Figure 21.8). The VCPs tend to be less rigid than most compression plates and stacking them greatly increases the strength of the construct [3]. Stacking two VCPs is another way of creating a repair that is stronger than when using a single compression plate of the same size. This is a good construct to use on femoral and tibial fractures in the appropriate-sized patients.

21.4 Postoperative Care

A bandage may be used to help attenuate postoperative swelling (except on the femur) for 3–5 days. A splint may be necessary, depending on the stability of the fracture repair. A complex fracture with open screw holes may best be protected with a splint for 2–4 weeks postoperatively. However, if a splint is not required, then it is best to avoid using one as they are not benign and require frequent visits to the hospital.

Restricted activity until the fracture has healed must be stressed to the owners. Follow-up radiographs should be taken every 4 weeks until there is sufficient bridging callus present to indicate that the fracture has healed.

Plates need only be removed if they are causing a problem. This will become evident by the patient's ongoing lameness and discomfort over the plate, or if a draining tract is present.

21.5 Plating Techniques for Various Long Bones

21.5.1 Humerus

The humerus is a difficult bone to approach. A plate is applied to the lateral side of the diaphysis. Most fractures will be located in the mid- to distal third of the diaphysis. Often the plate will need to be contoured to fit the lateral condyle and epicondyle in order to have enough screws in the distal fragment. This degree of contouring can be challenging (Figure 21.9). The humerus is one of the bones that fractures the least frequently and is best left in the hands of a trained surgeon if possible.

21.5.2 Radius

The plate is applied to the tensile side of the radius, which is the cranial surface (Figure 21.10). The approach is straightforward, especially for fractures in the mid- to distal portions of this bone. In very distal diaphyseal/metaphyseal fractures it can be more challenging to fit two screws in the distal fragment while avoiding the carpus. T-plates are designed specifically for these very distal fractures (Figure 21.11). Small hypodermic needles can be placed in the carpus to help identify its location at surgery. Fractures of the radius in toy breed dogs are among the more common fractures seen in private practice [4]. One of the common complications is some degree of stress protection (see Chapter 10). The author prefers to use a construct of lesser strength (single VCP, 1.5 or 2.0 thin DCP versus stacking VCPs or the locking plate system) and augment the repair for 2 weeks with a small tongue depressor splint followed by a soft padded bandage for 1 or 2 weeks.

21.5.3 Femur

The plate is applied to the tensile side of the femur, which is the lateral surface (Figure 21.12). The approach is straightforward although a little more complicated than for the tibia or radius because of all the muscles. A less experienced surgeon is encouraged to review the regional anatomy and consult the chapter on approaches to the bones in the text before performing the surgery. Instrumentation such as appropriate-sized retractors and reduction forceps (more than one of each are often useful)

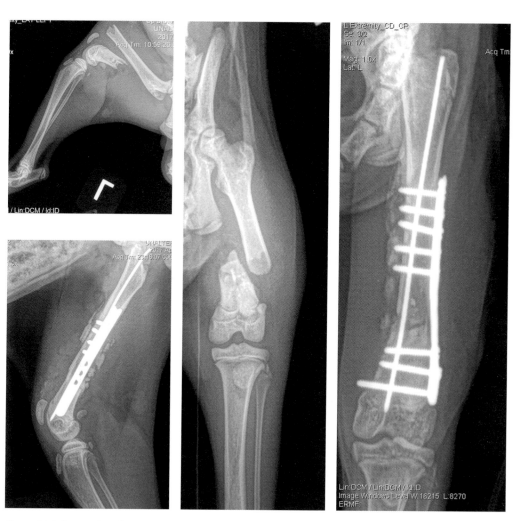

Figure 21.7 Pre- and 14 days postoperative radiographs of the left femur of a young cat. The fracture was stabilized using a pin–plate combination. Callus formation is already visible 14 days postsurgery.

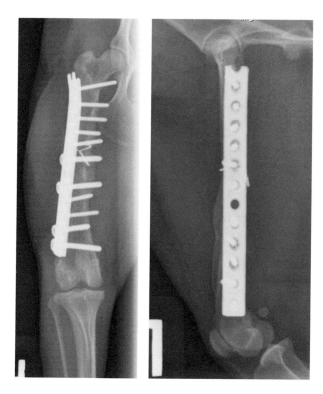

Figure 21.8 Two views of a healed femoral fracture in a Yorkshire terrier that was stabilized with staked veterinary cuttable plates.

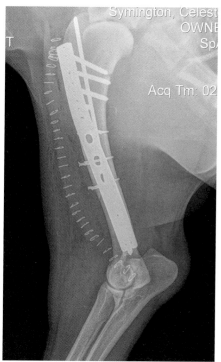
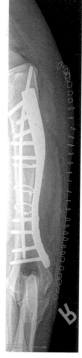

Figure 21.9 Postoperative radiographs of a humerus with the plate applied to the lateral side of the bone. Note the degree of contouring necessary for the plate to properly fit the bone.

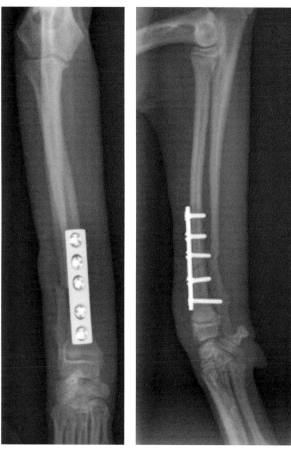

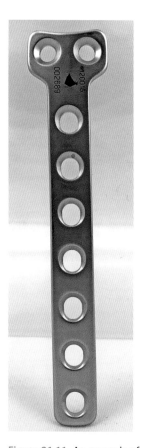

Figure 21.10 Postoperative radiographs of a radius with the plate applied to the cranial surface of the bone.

Figure 21.11 An example of a T-plate.

are necessary. A strong repair is indicated for diaphyseal femoral fractures. The smaller (2.0) plates are often not strong enough for some of the more complex fractures as well as to counteract the bending forces of a transverse fracture, so a stronger construct such as stack plating or a pin–plate combination is advised. A femoral fracture cannot readily be supported with a splint so it is important to select a construct that will offer sufficient strength.

21.5.4 Tibia

The plate is applied to the tensile side of the tibia, which is the medial surface (Figure 21.13). The approach to the medial side of the tibia is straightforward. Like the femur, the tibia needs a strong repair so an appropriate construct must be selected. For small dogs or cats that require a 2.0 plating system it may be wise to consider stacking the VCPs or using a pin–plate combination. The larger plating systems appear to be relatively stronger but, if there is doubt, then a pin–plate combination can be utilized. The tibia can be supported with an external splint for 2–4 weeks postoperatively if necessary.

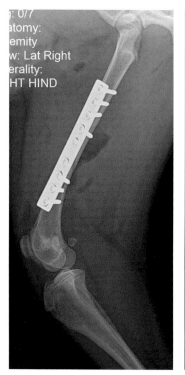
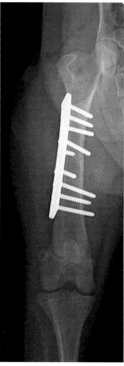

Figure 21.12 Postoperative radiographs of a femur with the plate applied to the lateral side of the bone.

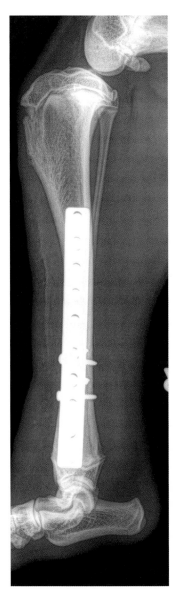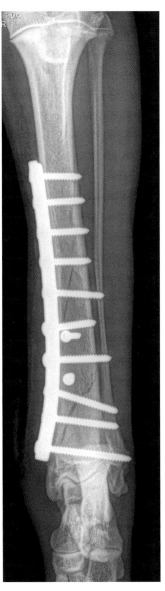

Figure 21.13 Postoperative radiographs of a tibia with the plate applied to the medial side of the bone.

References

1 DeCamp, C.E., Johnston, S.A., Déjardin, L.M., and Schaefer, S.L. (2016). *Brinker, Piermattei and Flo's Handbook of Small Animal Orthopaedics and Fracture Repair*, 5e. St Louis, MO: Elsevier.

2 Hulse, D., Hyman, W., Nori, M., and Slater, M. (1997). Reduction in plate strain by addition of an intramedullary pin. *Vet. Surg.* 26: 451–459.

3 Bichot, S., Gibson, T.W., Moens, N.M. et al. (2011). Effect of the length of the superficial plate on bending stiffness, bending strength and strain distribution in stacked 2.0–2.7 veterinary cuttable plate constructs. An in vitro study. *Vet. Comp. Orthop. Traumatol.* 24 (6): 426–434.

4 Roush, J.K. (2015). Pet health by numbers: Prevalence of bone fractures in dogs and cats. Today's Veterinary Practice July/August. Retrieved from: http://todaysveterinarypractice.navc.com/pet-health-by-the-numbers-prevalence-of-bone-fractures-in-dogs-cats

22

External Fixators

Kathryn Wander

Centro Veterinario Costa Ballena, Uvita de Osa, Puntarenas, Costa Rica

External skeletal fixation is a means of fracture stabilization using pins that are placed transversely into a bone, which are then held in place by extra-cutaneous fixation.

External fixators consist of three primary components (Figure 22.1):

1) Pins that are inserted transverse into the bone.
2) An external connecting bar to span the fixator pins.
3) Clamps or some other means to firmly connect the pins to the bar.

22.1 Case Selection

External fixators are very versatile. There are many different configurations that can be applied to different bones. They were first used on distal bones, such as the radius and tibia, since these bones are away from the body wall and have a smaller muscle mass. External fixators can also be used on the femur and humerus in certain circumstances, but there is a higher morbidity due to the muscle mass around these bones. External fixators are also used to stabilize mandibular fractures.

The cost of pins and clamps is generally lower compared with orthopedic plates and screws. Many times, the clamps can be reused from patient to patient—although with time the clamps may deteriorate and not hold as well.

External fixators are frequently used in birds and exotics. The external fixation can be extremely lightweight. The pins are ultimately removed, leaving the bird without extra metal to alter its balance or ability to fly.

External fixators can be used in areas of infection, open fractures, gunshot wounds, or degloving injuries. This allows the wounds to be managed properly while supporting the bones during the healing process.

External fixators also allow for destabilization as the fracture heals. Initially, the fracture may need extra support but, as the fracture starts to heal, pins can be removed in order to transfer more weight to the healing bone. This further induces additional bone healing if the pins are removed at the appropriate time.

22.2 Basic Rules of External Fixation

22.2.1 Pins

External skeletal fixator (ESF) pins may be the most critical component of the system, since the bone–pin interface is the limiting factor between success and failure. In the early conception of ESFs, smooth pins were used as fixator pins. These pins loosened rapidly, leading to failure of the fixation. Positive profile pins were introduced and have superior holding power to smooth pins or negative profile pins. Positive profile pins are pins with the thread machined onto the pin, so the thread diameter is larger than the pin diameter. Pin insertion techniques were changed to increase the holding power and strength of the positive profile pin. These pins are cost-effective and widely available (Figure 22.2).

Several types of ESF pins have been developed in different sizes (Figure 22.3). These include centrally and end-threaded pins. The centrally threaded pins are drilled through both the near and far cortices of the bone and connecting bars are attached on both sides of the limb. The end-threaded pins, or half-pins, are drilled into the near cortex and threads penetrate the far cortex without exiting the skin on the far side. A connecting bar is placed on only one side of the bone. Very small fixation pins are also available for use in birds, small mammals, and exotics.

There are some newer pins from IMEX, called Duraface™ pins, which are a negative profile pin that has

Fracture Management for the Small Animal Practitioner, First Edition. Edited by Anne M. Sylvestre.
© 2019 John Wiley & Sons, Inc. Published 2019 by John Wiley & Sons, Inc.

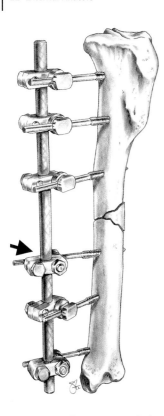

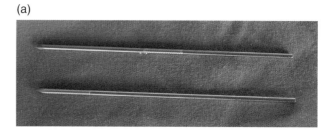

(a)

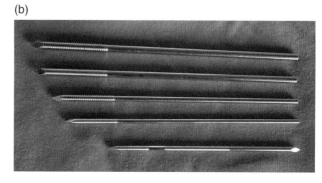

(b)

Figure 22.3 Examples of positive profile fixation pins used for linear external skeletal fixators. (a) End-threaded pins and centrally threaded pins. *Source:* Courtesy IMEX Veterinary Inc., Longview TX. (b) Positive profile pins in varying sizes.

Figure 22.1 Components of a linear external skeletal fixator. This illustration shows a Type I external skeletal fixator on the medial aspect of the tibia. Positive profile pins have been drilled into the bone connected to clamps, which are also connected to a bar. The part of the clamp that holds the pin is placed closest to the bone. *Source:* Courtesy IMEX Veterinary Inc., Longview TX.

(a)

(b)

(c)

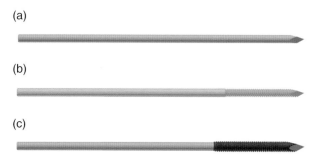

Figure 22.2 Examples of fixation pins used for linear external skeletal fixators. (a) Smooth pin; (b) negative profile pin; and (c) positive profile pin. *Source:* Courtesy IMEX Veterinary Inc., Longview TX.

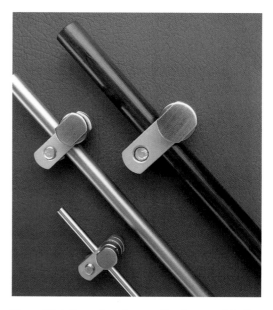

Figure 22.4 Examples of connecting bars used for linear external skeletal fixators. Carbon fiber (top, black), titanium (center), and stainless steel (bottom, small). *Source:* Courtesy IMEX Veterinary Inc., Longview TX.

similar properties to the positive profile pin, for those individuals who prefer to use negative profile pins.

22.2.2 Connecting Bars

There are many types of connecting bars. In the original Kirschner–Ehmer system, stainless steel bars were used. These bars were not very stiff. The development of titanium, aluminum, and carbon fiber rods has improved the stiffness and strength of ESF constructs (Figure 22.4).

22.2.3 Clamps

External skeletal fixation clamps come in different styles depending on the manufacturer. Newer clamps are stronger and more versatile, in that they can accommodate different size pins in the construct. Clamps are easily added or subtracted as needed. Most surgeons reuse ESF clamps as a means of decreasing costs. There

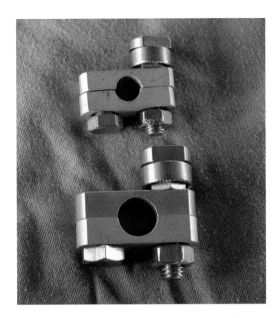

Figure 22.5 Examples of external skeletal fixator clamps.

is evidence that, over time, these clamps may lose some holding power, but it does not appear to be clinically significant (Figure 22.5).

Acrylic constructs using polymethylmethacrylate (PMMA) or epoxy putty have been used to make a connecting bar between ESF pin ends. This is a simple and economic alternative as it eliminates connecting bars and clamps. Using connecting bars of PMMA makes destabilization of the fracture more difficult, since the construct is difficult to cut. When using PMMA, it is usually easier to use a hanging leg technique for the tibia and the radius. By leaving the limb suspended from a pole or ceiling during the process, this leaves your hands free to manage the PMMA (Figure 22.6). When applying an external fixator to the tibia, the bone will usually come into better alignment if the assistant places the limb under tension while holding onto the calcaneus rather than the toes.

22.3 Fundamentals of Application

Proper application is essential to preventing complications.

Safe corridors are used to avoid placing pins through large muscle groups or neurovascular bundles.

Selection of the proper pin size is a function of the size of the bone as well as the size of the patient. The pin diameter should be no more than 20–25% of the bone diameter. Pins should be placed at least 1 cm away from the fracture. Fissures should be avoided as the drilling of a pin into a fissure line could cause additional fractures, resulting in loss of fixation. In general, pins should be placed along the entire length of the bone. This will reduce the load on the pins closest to the fracture.

Release incisions should be at least 1 cm in length.

Pilot holes are predrilled for pin placement. Direct placement of the positive profile pin with a high-speed drill leads to thermal necrosis, microfracture of the bone, and subsequent pin loosening. Low-speed predrilling of a pilot hole 10% smaller than the pin diameter eliminates these problems [1] (Figure 22.7).

The number of pins in each fracture fragment is important for adequate stability. A minimum of two pins are placed above and below the fracture, but three or four is better to avoid premature pin loosening. Three to four pins in each major fracture segment also increases the stiffness of the construct. Five or more pins in each segment provides no additional benefit. Selecting an appropriate ESF construct is also critical. Different frame constructs will be discussed; however, with the development of stronger pins, clamps, and bars, complex frame configurations and multiple bars and planes of application are not needed as frequently.

22.4 Fixators: Biomechanics/Constructs (Figure 22.8)

- Type IA – Unilateral uniplanar: Type IA fixators are usually applied to the medial side of the radius and tibia and the lateral surface of the humerus and femur. The fixation pins are referred to as half-pins because they only penetrate the skin on one side. These pins are driven through both cortices, but only penetrate the near skin surface.
- Type IB – Unilateral biplanar: Type IB fixators are applied most often to the tibia. On the tibia, the bars are placed on the medial and cranial surfaces of the bone.
- Type II – Bilateral uniplanar: Type II configurations are used primarily on the tibia and the radius because of the proximity of the body wall. These configurations are usually placed in the mediolateral plane.
- Type III – Bilateral biplanar: Type III fixators can only be applied to the tibia or radius due to the proximity of the body wall to the femur and humerus. Fractures requiring this type of construct are better left in the hands of a trained surgeon.
- ESF with intra-medullary (IM) pin tie-in.
- Humeral and femoral fractures are not usually stabilized with external fixators alone because of the proximity to the body wall. Type II and Type III constructs, which are the most stable, cannot be applied to these bones. To provide sufficient strength with complicated humeral and femoral fractures, an IM pin combined with a Type Ia external fixator can be used. Normally the number of fixation pins is limited to two pins placed above and two pins placed below the fracture.

(a)

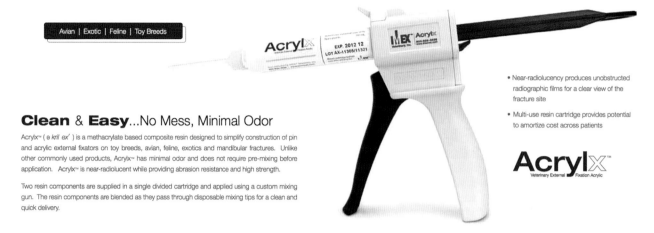

Avian | Exotic | Feline | Toy Breeds

Clean & Easy...No Mess, Minimal Odor

Acrylx™ (ə *kril ex'*) is a methacrylate based composite resin designed to simplify construction of pin and acrylic external fixators on toy breeds, avian, feline, exotics and mandibular fractures. Unlike other commonly used products, Acrylx™ has minimal odor and does not require pre-mixing before application. Acrylx™ is near-radiolucent while providing abrasion resistance and high strength.

Two resin components are supplied in a single divided cartridge and applied using a custom mixing gun. The resin components are blended as they pass through disposable mixing tips for a clean and quick delivery.

- Near-radiolucency produces unobstructed radiographic films for a clear view of the fracture site
- Multi-use resin cartridge provides potential to amortize cost across patients

Acrylx™
Veterinary External Fixation Acrylic

(b)

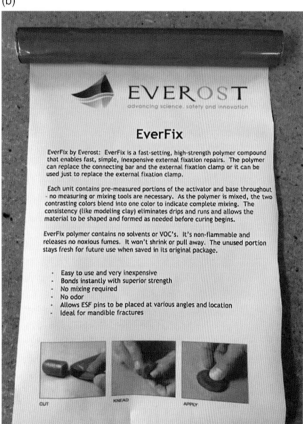

Figure 22.6 Examples of commercially available acrylic products. (a) IMEX Acrylx™. (b) EverFix™ putty from Everost.

- To provide additional strength, the IM pin exiting the femur or the humerus can be "tied in" to the Type Ia external fixator construct either with an acrylic splint or an additional short segment of external bar (Figure 22.9).

22.4.1 Acrylic Splints/Constructs

Application of acrylic bars (polymethymethacrylate) or epoxy bars is fairly simple. This is usually done with the limb hanging in proper alignment. Plastic tubing is generally used to hold the acrylic or epoxy while it solidifies.

(a)
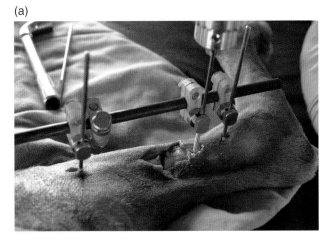
(b)
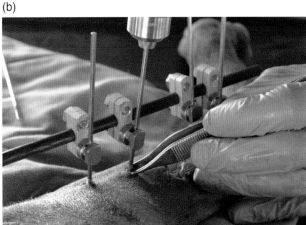

Figure 22.7 Pilot holes should be drilled through the clamps. (a) The IMEX clamps also allow for pin placement through the clamp. (b) Pins may also be placed at an angle through the clamps.

If postoperative radiographs show improper pin placement or malalignment of the fracture, it is more difficult to correct the problem.

22.4.2 Circular External Fixators

Circular external skeletal fixation (CESF) systems use pins of small diameter (1.5–2.0 mm) tension wires instead of rigid ones; this allows for controlled axial micro motion at a fracture or osteotomy site. The micro motion is not enough to compromise stability but will stimulate callus formation [2]. This technique is very versatile allowing fixation of very small bone fragments with the thin wires, dynamic distraction, or compression of bone fragments. While the CESF shares many common principles with conventional ESF, there is a significant learning curve to become proficient with this technique and therefore it will not be discussed in further detail.

22.5 Postoperative Care

Postoperative analgesia should be provided.

The fixator, pin–skin interface, and limb should be cleaned of any blood and debris. The pin–skin interface should be cleaned with an antiseptic solution.

A topical antibiotic ointment is first placed at the pin–skin interface to decrease microbial contamination and migration from the skin surface. Sterile gauze sponges should be wrapped around and between each pin.

A non-adherent padding is then placed between the fixator and the skin. Rinsed and dried surgical scrub sponges work well for this. If foam is used, slits should be cut in the foam to facilitate placement around the fixation pins.

The limb and fixator are then wrapped in cast padding or cotton beginning at the digits and extending proximal to the fixator.

This bandage absorbs exudate from the release incision and decreases postoperative swelling. The compression also reduces motion between the skin and the fixator pins. Excessive motion can cause increased drainage and potential loosening of the pins.

A compressive bandage is kept in place until postoperative swelling has subsided.

The initial bandage is changed 24–48 hours after surgery. Another compressive bandage is then placed. After approximately 1 week, gauze packing can be discontinued.

After the compressive bandage is no longer needed, another bandage is placed over the fixator to protect the construct as well as the owners and the animal from damage or injury due to impact or entrapment of the frame on other objects. After the animal is released from the hospital, postoperative examinations should be performed every 2 weeks for the first 6 weeks. The pin–skin interface is examined for drainage or irritation. The outer bandage is changed every 2 weeks. Dogs are maintained on postoperative cephalexin for 2 weeks while the skin incisions heal around the pins. If drainage is seen around any of the pins, this could be a sign of infection or loosening of a pin. A radiograph is taken 6 weeks postoperatively to assess bone healing. If there is sufficient healing, a very stable construct, such as a Type III, may be destabilized to allow more transfer of weight into the fracture to speed healing of the fracture. The entire fixator is removed once the bone has healed. This is usually 12–16 weeks after surgery, but depends on the patient age, activity, and the type of fracture [3]. Once all of the pins are removed, the dog should continue with reduced

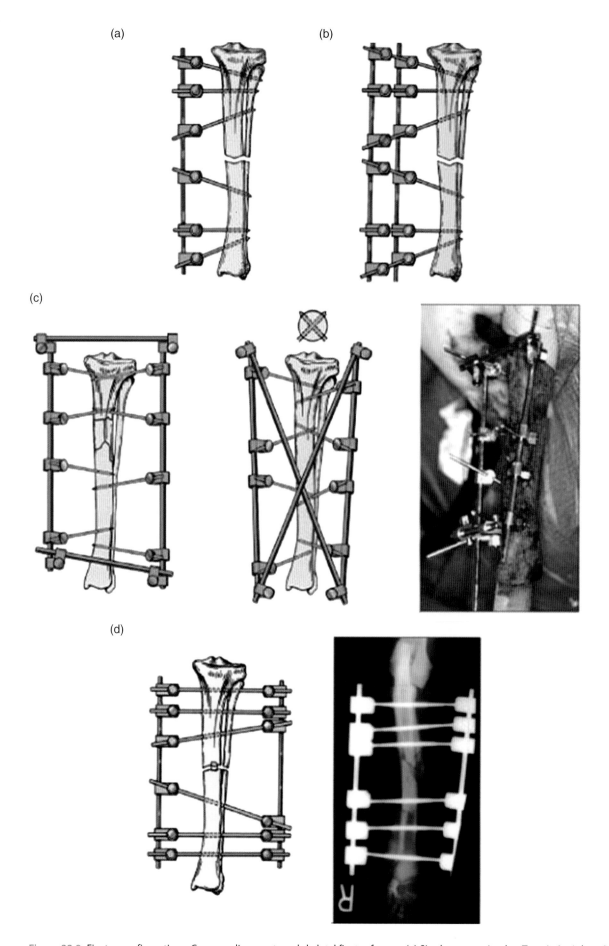

Figure 22.8 Fixator configurations. Common linear external skeletal fixator frames. (a) Single connecting bar Type Ia (uniplanar). (b) Double connecting bar Type Ia (uniplanar). (c) Type Ib (unilateral biplanar). (d) Type IIa (bilateral). (e) Type IIb (bilateral). (f) Type III (bilateral biplanar). (g) Double clamp Type Ia. Note how the non-threaded pins are placed at a 70° angle. *Source:* From [4].

(e)

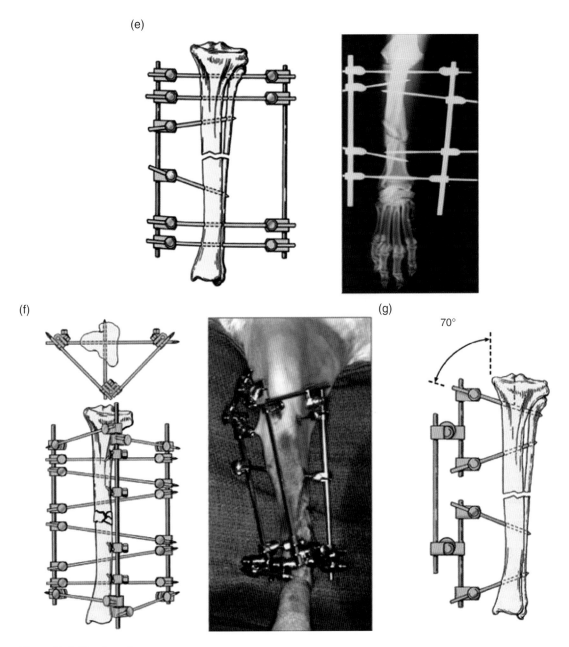

(f)

(g)

Figure 22.8 (Continued)

activity for another 3–4 weeks while the pin holes in the bone start to heal.

22.6 Complications

Normally, the pin tracts will produce a small amount of serous discharge for the first few days. This is then followed by the formation of a dry scab. If drainage persists, increases, or becomes purulent or serosanguinous, the surgeon must determine the source of the problem. Cleaning of the pin tracts with chlorhexidine or povidone iodine solution is usually indicated. Systemic antibiotics may be required in some cases. Persistent pin drainage, especially accompanied by lameness, is almost always a sign that one or more pins are loose and must be removed.

(a)　　　　　　(b)

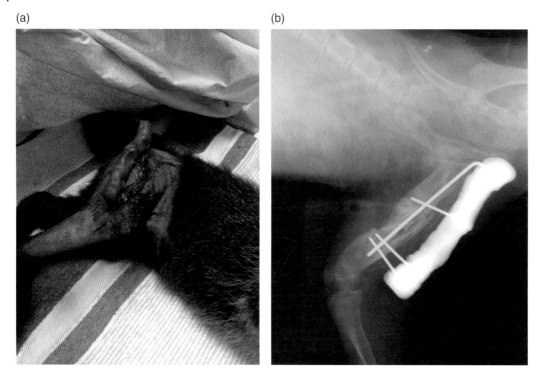

Figure 22.9 Example of a Type I external skeletal fixator with a tie-in placed on the femur of a coatimundi using EverFix™ from Everost (a). Radiographs show healing at 6 weeks, just prior to removal (b).

22.7 Preferred Technique for Various Long Bones

22.7.1 Tibial Fractures

In general, the author places Type IB fixators on most tibia fractures. Three pins are placed above and below the fracture. For a straightforward two-piece fracture, the author will place two pins above and two pins below the fracture on the medial aspect of the bone and then one to two pins above and one to two below the fracture in the cranial plane.

22.7.2 Humeral Fractures

The author likes to use a Type I fixator with an IM pin tied into the fixator. In smaller animals, the IM pin can be bent to a 90° angle, so it is easily incorporated into the Type I fixator. The author prefers to use acrylic (PMMA) fixators for this application so they do not interfere with normal daily activity, but manufactured Kirshner–Ehmer clamps also work well. The addition of the IM pin provides additional stability to bending forces (Figure 22.10).

22.7.3 Femoral Fractures

The author prefers to plate femoral fractures. If there is a cost issue and the owner cannot afford a plate and screws, the author will use a Type I fixator with an IM pin for a simple two-piece fracture or an IM pin and cerclage. Severely comminuted fractures or fractures with multiple fissures should be stabilized by a trained surgeon.

22.7.4 Radial Fractures

The author does not place fixators on the radius of dogs weighing less than 10 lb (4.5 kg). These dogs have decreased blood supply to the distal radius and will heal with fewer complications with a plate/screw technique. Type II fixators can be used on severely comminuted fractures of the radius in dogs >15 kg. The pins are placed using a hanging leg technique to maintain alignment of the limb.

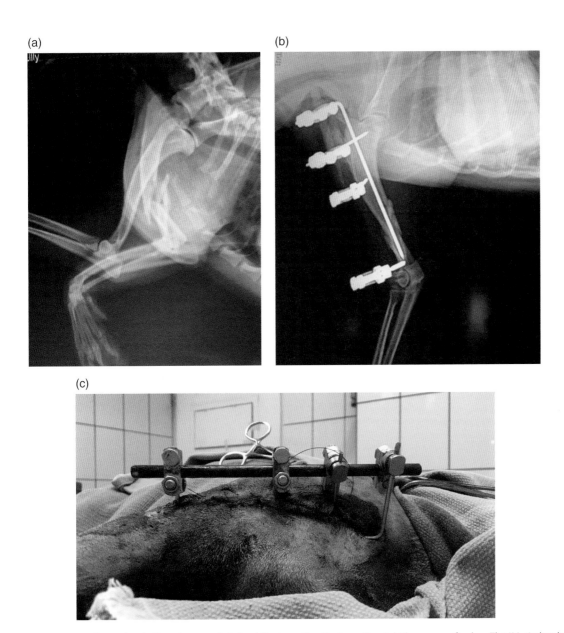

Figure 22.10 Example of a Type I external skeletal fixator with a tie-in on the right humerus of a dog. The IM pin has been bent to a 90° angle and connected to the Type I fixator. (a) Preoperative radiographs. (b) Postoperative radiograph. (c) Postoperative picture prior to applying a bandage to cover the apparatus.

References

1 DeCamp, C.E., Johnston, S.A., Dejardin, L.M., and Schaefer, S.L. (2016). *Brinker, Piermattei, and Flo's Handbook of Small Animals Orthopedics and Fracture Repair*, 5e. St. Louis, MO: Elsevier.

2 Lewis, D.D., Lanz, O.I., and Welch, R.D. (1998). Biomechanics of circular external skeletal fixation. *Vet. Surg.* 27: 454–464.

3 Fossum, T.W. (2002). *Small Animal Surgery*, 2e. St. Louis, MO: Mosby.

4 Tobias, K.M. and Johnston, S.A. (2012). *Veterinary Surgery Small Animal*. St Louis, MO: Elsevier/Saunders.

23

Repair of Physeal Fractures

Thomas W.G. Gibson

Ontario Veterinary College, University of Guelph, Guelph, Ontario, Canada

Treatment of fractures in the immature veterinary patient can be both challenging and very rewarding. As with all fractures the goal of treatment is return to full function with early, active, pain-free movement and full weight bearing. In the case of immature animals, success is most often achieved when fractures are diagnosed and treated quickly following injury. This is largely due to the fact that immature animals will begin the healing process quickly. This rapid healing is a distinct advantage when treating fractures in immature animals as the fractured bone will quickly assume load sharing responsibilities with the orthopedic implants used in the repair postoperatively. In some cases, this characteristic will make some fractures amenable to external coaptation as a definitive treatment. This rapid healing can also be a curse when fractures in immature animals are misdiagnosed or definitive treatment is delayed for some reason. The rapid production of fibrous tissue and callus at the site of the fracture can interfere with surgical reduction and alignment when definitive internal fixation is attempted. In some cases when treatment is delayed, the fracture may heal in a malaligned fashion requiring correction of rotation and alignment by osteotomy.

Simple, inexpensive instrumentation is required for internal fixation using crossed pin and pin and tension band techniques (Figure 23.1).

23.1 Physeal Fractures

Physeal fractures constitute up to 30% of appendicular fractures in immature dogs [1]. Salter–Harris (SH) I and II are the most common types of fractures, representing 77% of physeal fractures [1]. Physeal fractures or "slipped physes" can occur throughout the immature skeleton due to the presence of cartilaginous growth plates. This typically occurs through the zone of hypertrophy of the physis, as this cartilaginous zone is much weaker than the adjacent bone and attached ligamentous structures. In cases of minor trauma, this separation usually does not affect the zone of proliferation and should not affect future growth. When injury is severe or compression of the zone of proliferation of the physis occurs, partial or complete premature closure of the physis can occur, resulting in abnormal growth and the possibility of angular limb deformities. The extent of this injury to the growth plate cannot be predicted at the time of injury or fixation so it becomes critical to counsel owners regarding the need for diligent monitoring, the requirement for recheck examinations and/or radiographic assessment, and the potential for additional surgical procedures in the future.

In most cases, physeal fractures are not amenable to conservative management using external coaptation. External casts or splints may be used successfully in physeal fractures (SH I or II) distal to the stifle and elbow if the animal's conformation allows adequate cast or splint placement. Chondrodystrophic breeds are problematic as are breeds with large thigh muscle mass like mastiffs. Long, slender-legged breeds are ideal. The conditions for successful use of coaptation include anatomical location, as mentioned, as well as the ability to adequately reduce the fracture, and keep it reduced until healing occurs. Closed reduction may result in physeal damage due to shearing forces and may also lead to less than perfect alignment resulting in rotational and/or angular deformities. This approach should also be avoided where muscle traction may lead to displacement of the fracture fragment. SH III and IV fractures are articular and require precise anatomical reconstruction. Conservative management is contraindicated [2].

The majority of physeal fractures are repaired using open reduction and internal fixation (ORIF). These repairs usually involve different configurations of Kirschner wires (K-wires). The veterinary literature contains very few reports of the success of surgical

Fracture Management for the Small Animal Practitioner, First Edition. Edited by Anne M. Sylvestre.

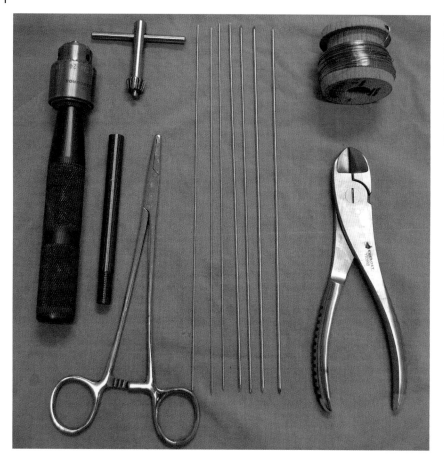

Figure 23.1 Simple instrumentation is required for internal fixation using crossed pin and pin and tension band techniques. (left to right) Jacobs chuck with key and protective sleeve, pin box with an assortment of Kirschner wires and Steinmann pins, pin and wire cutters, orthopedic wire, and pin pullers/wire twisting pliers. A pin bender (not shown) may also be a useful piece of equipment.

outcome of these repairs but the majority report good to excellent function following ORIF. Damage to the physis may result in poor physeal function following surgical repair and result in growth abnormalities [3].

Practitioners managing physeal fractures in immature patients need to be well versed in the Salter–Harris classification system for describing the fracture, for deciding on the ideal method of fixation, and for providing a prognosis. Because of the very distal location of most physeal fractures, the use of K-wires or small Steinman pins placed in a crossed fashion is the most common internal fixation method.

23.1.1 Crossed Pin Technique

A useful way of counteracting rotational forces when treating physeal fractures with intra-medullary fixation is by using crossed pins (K-wires or Steinman pins depending on patient size). Crossed pinning is accomplished by reduction of the fragment followed by driving pins in a normograde fashion on either side across the fracture and exiting through the opposite cortex. The pins should completely exit the opposite cortex but not be left long enough to interfere with soft tissues. In many cases in immature animals the epiphyseal fracture

fragment is very small and immediately adjacent to the joint. A small-gauge hypodermic needle to locate the joint is useful to ensure that the starting point for the pin is outside of the joint. If there is any obliquity to the fracture, driving the pin from the side that will cross the fracture as close to perpendicular as possible will help eliminate shear and loss of reduction when the second pin is driven. The pins must be placed at an angle that results in the pins crossing within the medullary cavity above the fracture line to ensure rotational stability of the repair. The pins should be trimmed flush with the cortex of the epiphyseal fragment using pin cutters. As the immature bone in these patients is very soft, bending of the pins may result in additional fracture of the small epiphyseal fragment and is usually not recommended. On occasion, normograding pins will result in the pin deflecting off the endosteal surface of the trans cortex and failing to purchase and exit the opposite cortex. This is described as placing a pin in a dynamic or "Rush" fashion. In most cases dynamic pinning of one or both pins will result in adequate stabilization if the fragment is well reduced and interdigitates at the fracture ends. Small diameter K-wires should be used: 0.035–0.045″ in toy and small dogs, 0.045–0.062″ for small and medium-sized dogs, and 1/8″ pins are adequate for larger dogs.

23.2 Avulsion Type Physeal Fractures

Avulsion fractures involve the bony attachment of a ligament or tendon. An apophysis is a normal bony outgrowth that arises from a separate ossification center and fuses with the bone in the course of time. The apophysis is also a site of tendon or ligament attachment. Similar to physeal fractures, when excessive forces are present the immature center of ossification is weaker than the tendons and ligaments resulting in avulsion fractures of these bony protuberances. The common locations for this type of fracture are the tibial tuberosity, the greater trochanter, the greater tubercle, and olecranon process. As these fractures are the result of excessive tensile forces, any surgical repair will have to overcome these forces to maintain the stability of the avulsed fragment. In most cases this will be accomplished by a pin and tension band or lag screw repair.

23.2.1 Tension Band Wiring Technique

The goal of tension band wiring is to overcome and actually convert distraction forces caused by muscle pull into compression at the fracture/osteotomy site. Sharp reduction forceps may aid in maintaining reduction but be careful not to split the fragment by applying too much pressure. Two parallel K-wires (0.035, 0.045, 0.062, or 0.8–2.0 mm) are placed relatively perpendicular to the fracture/osteotomy with the pins at the periphery of the cut. This orientation will best facilitate inter-fragmentary compression and limit interference with the tendon. If possible, the K-wires should engage the opposite cortex. Holes are drilled transversely through the bone's main shaft, distal and parallel to the fracture/osteotomy. The distance between these holes and the fracture or osteotomy is roughly equal to the distance from the fracture/osteotomy to the tip of the apophysis.

A wire (22, 20, or 18 gauge or 0.8, 1.0, or 1.2 mm) is passed through the hole in the shaft, crossed on the lateral cortex and under the tendon, as close to the K-wires as possible. Although some authors feel twisting the wire on only one side of the figure-8 pattern is adequate, forming a knot on both sides gives more even tightening. To simplify this, the two separate wires can be used to form the figure-8. One wire is passed through the distal hole and crossed on the lateral cortex, and a shorter wire passed under the tendon next to the pins. The ends of the separate wires are twisted together and tightened by alternating between the two knots until both are secure. The K-wires are then bent laterally 90°, cut off leaving 3–5 mm, and rotated medially to minimize skin irritation. Although these implants may be left in place indefinitely, figure-8 wire breakage or loosening and migration of the K-wires are not uncommon. In this situation removal of both pins and figure-8 wire is recommended.

23.3 Repair Techniques for Various Physeal Fractures

23.3.1 Proximal Humerus

These repairs are performed through a craniolateral approach to the proximal humerus. Due to the epiphyseal attachment of the dome-like humeral head to the glenoid of the scapula, the epiphyseal fragment usually remains in place and the remainder of the humerus is displaced caudolaterally. The interdigitation of the dome-like physis adds relative stability to the fracture repair once reduction is accomplished. Parallel K-wires are placed proximally to distally through the greater tubercle to secure the epiphysis in place. Addition of a tension band wire can add to stability. This fracture can also be stabilized by a single lag screw placed in a similar orientation.

23.3.2 Proximal Ulna

A caudal surgical approach to the ulna allows reduction of the fracture fragment and stabilization by placing two K-wires through the fragment, across the fracture line, and into the proximal ulna. Engaging the trans cortex with these pins will add strength to the repair. A transverse hole is drilled with a drill bit or K-wire through the ulna distal to the fracture line. A figure-8 wire is placed to counteract triceps pull and provide compression of the fracture. Pins are bent and rotated to prevent wires from slipping off the olecranon and to minimize soft tissue irritation.

23.3.3 Proximal Radius

Fractures of the proximal radius are generally reduced with the elbow flexed. SH I fractures are stabilized using a crossed pin technique with a K-wire driven from the proximolateral surface of the radial head near the articular surface, across the fracture, and into the medial cortex of the radius. The second K-wire is inserted from medial to lateral to improve stability.

23.3.4 Distal Radius

Fractures of the distal physis have little soft tissue coverage and may be repaired in a closed fashion with fluoroscopic guidance. Open reduction and repair with cross pins may require small bilateral incisions laterally and medially. This will facilitate adequate exposure ensuring adequate fracture reduction and allow placement of pins in a crossed fashion originating in the radial and ulnar styloid processes and crossing above the physeal fracture line. Careful levering of the distal fracture fragment with a small, thin periosteal elevator is often the most effective way to gently reduce the fracture and avoid damage to the physis.

23.3.5 Greater Trochanter

Internal fixation is accomplished by a craniolateral approach to the hip joint, reduction of the fracture, and stabilization. Stabilization is typically achieved using parallel K-wires placed perpendicularly to the fracture line and augmented with a tension band using orthopedic wire. Alternatively a lag screw combined with an antirotational K-wire can be used. Use of a screw should be reserved for larger dogs due to the risk of fracturing the small, avulsed fragment during screw placement.

23.3.6 Distal Femur

A lateral approach to the distal femur/stifle region is performed. With the stifle in flexion and the hock extended, traction is applied cranially to the proximal tibia, taking advantage of the soft tissues attached to the femoral condyles to pull the distal fragment cranially to achieve reduction. Fortunately the presence of the four metaphyseal pegs in the physis provides some innate stability of the distal fragment and can be used to confirm that the fracture is accurately reduced. Some surgeons recommend over-reduction of the distal fragment in relation to the proximal fragment to increase implant purchase in the small distal fragment. It is debatable if this is superior to normal reduction as some of the innate stability is lost with over-reduction. Stabilization consists of crossed placement of at least two K-wires or Steinmann typically in a normograde fashion. Pins should be started medial and lateral to the femoral trochlea avoiding the articular cartilage. The lateral pin is started just caudal to the origin of the long digital extensor muscle and directed proximally at a 30–40° angle. The medial pin is initiated in approximately the same location from the medial side. Pins are advanced to the fracture; reduction (or over-reduction) is confirmed and then they are driven alternately in a proximal direction across the fracture to engage the trans cortex. As described above, pins must cross above the fracture

to provide maximum stability. On occasion one or both pins will "Rush" or deflect off the inner trans cortex resulting in dynamic rather than crossed pin placement. Both crossed and dynamic pinning have been shown to provide adequate stability.

23.3.7 Tibial Tuberosity

Open reduction and stabilization consists of a craniolateral approach to the tibial tuberosity. With the stifle extended the fragment is reduced and two K-wires or pins are placed side by side through the fragment and into the proximal tibia. Reduction can be facilitated using sharp reduction forceps, but care must be taken to avoid splitting or crushing the soft, immature bone. This author's preferred method is to drive the first pin through the fragment and use the Jacobs chuck to manipulate the fragment. In small patients with minimal displacement, two K-wires may be sufficient to stabilize the fragment. In most cases a pin and tension band is recommended.

23.3.8 Proximal Tibial Physis

In most cases an open reduction is chosen through a craniolateral approach. Traction on the metaphysis of the tibia along with careful levering of the fragment usually is all that is required for accurate reduction. Once reduced, K-wires or small Steinmann pins are placed medially and laterally on the non-articular surface of the epiphyseal fragment, across the physis, and into the tibial metaphysis, crossing distal to the fracture line as previously described. In many cases these two pins are all that is required, but a third pin may be placed in the tibial tuberosity for additional stability.

23.3.9 Distal Tibial Physis

A medial approach is preferred allowing gentle traction and levering to reduce the epiphysis. Pins are inserted in the medial malleolus (tibia) and the lateral malleolus (fibula) across the fracture and into the tibial metaphysis and through the trans tibial cortex. As the epiphyseal fragment is small and the malleoli extend distally to the actual joint space, pins must be angled to avoid penetrating the joint. This acute angle will sometimes result in one or both pins being placed in a dynamic fashion.

References

1 Maretta, S.M. and Schrader, S.C. (1983). Physeal injuries in the dog: a review of 135 cases. *J. Am. Vet. Med. Assoc.* 182: 708–710.

2 Prieur, W.D. (1989). Management of growth plate injuries in puppies and kittens. *J. Small Anim. Pract.* 30: 631–638.

3 Kim, S.E., Hudson, C.C., and Pozzi, A. (2012). Percutaneous pinning for fracture repair in dogs and cats. *Vet. Clin. North Am. Small Anim. Pract.* 42: 963–974.

Recommended Reading

De Camp, C., Johnston, S.A., Déjardin, L.M., and Schaefer, S.L. (2016). *Brinker, Piermattei and Flo's Handbook of Small Animal Orthopedics and Fracture Repair*, 5e. St Louis, MO: Elsevier.

Fossum, T.W. (2013). *Small Animal Surgery*, 4e. Maryland Heights, MO: Mosby.

Johnson, K.A. (2014). *Piermattei's Atlas of Surgical Approaches to the Bones and Joints of the Dog and Cat*, 5e. Philadelphia, PA: Saunders.

Johnson, A.L., Houlton, J.E.F., and Vannini, R. (2006). *AO Principles of Fracture Management in the Dog and Cat*. Stuttgart, Germany: AO Publishing/Thieme.

Tobias, K.M. and Johnson, S.A. (2012). *Veterinary Surgery: Small Animal*. Philadelphia, PA: Saunders.

24

Fractures of the Jaw
Teresa Jacobson

Sitara Animal Hospital, Lake Country, British Columbia, Canada

Jaw fractures occur commonly in cats and dogs as a result of vehicular trauma, falls from heights (especially in cats), blunt force trauma from being hit with, or by, objects (e.g. golf clubs, baseball bats), dog fights (especially in the big dog versus little dog scenario), and/or an altercation with another animal (e.g. kicked by horse). Jaw fractures also occur secondary to periodontal disease, dentigerous cysts, and neoplasia, and iatrogenically during extractions.

24.1 Anatomical Considerations

Jaw fractures, unlike fractures everywhere else in the body, have the added complication of tooth involvement. The jaw is divided into the maxilla and the mandible. The upper jaw, the maxilla (Figures 24.1 and 24.2), contains the maxillary, incisive, palatine, zygomatic, lacrimal, frontal, and nasal bones [1]. The nasal cavity, the infraorbital bundle, the palatine vessels, the cranial nerves, the orbit, and the maxillary recesses make fractures of the maxilla particularly challenging [2].

The lower jaw (Figure 24.3) consists of paired bones, the left and the right mandibles joined at the rostral aspect by a ligamentous or cartilaginous union, making a separation of the rostral mandible a ligamentous separation rather than a fracture [2]. The dorsal two-thirds of the mandible contain the roots of the mandibular teeth and the ventral one-third contains the mandibular canal with its corresponding mandibular vein, artery, and nerve bundle. The rostral aspect of the mandible contains the body (cranial horizontal part) and the ramus (caudal horizontal aspect) of the mandible contains the coronoid, the condylar, and the angular process [3]. The mandible has two sides that must be identified for fracture repair: the compression side of the mandible, the ventral or alveolar border, and the tension side of the mandible where the teeth are located [4]. The large masticatory muscles that close the jaw are the masseter, temporalis, and pterygoideus, which pull the caudal mandible in a dorsal fashion [5, 6]. The digastricus and sublingual muscles in the rostral aspect of the jaw pull the rostral mandible in a caudoventral motion to open the jaw [5, 6]. Fractures of the mandible are often referred to as favorable or unfavorable depending on whether the fracture line extends in the caudodorsal direction—a favorable fracture line (Figure 24.4)—or in the caudoventral direction—an unfavorable fracture (Figure 24.5). When there is an unfavorable fracture the thick masticatory muscles that close and open the jaw pull the fracture apart and make the fracture repair more challenging [5]. A favorable fracture may be stabilized with a simple tape muzzle or a simple intra-osseous wire. An unfavorable fracture will require more invasive techniques such as intra-osseous wires, interdental wiring with acrylic reinforcement, or referral for repair with mini plates [5]. Fractures of the maxilla are less common than fractures of the mandible. The maxilla is a "box" so when there is a maxillary fracture there is usually more than one. The average number of maxillary fractures is five and it is common to have epistaxis as a clinical sign when there is a fracture of the maxilla. The compression side of the maxilla is the nasal chamber. Complications with maxillary fractures include airway obstruction due to nasal sinus obstruction from the fracture itself or due to the epistaxis.

24.2 Jaw Fracture Management

Oral fracture repair requires a skilled clinician with adequate magnification and good lighting, diagnostic intraoral and extra oral radiographs to assess the extent

Fracture Management for the Small Animal Practitioner, First Edition. Edited by Anne M. Sylvestre.
© 2019 John Wiley & Sons, Inc. Published 2019 by John Wiley & Sons, Inc.

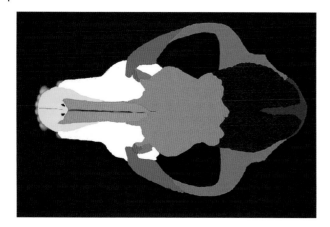

Figure 24.1 Bones of the maxilla in a dorsal view. Yellow = incisive bone, teal = nasal bone, white = maxilla bone, green = zygomatic bone, brown = temporal bone, pink = frontal bone, gray = palatine bone, orange = lacrimal bone, purple = parietal bone, red = occipital bone.

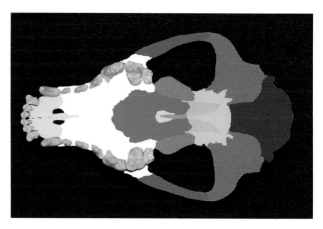

Figure 24.2 Bones of the maxilla in a ventral view. Yellow = incisive bone, white = maxilla bone, green = zygomatic bone, brown = temporal bone, pink = frontal bone, gray = palatine bone, purple = parietal bone, red = occipital bone, beige = vomer bone, lavender = pterygoid bone, blue = basisphenoid bone.

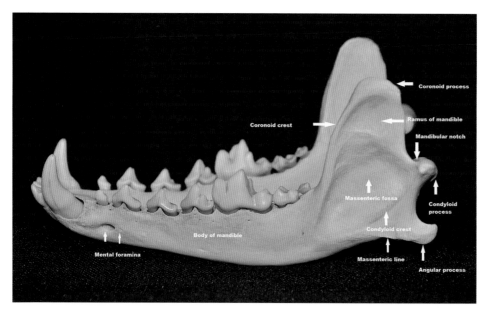

Figure 24.3 The mandible with arrows indicating the mental foramina, the body of the mandible, the mesenteric line, the angular process, the condyloid crest, the masseteric fossa, the mandibular notch, the coronoid crest, the coronoid process, the condyloid process, and the ramus of the mandible.

of injuries, financial commitment of the owner, and special consideration for anesthesia and for patient feeding and care postoperatively.

24.2.1 The Principles of Jaw Fracture Management

The patient must be handled gently and no harm must be done with every step of the treatment.

The patient is stabilized, treated for shock and other life-threatening injuries.

Awake examination of the patient's head includes:

- evaluation for soft tissue injuries;
- bleeding from the ears, nose, and oral cavity;
- assessment of the eyes for trauma;
- assessment of dental occlusion [7].

The goal is for a return to normal occlusion/function so there can be normal mastication as soon as possible.

Soft tissues are handled gently to preserve, protect, and minimize morbidity.

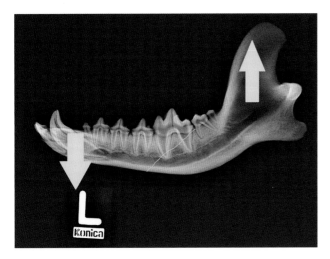

Figure 24.4 The arrows depicting the pull of the muscle on the mandible. The forces of the muscles will actually assist in maintaining the fracture reduction. This is considered a "favorable" fracture. The fracture line runs from ventral on the rostral mandible to dorsal on the caudal mandible.

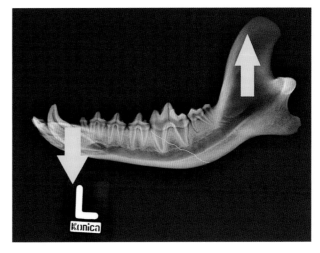

Figure 24.5 Arrows depict the external muscle forces on the fracture site. The forces on this "unfavorable" fracture will pull the rostral portion of the jaw ventrally and the caudal portion of the jaw dorsally. The external forces will not assist in maintaining fracture reduction. The fracture line runs from dorsal on the rostral mandible to ventral on the caudal mandible.

Tooth roots are avoided, as well as the mandibular neurovascular bundle, the maxillary vessels and nerves, and the eye (which is very vulnerable especially in small dogs and cats with maxillary fractures). The hardware is kept to a minimum (the fewer implants, the better).

The forces on the fracture line are neutralized to stabilize the jaw and promote boney union.

The patient and client must be supported with attentive and intensive aftercare (that means daily telephone calls if necessary and at least weekly recheck examinations).

24.2.2 Intubation Considerations for the Fracture Repair

When the patient has been adequately stabilized for anesthesia and an appropriate anesthetic plan has been formulated, the next step is to consider maintenance of occlusion. With jaw fracture repair it is essential to maintain normal occlusion. To assess occlusion it is necessary to open and close the jaw as many times as necessary to get the job done. This can be done by extubating and re-intubating the patient, but this method is time-consuming and increases anesthetic risk for the patient, especially in cats, where there is a risk of laryngeal spasm. It is critical to keep the mouth and, especially, the laryngeal area free of blood, debris, and packing if the patient is to be extubated and intubated multiple times. This method, along with increased anesthetic risk, will add time to the overall procedure as well as increasing the anesthetic time for the patient and normal occlusion may not be maintained after re-intubation [8, 9]. One alternative is to use a short endotracheal tube, cut so that when disconnected from

the anesthetic gas line it is entirely within the mouth, allowing the jaw to close and assess normal occlusion. The cost is minimal as the endotracheal tube is cut to fit that specific case.

Another alternative is to intubate the patient initially via pharyngostomy. This method allows the clinician to manipulate the oral cavity without risk of interfering with the endotracheal tube and allows for normal closure of the jaw to assess normal occlusion during the fracture repair procedure. Placement of the pharyngotomy tube requires some knowledge of the anatomical landmarks. It is necessary to know where the carotid arteries, the linguofacial vein, vagosympathetic trunk, and recurrent laryngeal nerves are located [8]. The site for pharyngostomy endotracheal tube placement is more rostral than the site used for pharyngostomy feeding tube placement. This is an important point. Performing a pharyngostomy requires training: text books are not meant to teach technique. Technique is taught in "hands on" wet labs.

24.2.3 Feeding Plan Post Jaw Fracture Repair

The goal of the jaw fracture repair is to return the patient's mouth to normal function as soon as possible. It is amazing that many patients will lap gruel immediately postoperatively or within a day of jaw fracture repair. Many patients will need, or benefit from, alternative feeding methods while the jaw is in the healing process. Feeding tube placement should be considered prior to surgical manipulation and placed during the anesthesia for the initial fracture repair. It is not ideal to repair the jaw and then re-anesthetize the patient to place a feeding tube when it is discovered that the patient is not eating well, or not at all, with the appliance or repair that was implemented for the jaw fracture. It is especially critical if the patient is going to have the canines bonded as part of the fracture stabilization procedure. There are three options for feeding tube placement: nasogastric, esophageal, and gastrostomy. The nasogastric feeding tubes tend to cause more patient discomfort during and in between feedings than an esophageal feeding tube. The pressure that can be applied and the volume fed through a nasogastric feeding tubes are less due to the smaller diameter of the tube required to fit through the nose, especially noted in cats. This will require that the client take longer to feed the patient through the nasogastric feeding tube when compared with an esophageal feeding tube. The placement of a gastrostomy feeding tube requires more skill than placement of a nasogastric or esophageal feeding tube. Placement of an esophageal feeding tube is simple and takes less than 5 minutes to accomplish.

The materials required for placing a feeding tube include:

- An appropriate sized feeding tube, French red rubber will do but a silicone feeding tube is preferred.
- Sterile surgical gloves.
- A scalpel blade (#15).
- Scalpel handle.
- Large curved (Kelly) hemostat.
- Non-absorbable polypropylene suture 2/0 or 3/0.
- Kitty Kollar™ and absorbent pads (Vet Wrap and cling can be used as an alternative).

The appropriate sizes of feeding tubes are: 10–12 French (F) for cats and small dogs, 16–18 F for 10–15 kg and 18–20 F for greater than 20 kg [8]. A French red rubber tube is adequate but they tend to harden over time with exposure to salivary secretions, making them much less flexible and presumably less comfortable for the patient if they are left in for long-term use (6–8 weeks or longer). A better option is a silicone feeding tube, which maintains its softness in the presence of salivary secretions.

As mentioned earlier, the site for pharyngostomy endotracheal tube placement is more rostral than the site used for pharyngotomy feeding tube placement. This is an important point as the placement of a feeding tube at the rostral location in front of the epihyoid may cause entrapment of the epiglottis and thus possible airway obstruction of the patient.

Figure 24.6 details the placement of an esophageal feeding tube. The feeding tube is premeasured by holding the tube against the cat or dog from the ear to the 8th or 13th rib (some controversy exists as to whether the tube should terminate in the mid-esophagus or just before the cardia in the stomach) [10]. The landmarks for placement of an esophagostomy feeding tube are similar to the landmarks for the pharyngostomy site for the pharyngotomy endotracheal tube. Just to review, the important anatomical features are the carotid arteries, the linguofacial vein, vagosympathetic trunk, and recurrent laryngeal nerves [8, 9]. The feeding tube placement is radiographed to ensure correct placement and to be sure there are no surprises such as calculus or tooth fragments in the esophagus that may be lodged as a complication of the initial trauma. Placement of a feeding tube should always be considered in the case of combination maxillary and mandibular fractures. It is easier to remove a feeding tube that is no longer in use after stoma formation in 10 days than it is to place a feeding tube with a second anesthetic after the jaw fracture repair has been completed and the patient is not eating well. The esophageal feeding tubes are generally well tolerated by the patient and relatively easy for the client to manage as well. The esophageal feeding tube is secured by using non-absorbable suture such as nylon in a Chinese finger tie or by adhesive tape around the feeding tube and sutures placed through the tape. The tube is further secured by the use of a Kitty Kollar which comes in a multitude of sizes for appropriate patient fit and comfort. Often the patient will tolerate the esophageal feeding tube with the Kitty Kollar on without the additional use of an Elizabethan collar making the patient's return to normal function more immediate. If a Kitty Kollar is not available, the feeding tube may be bandaged in using conform and Vet Wrap.

24.3 Pain Management

Pain management in jaw fracture repair is crucial pre-op, intra-op, and postoperatively. Multi-modal analgesia must be applied to prevent pain in the patient. The use of non-steroidal anti-inflammatories, opioids, intraoral regional nerve blocks, and general anesthesia is necessary in our animal patients to provide adequate pain control. Intraoral regional nerve blocks can increase patient safety, allow earlier discharge, decrease costs, are good for client relations, and decrease patient morbidity [11]. Placing intraoral nerve blocks before beginning treatment helps prevent "wind-up." The use of oral regional nerve blocks allows the anesthetist to decrease the vaporizer settings, which allows for optimal cardiac output, respiratory rate, blood pressure, and tissue perfusion and oxygenation [11, 12].

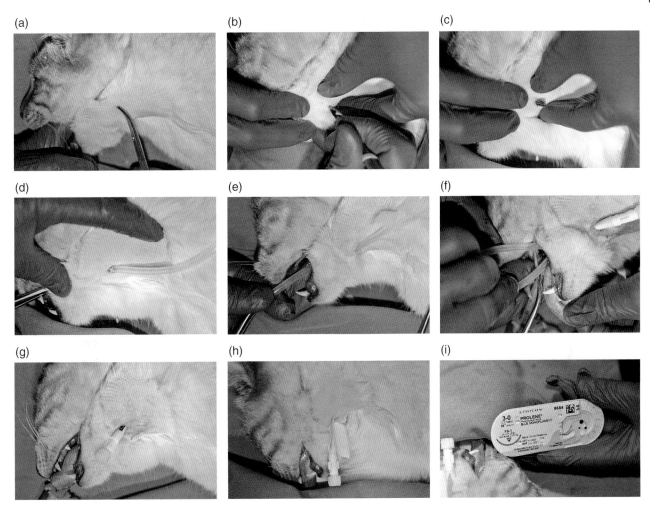

Figure 24.6 Placing an esophageal feeding tube. A large curved hemostat (Kelly) is placed into the oral cavity ventral to the caudal angle of the mandible, behind the wing of the atlas and caudal and dorsal to the thyrohyoid bone, which can be palpated digitally with the index finger from the pharynx. A hemostat indicates the point where the tip of the Kelly is palpable (a). An incision is made over the palpable tip of the Kelly hemostat, just large enough to allow the passage of the esophageal feeding tube (b). The tip of the large hemostat (Kelly) is pushed through the incision (c). The end of the feeding tube is grasped with the Kelly hemostat and pulled into the oropharynx and mouth (d and e). The feeding tube is reversed back on itself using the hemostat to force it back down the pharynx carefully past the endotracheal tube into the esophagus (f). The feeding tube needs to be in a straight line from the incision on the neck toward the stomach (g). The feeding tube is secured with tape or a Chinese finger trap tie (h). Using a colored non-absorbable suture allows easier location of the sutures for removal at a later date (i). If using tape to secure the feeding tube, the tape is sutured to the skin with non-absorbable suture (j). A radiograph is taken to confirm the location of the feeding tube between the eighth and ninth ribs (k). An absorbent Kitty Kollar pad is placed around the feeding tube; a make-up removal pad can easily be used by making a central hole in it (l). A Kitty Kollar is placed over the feeding tube and the absorbent pad (m). The finished result of placement of an esophageal feeding tube in a cat (n).

24.4 Maxillofacial Fracture Repair

There are many different non-invasive jaw fracture repair techniques that can be utilized to repair jaw fractures. The use of tape muzzles or commercial nylon muzzles is suitable and sufficient for certain jaw fractures in some patients. Nylon or tape muzzles are also a nice additional support for other types of jaw fracture repair.

Interdental bonding, interdental wiring, and acrylic reinforcement are other options for jaw fracture repair that are relatively inexpensive and not as technically challenging as some of the more invasive methods of jaw fracture repair, and are considered adequate in many jaw fracture cases. There are four types of interdental wiring that can be used along the maxilla and mandible when the stabilization of the jaw is required. They are: the Ivy loop; the Stout's multiple loop, Essig's,

(j)

(k)

(l)

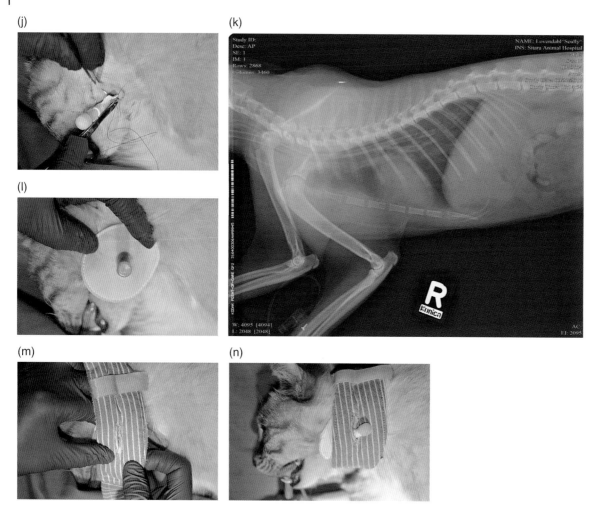

(m)

(n)

Figure 24.6 (Continued)

and the Risdon techniques with acrylic re-enforcement. When there is symphyseal separation, symphyseal wiring can be used. Direct osseous wiring can also be used as a primary or secondary fracture repair technique. Some of these techniques are described in detail below. Inter-arcade bonding can be used for maxillomandibular fixation; also acrylic splint techniques for edentulous patients with maxillary or mandibular fractures.

Other methods of fracture repair can be used, such as mini plates and screws, and are not discussed in this chapter as they require extensive training and can easily cause iatrogenic trauma in the hands of the inexperienced. The use of external fixators is a bad choice for maxillofacial fracture repair because of the short width of the mandible and maxilla.

The following materials are required for non-invasive fracture repair techniques:
- The ability to obtain diagnostic intraoral and extraoral radiographs.
- A high-speed hand piece (to assist in implant placement and tooth extraction if necessary).
- Low-speed polisher and flour pumice for polishing.
- Sterile surgical gloves.
- Orthopedic wire (20, 22, or 24 gauge) depending on the size of the patient.
- 18 or 20 gauge needles (needle must be larger than the wire).
- Wire twisters (an old pair of needle drivers will do this job adequately).
- Wire cutters (a pair with a fine narrow nose from a hardware store will do the job).
- Scalpel blade and handle to incise the soft tissues (prevents burrs or wires from twisting tissue).
- Periosteal elevators are also necessary to lift soft tissues gently from bone and expose the fracture sites when necessary.
- Phosphoric acid tooth etching material.
- Cold curing acrylic material, cartridges, mixing tips, and a delivery gun for the acrylic.

- Flowable composite and a light cure gun (not absolutely necessary if using dual cure composite but helpful and handy to have).
- Diamond burrs or a Goldie burr.

It is essential to have the ability to obtain intraoral radiographs and larger conventional extra oral radiographs as well. Skulls are useful tools to assist in restoration of normal occlusion and to assist the clinician in avoiding the vital structures such as tooth roots, vessels (the foramen are essential landmarks), and the orbit. It is very helpful to also have flowable light cure composite and a light cure gun if bonding of the canines is going to be part of the jaw fracture repair.

The oral cavity is not sterile and this is also a complication that must be dealt with when treating maxillary and mandibular fractures. Chlorhexidine gluconate rinses at a concentration of 0.12% are bactericidal, have a broad spectrum of antimicrobial activity, bind well to the oral tissues including tooth surfaces, and can remain effective as an antimicrobial for up to 12 hours [13]. It is useful and recommended to rinse the mouth and the fracture site in preparation for oral fracture repair.

First, full-mouth intraoral radiographs are obtained to assess the roots of the teeth and the alveolar bone in which they normally are anchored. Then, a complete dental cleaning and polishing needs to be performed on the teeth using an ultrasonic scaler and hand instruments followed by polishing with flour pumice in order to prepare the teeth for jaw fracture repair. Polishing without fluoride is important as fluoride will interfere with the bonding of many dental materials.

24.5 Methods of Maxillofacial Fracture Stabilization

24.5.1 Tape or Nylon Muzzles (Figure 24.7)

Tape muzzles are quick and easy to fit on the patient because they are custom-made for the case. It is good to have several sizes of white adhesive tape on hand for this purpose; 0.5-in., 1-in., and 2-in. widths to fit the smallest of puppies to the largest of dogs. When done correctly no tape is stuck to the patient, all the sticky sides are in and stuck to each other. Long hair is clipped away from the muzzle and the face to allow for the tape muzzle to fit well and to make home care easier for the patient and the client. The first tape is placed around the muzzle with the sticky side facing out leaving a gap of 0.5–1 cm for the mouth to open so the patient can lap up gruel [4]. An important consideration is the size of the patient when leaving the gap: a small dog and cat need less, a large dog needs more. The canine teeth cusps should just overlap

and the incisors should be separated. Often the size (the diameter) of the patient's endotracheal tube is the perfect gap. The second tape is cut twice the measured distance from the left upper canine behind the ears to the right upper canine. The tape is placed sticky side out and positioned behind the middle of the patient's head between the ears. It is attached to the tape at the muzzle. A third tape is placed around the muzzle with the sticky side to the first muzzle tape: this will secure the second tape that goes behind the ears. The tape that came from behind the ears is now stuck back on itself along the sides of the muzzle toward the ears. Another tape (the fourth tape) is then placed around the muzzle to reinforce the muzzle component. Sometimes an additional tape is required from the dorsal aspect of the nose tape up between the eyes attached to the tape behind the ears for better stability [4]. It is advisable to create at least three tape muzzles so that they can be replaced when they get excessively soiled. There are also a wide range of shapes and sizes of commercial nylon muzzles available on the market and, as long as they fit the patient adequately providing support and the ability for the patient to lap up a gruel, they are quick and easy to use and easy to wash (Figure 24.8). Tape or nylon muzzles can be used for emergency initial fracture support, for primary fracture support of minimally displaced fractures, for fractures in young growing patients, or for additional support of other fracture repair techniques. The oral cavity has a very rich vascular supply and therefore does not always require rigid fixation for adequate fracture healing [5]. Complications of tape muzzle or a nylon muzzle are aspiration due to vomiting, thermoregulatory and respiratory difficulties due to the inability to pant, dermatitis from moisture and muzzle contact, and failure of the fracture to heal.

Cats rarely tolerate a tape muzzle and patient selection for a tape muzzle in the cat is critical [14]. An alternative to a tape muzzle in the cat is the use of suture and buttons: the modified labial button technique [15].

24.5.2 Osseous Wiring Techniques for Maxillofacial Fracture Repair

There are three types of osseous wiring techniques: circumferential, trans-osseous (inter-fragmentary), and trans-circumferential.

24.5.2.1 Circumferential (or Symphyseal Wiring Technique) (Figure 24.9)

This technique is used for simple ligamentous symphyseal separation, commonly seen in cats. A small incision is made on the ventral midline of the mandible at the level of the mandibular canine teeth just caudal to the symphysis. A 20 gauge needle is passed through the

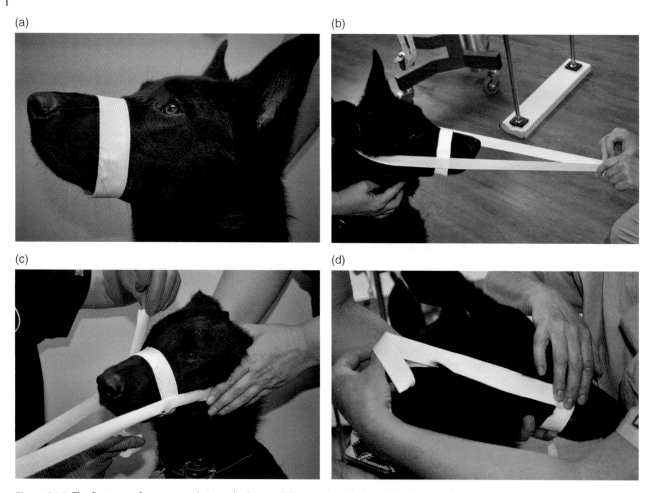

(a) (b) (c) (d)

Figure 24.7 The first tape of a tape muzzle is applied around the muzzle with the sticky side away from the patient (a). It is important to allow the patient a 5–10-mm gap, depending on the size of the patient, so they can lap up gruel. The second tape is placed non-sticky side against the hair and is twice as long as the length of the tape from canine to canine (b). The third tape is placed over the muzzle tape to secure the tape from behind the head (c). The long ends of the second tape are then secured back to the side of the dog's face and around the back of the head (d and e). The finished tape muzzle should fit comfortably and allow the patient the ability to easily lap gruel (f, g and h).

incision on the mandible close to the most caudal edge of the mandibular symphysis along the frenulum into the oral cavity. Then one-half of an appropriate gauge orthopedic wire is passed subcutaneously from the oral cavity into the 20 gauge needle to exit on the mandible through the same incision near the caudal aspect of the mandibular symphysis just caudal to the crowns of the canines [16]. The same procedure is repeated on the opposite side with the other mandible. Then the two ends, at the ventral aspect of the mandibles, are twisted together. It is important not to twist the wires too tight. It is normal for there to be some movement at the mandibular symphysis: it's a joint. The goal is to provide stabilization not rigid fixation. The ends of the twisted wire are then covered with a small amount of acrylic or flowable composite material and light cured to prevent the twisted wire end causing the patient discomfort. The length of time support is required for a ligamentous injury is less than

that required for fracture repair. Around 3–4 weeks is generally sufficient for mandibular symphyseal ligamentous separation, at which point the wire is removed.

24.5.2.2 Trans-Osseous (Inter-Fragmentary) Wire
A horizontal inter-fragmentary wire is a useful method when trying to stabilize a "favorable" fracture of the body of the mandible (Figure 24.10). A small incision is made with a scalpel and a round burr is used to create holes for the wire; or a chuck and a K-wire can be used to make the holes, being extremely careful not to damage tooth roots or the mandibular canal. The use of a K-wire makes it easier to feel tooth roots than a drill. Inter-fragmentary wires can be used alone or with the addition of acrylic on the teeth involved to stabilize fracture fragments. A figure-8 inter-fragmentary wire can be used to stabilize a butterfly fragment (Figure 24.11). Inter-fragmentary wiring techniques can be used in the caudal mandible as

(e)

(f)

(g)

(h)

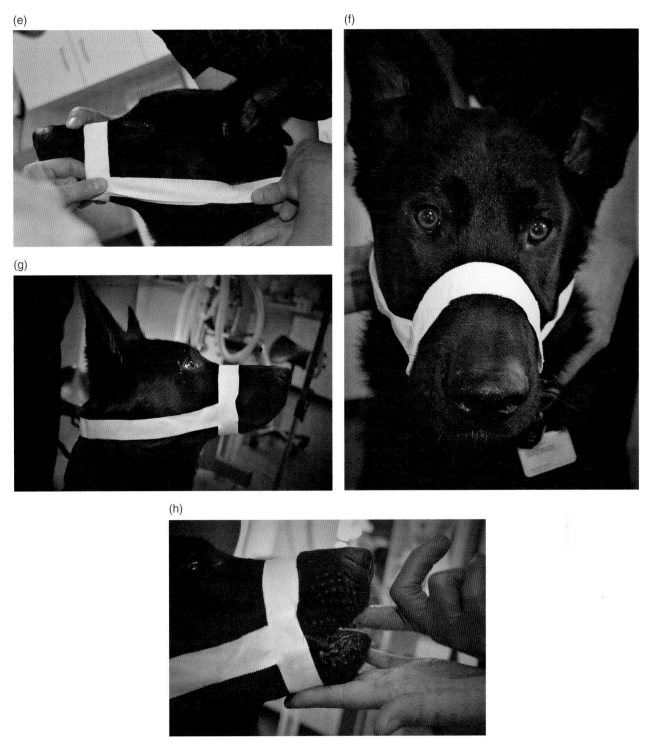

Figure 24.7 (Continued)

well (Figure 24.12). The techniques can be used, along with variants of the intra-osseous wires, to stabilize multiple fragments as well (Figure 24.13).

Sloping the drill/K-wire holes toward, but not into, the fracture site will help to compress the fracture site when the wires are tightened. The holes are drilled 5–10 mm away from the fracture site and oblique to it. The wire is passed from outside to inside. A large loop is used to decrease bending and kinking of the wire. The wire is passed until the kink is through (this means long wires

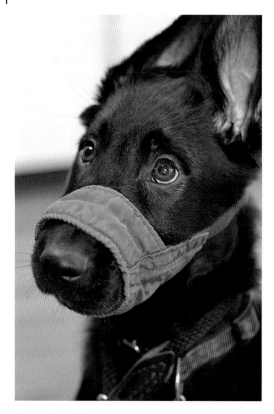

Figure 24.8 Nylon muzzles are inexpensive and easy to clean. They must be adjusted to fit the patient so that the patient can lap up gruel.

are necessary). Details on how to properly twist a cerclage wire are found in Chapter 20. The wire must be tight and this can be accomplished by placing an instrument on the side the wire is being twisted on and putting some "lift" pressure on it and then releasing as it is twisted. When the twisting is complete the wire is bent toward the apex of the teeth; twisting and bending is done in one motion. The wires need to cross perpendicular to the fracture line. The least amount of wires possible should be used to achieve fracture stabilization. All wires should be placed before tightening. When repairing a fracture with several wires, the wires are tightened from caudal to rostral.

24.5.2.3 Trans-Circumferential Wiring

This technique can be used when large amounts of edema are present or when an edentulous case exists. Interdental wiring for edentulous patients is definitely more challenging but also easily done to provide a stable jaw repair when no teeth remain for support. The acrylic splint is made for the length of the jaw to be stabilized and then secured to the jaw using multiple cerclage wires. Acrylic is laid along the edentulous portion of the jaw that needs to be stabilized. It is necessary to have at least one cerclage wire on either side of the fracture site.

Incorporation of the wire into the splint is necessary for a stable repair. This wiring technique can also be used between the roots of the mandibular 09 in a dog under the ventral aspect of the mandible in an "unfavorable" fracture of the body of the mandible.

24.5.3 Intra-Dental Wiring Techniques with Acrylic Reinforcement

This technique is less challenging than other techniques, requires minimal equipment, is quick, maintains normal occlusion, and is minimally invasive therefore less likely to cause iatrogenic trauma [4]. All reinforcement with acrylic requires a clean prepared mouth. In a clean mouth where the teeth have been polished with flour pumice, acid etch is applied according to the manufacturer's directions. For example 37% phosphoric acid should be applied evenly to the area of tooth meant to be bonded together and left on for 15–20 seconds, then rinsed well for at least twice as long as the area was etched, and then air dried. Then primer and sealer should be applied to the acid-etched area of the teeth to be bonded again according to the manufacturer's instructions. Both the primer and adhesive are light cured according to the manufacturer's instructions. The teeth are then ready for the application of acrylic. Removal of the acrylic after the fracture has healed requires the use of a pear shaped burr such as a #330 or a round burr to make cuts in the acrylic carefully to avoid causing damage to the teeth. The acrylic is then removed gently using extraction forceps. The wire is removed with wire cutters and the teeth are cleaned and polished post-appliance removal.

24.5.3.1 Ivy Loop Technique (Figure 24.14)

The Ivy loop technique is suitable for non-displaced stable fractures of the maxilla or the mandible. The Ivy loop technique is used to wire two teeth together. It is best for the loops to be on the lingual side of the mandible but often in small patients such as Yorkshire terriers this is not possible so the loops will be on the buccal side. The mandible of a large dog is best done with the loops on the lingual side. In the maxilla the loops are *always* on the buccal side because this interferes the least with occlusion. The placement of the wire is done by taking a length of wire three times as long as the length of jaw to be wired. There will be a working end of the wire and a stationary end. The stationary end remains straight on the opposite side of the working wire. The stationary wire is on the buccal side of the maxilla and preferably on the lingual side of the mandible when the size of the patient permits. For the mandible in a small patient, a 20 gauge needle with 22 gauge orthopedic wire threaded through it, is placed from the lingual aspect of the tooth,

(a)

(b)

(c)

(e)

(d)

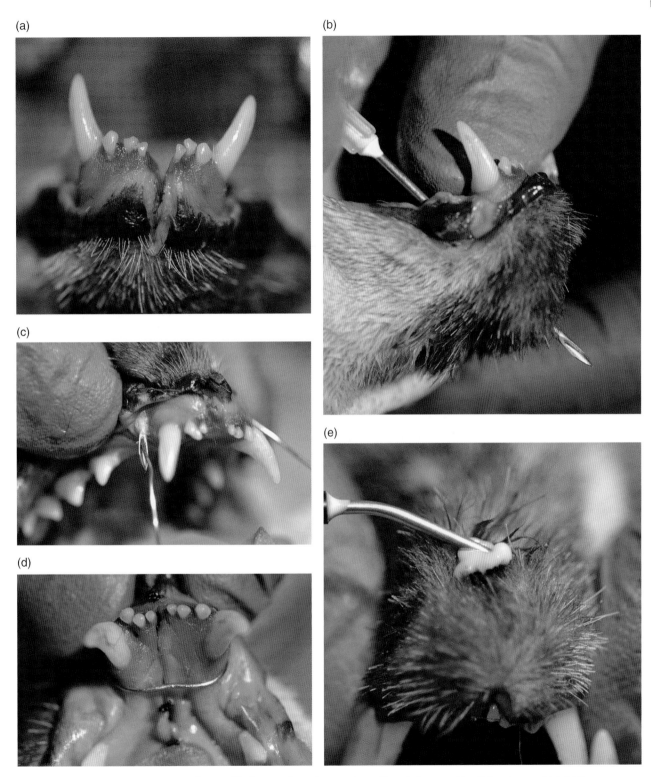

Figure 24.9 A common presentation of a mandibular symphyseal separation with soft tissue and tooth involvement (a). A 20 gauge needle is inserted just caudal to the crowns of the mandibular canines through a small skin incision on the ventral mandible (b). The process is repeated on the other side to pass the wire around the mandibular symphysis (c). The wire is tightened just enough to appose the mandibles (d). The twisted knot on the ventral mandible is covered with a small amount of flowable composite or acrylic to prevent discomfort or trauma to the patient from the wire ends (e).

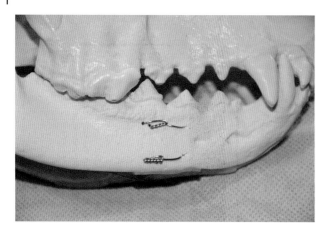

Figure 24.10 Two inter-fragmentary wires placed to stabilize this mandibular body fracture with care and attention taken to avoid tooth roots and the mandibular canal.

through the distal interdental space in the tough attached gingival tissue, around the buccal surface of the tooth, and then back through the 20 gauge needle at the mesial interdental surface of the tooth. The working end of the wire is passed under and over the stationary end of the wire, then passed back through the interdental space of the tooth. A small loop is left on the buccal surface of the mandible that will be used to twist and tighten the wire down to the tooth. The loop needs to be secured with a few twists at this point but not fully tightened down until the two teeth have been wired. The working end of the wire is then moved onto the next tooth and the procedure is repeated for the second tooth. After the two teeth are wired, the working end and the stationary end are twisted together on the buccal surface to minimize post jaw fracture repair. The small loop is now tightened around the teeth to fit snuggly. The 20 gauge needles

(a) (b)

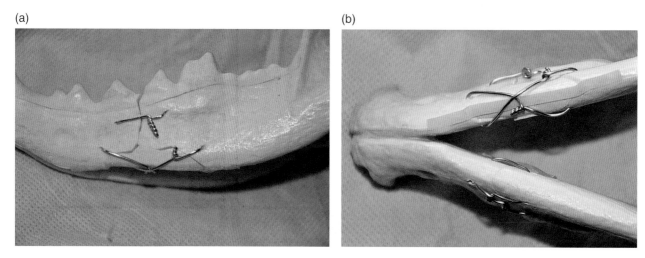

Figure 24.11 Inter-fragmentary wires used to stabilize a mandibular fracture and replace a butterfly fragment. Lateral (a) and ventral (b) views.

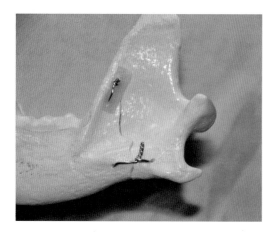

Figure 24.12 Inter-fragmentary wires used to stabilize a fracture in the caudal mandible.

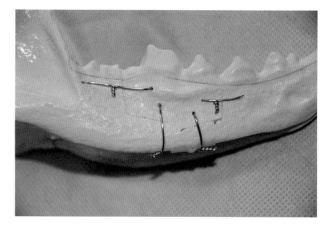

Figure 24.13 The use of multiple inter-fragmentary intra-osseous wires to stabilize a mandibular fracture.

(a)

(b)

(c)

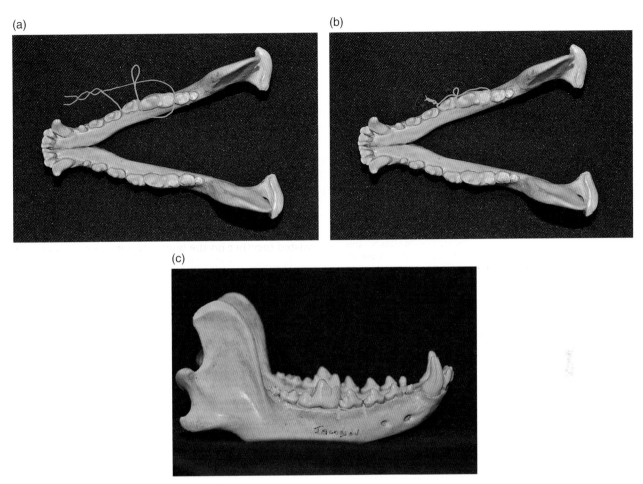

Figure 24.14 Ivy loop technique. Placement of the wire begins around the first tooth by passing the wire distally through the interdental space and then back through the mesial interdental space of the same tooth (a). One-half of the wire is stationary and one-half is a working end. A loop is left on the buccal surface and is not tightened until all the wire has been placed. Wires are tightened at each loop when all the wire has been placed (b). Wires are bent to face away from the dental arcade (c). It is best for the loops to be on the lingual side of the mandible but often in small patients such as Yorkshire terriers this is not possible so the loops will be on the buccal side. The mandible of a large dog is best done with the loops on the lingual side. In the maxilla the loops are *always* on the buccal side because this interferes the least with occlusion.

need to be changed frequently as they get dull and bend quickly. The wires must be handled gently to avoid excessive kinks and bends as these will make them more difficult to tighten later.

24.5.3.2 The Stout Loop Technique

This technique is more commonly used in fracture repair. This technique follows the same principle as the Ivy loop technique but it includes more than just two teeth (Figure 24.15). It is normally considered sufficient to include two teeth on either side of the fracture line to provide adequate stabilization. The working end is passed around multiple teeth just as previously described in the Ivy loop technique. Stout loop wires should be avoided around avulsed teeth.

24.5.3.3 The Use of Acrylic to Re-enforce the Wire Appliance

Teeth and wire that require acrylic reinforcement must be acid-etched before acrylic application to improve the adhesion of the acrylic. Phosphoric acid is applied according to the manufacturer's instructions, rinsing well as indicated by the manufacturer. The most important thing to remember with the application of acrylic is that it must not interfere with the normal bite and normal mastication of the patient. Interference is avoided in mandibular fractures by not placing acrylic higher than the height of the mandibular first molar (Figure 24.16). Acrylic should not be placed on the buccal surface of the mandibular molars as it will interfere with normal occlusion. The acrylic splint is reinforced lingually on

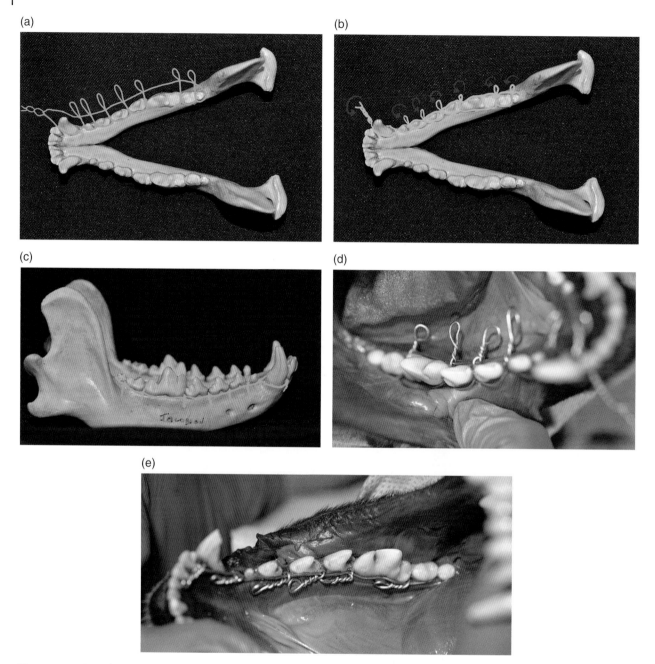

Figure 24.15 Stout loop technique. Placement of the wire begins around the first tooth by passing the wire distally through the interdental space and then back through the mesial interdental space of the same tooth. One-half of the wire is stationary and one-half is a working end. A loop is left on the buccal surface and is not tightened until all the wire has been placed. Each tooth to be included in the splint is wired in the same manner (a). Wires are tightened at each loop when all the wire has been placed (b). Wires are bent to face away from the dental arcade (c). The Stout loop technique on the right mandible before the addition of acrylic reinforcement (d and e).

the mandible to prevent interference during occlusion [17]. Acrylic can be placed lingually and buccally mesial to the mandibular first molar, *but* distal to the mandibular first molar acrylic is to be placed lingual only or the occlusion of the patient will be compromised. The acrylic is used to cover the wires on the entire length of the appliance lingually on the mandible. As long as the acrylic material is still viscous it can be added and it will bond. When the cold cure acrylic material is cured it can be easily contoured with a diamond burr or a Goldie burr so that it is smooth and there are no areas that will irritate the soft tissues of the patient. There should be a minimal amount of acrylic on the gingiva and no acrylic on the mucosa to minimize soft tissue irritation.

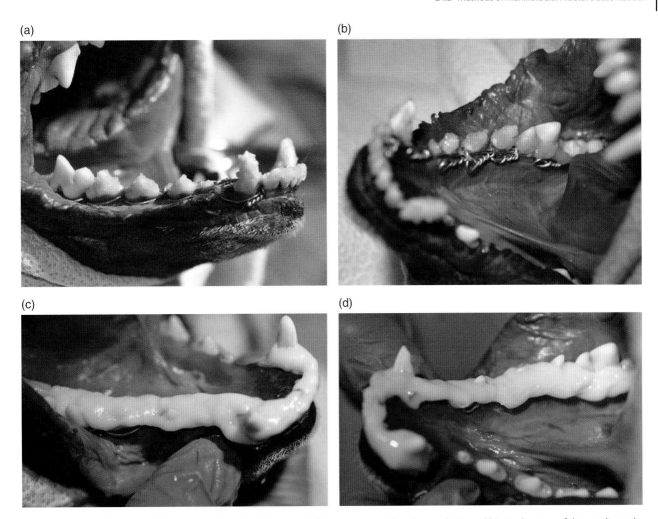

Figure 24.16 Applications of the phosphoric acid-etching material prior to applying the acrylic (a and b). Application of the acrylic to the left mandible with care taken to avoid causing a malocclusion due to improper placement of acrylic (c and d).

24.5.4 Bonding the Maxillary to the Mandibular Canines

This technique is used for stabilization of fractures of the caudal mandible, bilateral mandibular fractures, or fractures of the temporal mandibular joint. The mandibular and the maxillary canines are bonded to each other allowing for enough space for the patient to lap up a gruel of food and water. These cases should always have a feeding tube placed at the time of the initial surgical jaw fracture repair. It is important not to leave in rigid fixation for longer than 3–5 weeks, to prevent temporomandibular joint (TMJ) ankyloses [18]. There can be complications such as aspiration pneumonia if there is vomiting as the patient cannot swallow well. This is a perfect time to intubate first then place a pharyngostomy endotracheal tube to allow the clinician to work in the oral cavity without the interference of the oral endotracheal tube. In a clean mouth polished with flour pumice, acid etch is applied according to the manufacturer's

directions. As mentioned previously, 37% phosphoric acid should be applied evenly to the area of tooth meant to be bonded together and left on for 15–20 seconds, then rinsed well for at least twice as long as the area was etched, and then air dried. Then primer and sealer should be applied to the acid-etched area of the teeth to be bonded again according to the manufacturer's instructions. Both the primer and adhesive should be light cured according to the manufacturer's instructions. The animal's occlusion is reduced to where both the canine teeth slightly overlap. The gap between the incisors needs to be around 10 mm in the cat and 10–15 mm in the dog depending on the size of the dog. If the gap is wider than this in the cat, it is difficult for them to swallow [19]. A light cure or dual cure composite is applied to both crowns and the bridge between the crowns. The composite should be applied from the tips of the coronal portion of the tooth to three-quarters of the entire tooth. Light cure is preferred, as it is quicker, according to the manufacturer's instructions. The composite is applied in layers of no more than 2 mm, and each layer is light cured. Final smoothing of the composite bonding material can be done with a diamond finishing burr or a Goldie burr. Removal of the composite after the fracture has healed requires the use of a pear shaped burr such as a #330 or a round burr to make cuts in the composite carefully to avoid causing damage to the teeth. The composite is then removed gently using extraction forceps. The teeth are clean and polished post composite removal.

Removal of the composite for the maxillomandibular bonding requires planning as the patient will be anesthetized without access to oral intubation. It is important to be organized before anesthetizing the patient to be as quick and safe as possible. A cutting (the author uses a pear shaped 330) burr on a high-speed hand piece will be necessary, as well as an elevator and the endotracheal tube for the patient. The composite bridge is scored between the canines on the right and left and then an elevator is used to gently force the composite apart. The patient is then intubated and the remaining composite can be removed by chipping away at the composite using extraction forceps or tartar removal forceps. The final removal of any remaining composite can be done using a hand-scaler. The teeth need to be completely scaled and polished after the composite removal.

24.6 Bone Grafts

Placement of bone allografts, if there are bone defects, can be used to improve the quality and aid in regeneration of bone in the defect. If an allograft is cost-prohibitive a synthetic demineralized bone graft can be placed in the defect in the fracture site after surgical alignment to assist in the clinical repair of lost bone [20–24]. It is important to have walls to place the bone graft into or the granulation tissue will fill in the defect before the bone has a chance to mineralize. These cases are often best left in the hands of a specialist.

24.7 Teeth in the Fracture Line

In acute blunt force trauma there may not always be radiographic evidence to help the clinician judge the vitality of the tooth involved in a jaw fracture. Teeth involved in a jaw fracture are always assessed for use as a critical part of the non-invasive repair techniques for jaw fracture repair and should be evaluated at a later date for vitality and possible endodontic or exodontic therapy. Some teeth in the fracture line may not die and require no follow-up endodontic or exodontic therapy. Therefore,

removal of teeth in the immediate area of the jaw fracture is no longer advocated unless they are periodontally affected. It is important to let the jaw fracture heal and reassess the teeth at a later date, up to 3–6 months after the fracture repair. If there are no clinical signs of oral pain or teeth with pulpal exposure and there are no clinical or radiographic changes consistent with tooth death, the teeth should be monitored clinically and radiographically every 6–12 months. If there are teeth with pulpal exposure they should be treated with emergency endodontic therapy at the time of the fracture repair or within 2 weeks of the primary fracture repair [25].

A tooth is deemed not to be salvageable in a maxillofacial fracture if it has extensive periodontal disease and it should be extracted before fracture repair is attempted [25]. If a tooth has a complicated crown fracture, complicated crown root fracture, is non-vital, or avulsed, it should be maintained for the use of stabilization of the jaw and treated with emergency endodontic therapy immediately or exodontic therapy at a later date. If the fracture line extends from the gingival margin to the apex of the tooth, the tooth should be extracted or hemi-sectioned [25] (Figure 24.17). A hemi-sectioned tooth requires endodontic therapy and this treatment is best left in the hands of a dental specialist. After fracture repair is complete, a complicated crown fracture, complicated crown root fracture, or non-vital tooth must be

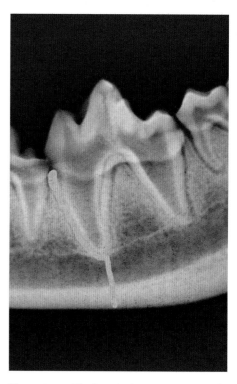

Figure 24.17 The fracture lines create a communication between the apex and the oral cavity. The treatment options are a hemi-section with endodontic therapy or extraction.

re-evaluated and treated. If endodontic therapy is not the best treatment option for the affected tooth or an option for the client, then exodontic therapy is necessary to provide the patient with a comfortable and healthy mouth.

24.8 Antibiotic Therapy in Maxillofacial Fracture Repair

The use of antibiotics is a choice the educated veterinary clinician should make on a case-by-case basis. It is suggested in the literature that antibiotic therapy is recommended for cases that involve open fractures [3, 26] and that long-term antibiotic use be reserved for those cases that have clinical or radiographic evidence of osteomyelitis [26].

24.9 Irrigation of the Appliance

Chlorhexidine solution at 0.12% may be used to irrigate the intraoral splint to remove food debris [26]. Chlorhexidine is bactericidal at this concentration but is not appealing to the taste buds of dogs and cats, or humans for that matter. It is an excellent solution for rinsing the mouth to decrease the bacterial load during oral surgery while the patient is anesthetized, but for the awake animal it tastes alarmingly disgusting, particularly for cats. For this reason one may tend to opt for simpler

home care solutions such as saline, as the patients tend to fuss less about this solution orally, thus client compliance is better. Twice daily oral rinsing is extremely important for keeping debris at a minimum and minimizing halitosis and mucositis due to oral bacteria, which can be severe in the days and weeks following facial fracture repair. This also helps to maintain the normal human–animal bond at home, which can be so severely disrupted in the face of a traumatic facial injury. Discharge instructions are not worth the paper they are written on if the client will not be able to follow the home care program recommended for the patient. Daily, gentle face, chest, and leg washing is necessary especially in cats to maintain their normal hygiene and make them comfortable and content.

24.10 Recheck Examinations

An awake oral recheck examination of a fracture repair should ideally occur every 7 days to evaluate the patient's return to normal function, to assess the soft tissue repair, and to address any ongoing concerns that the owner may have. An anesthetized recheck examination should occur 6–8 weeks post fracture repair [26]. Unless the canines are bonded, they should be assessed at 4 weeks due to the risk of TMJ damage. At the anesthetized recheck examination, if the fracture site appears to be clinically stable and there are radiographic signs of bony union at the fracture site, the appliance may be removed.

References

1 Evans, H.E. and Christensen, G.C. (2013). The skeleton: the skull. In: *Miller's Anatomy of the Dog*, 4e (ed. H.E. Evans and A. de Lahunta), 84–113. Philadelphia, PA: WB Saunders.

2 Boudrieau, R.J. and Verstraete, J.M. (2012). Principles of maxillofacial trauma repair. In: *Oral and Maxillofacial Surgery in Cats and Dogs* (ed. J.M. Verstraete and M.J. Lommer), 233. Philadelphia, PA: WB Saunders.

3 Woodbridge, N. and Owen, M. (2013). Feline mandibular fractures: A significant surgical challenge. *J. Feline Med. Surg.* 15: 211–218.

4 Gorrel, C., Penman, S., and Emily, P. (1993). Jaw fractures. In: *Handbook of Small Animal Oral Emergencies*, 37–45. New York: Pergamon Press.

5 Wiggs, R.B. and Lobprise, H.B. (1997). Oral fracture repair. In: *Veterinary Dentistry Principles and Practice* (ed. R.B. Wiggs and H.B. Lobprise), 259–279. Philadelphia, PA: Lippincott-Raven.

6 Eickoff, M. (2012). How I approach fractures of the maxilla and mandible in cats. *Vet. Focus* 22 (3): 17–22.

7 Hennet, P. (2014) Diagnostic approach to the feline maxillofacial trauma. 39th World Small Animal Veterinary Association Congress Proceedings, pp. 632–634. World Small Animal Veterinary Association, Cape Town, South Africa.

8 Lantz, G. (2012). Pharyngotomy and pharyngostomy. In: *Oral and Maxillofacial Surgery in Cats and Dogs* (ed. J.M. Verstraete and M.J. Lommer), 545. Philadelphia, PA: WB Saunders.

9 Smith, M.M. (2004). Pharyngostomy endotracheal tube. *J. Vet. Dent.* 21 (3): 191–194.

10 Wooden, J. (1987). Intubation. In: *Manual of Clinical Procedures in the Cat and Dog* (ed. S.E. Crow and S.O. Walshaw), 162–166. Philadelphia, PA: J.B. Lippincott Company.

11 Rochette, J. (2005). Regional anesthesia and analgesia for oral and dental procedures. In: *Veterinary Clinics of North American Small Animal Practice Dentistry* (ed. S.E. Holmstrom), 1041–1058. Toronto: Veterinary Clinics of North America Small Animal Practice Elsevier Inc.

12 Steffey, E.P. and Howland, D. Jr. (1977). Isoflurane potency in the dog and the cat. *Am. J. Vet. Res.* 38 (11): 1833–1836.

13 Robinson, J.G.A. (1995). Chlorhexidine gluconate – the solution for dental problems. *J. Vet. Dent.* 12 (1): 29–31.

14 Somrak, A.J. and Manfra-Marretta, S. (2015). Management of temporomandibular joint luxation in a cat using a custom-made tape muzzle. *J. Vet. Dent.* 32 (4): 239–246.

15 Goodman, A.E. and Carmichael, D.T. (2016). Modified labial button technique for maintaining occlusion after caudal mandibular fracture/temporomandibular joint luxation in the cat. *J. Vet. Dent.* 33 (1): 47–52.

16 Legendre, L. (1998). Use of maxillary and mandibular splints for restoration of normal occlusion following jaw trauma in a cat: a case report. *J. Vet. Dent.* 15 (4): 179–181.

17 Hall, B.P. and Wiggs, R.B. (2005). Acrylic splint and circumferential mandibular wire for mandibular fracture repair in the dog. *J. Vet. Dent.* 22 (3): 170–175.

18 Soukup, J.W. and Snyder, J.S. (2014). Traumatic dentoalveolar and maxillofacial injuries in cats. Overview of diagnosis and management. *J. Feline Med. Surg.* 16: 915–927.

19 Moores, A.P. (2011). Maxillomandibular external skeletal fixation in five cats with caudal jaw trauma. *J. Small Anim. Pract.* 52: 38–41.

20 Mellonig, J.T. (1991). Freeze-dried bone allografts in periodontal reconstructive surgery. *Dent. Clin. North Am.* 35 (3): 505–521.

21 Reynolds, M.A., Aichelmann-Reidy, M.E., Branch-Mays, G.L. et al. (2003). The efficacy of bone replacement grafts in the treatment of periodontal osseous defects. A systematic review. *Ann. Periodontol.* 8 (1): 227–265.

22 Farina, N.M., Guzon, F.M., Pena, M.L. et al. (2008). In vivo behaviour of two different biphasic ceramic implanted in mandibular bone of dogs. *J. Mat. Sci: Mat. Med.* 19: 1565–1573.

23 Habibovic, P. and de Groot, K. (2007). Osteoinductive biomaterials: properties and relevance in bone repair. *J. Tissue Eng. Regen. Med.* 1: 25–32.

24 Bongio, M., van den Beucken, J.J.J.P., Leeuwenburgh, S.C.G. et al. (2010). Development of bone substitute materials: from "biocompatible" to "instructive". *J. Mat. Chem.* 20: 8747–8759.

25 Schloss, A.J. and Manfra-Marretta, S. (1990). Prognostic factors affecting teeth in the line of mandibular fractures. *J. Vet. Dent.* 7 (4): 7–9.

26 Legendre, L. (2003). Intraoral acrylic splints for maxillofacial fracture repair. *J. Vet. Dent.* 20 (2): 70–78.

25

Approaches to the Long Bones

Anne M. Sylvestre

Focus and Flourish, Cambridge, Ontario, Canada

Bones have an endosteal blood supply that comes from the nutrient artery and vein. These vessels supply the marrow by entering the compact bone through the nutrient foramen. Upon reaching the medullary cavity, they repeatedly subdivide to serve the marrow and adjacent endosteum and cortical bone. This supply can be damaged at the time of the fracture; it also can easily be damaged when an intra-medullary pin is placed. Bones also have periosteal arteries and veins. These vessels typically arise from the overlying muscles on the bone. Therefore, they may be numerous in some bones (femur) and fewer in others (phalanges), but they are typically quite small. They can become damaged at the time of the trauma and during the surgical approach. A fractured bone that has a good blood supply will heal well. Therefore, when approaching a bone for fracture repair, it is important to minimize dissection and maintain most of the soft tissue attachments to the fragments, thereby preserving as much of the vasculature as possible.

In this chapter the surgical approaches for the more common diaphyseal fractures of the four major long bones are described. The reader is strongly encouraged to refer to *Piermattei's Atlas of Surgical Approaches to the Bones and Joints of the Dog and Cat* for a comprehensive description of approaches to other areas of these bones [1].

25.1 Approach to the Diaphysis of the Humerus

The lateral approach to the humeral diaphysis allows for the patient to be comfortably positioned in lateral recumbency. The entire bone can be exposed, which is important for fractures that require positioning the plate further proximal on the bone; the lateral approach also makes it possible to combine plating with an intramedullary pin. The disadvantages of the lateral approach

include: aggressive plate contouring is often necessary, the brachialis muscle must be retracted, and the radial nerve must also be identified and protected. As with all surgeries, a full understanding of the regional anatomy is important.

25.1.1 Patient Position

The patient is positioned in lateral recumbency with the affected limb up. Free draping of the limb is important, with the paw and antebrachium wrapped in a sterile drape.

25.1.2 The Surgical Approach (Figure 25.1)

The skin is incised over the lateral aspect of the humerus. The incision should be most of the length of the bone: a small approach will simply make identification of the relevant anatomical landmarks more difficult. The subcutaneous connective tissues are incised in the same plane as the skin. Underneath the skin and within the prominent superficial fascia is located the cephalic vein and its branches: the omobrachial and axillobrachial veins. These veins are dissected free from the surrounding fascia, ligated, and transected to improve the exposure. With the vessels out of the way, the lateral head of the triceps muscle is readily visible as are the radial nerve and brachialis muscles. The brachialis muscle is elevated from the underlying humeral fracture. Once the muscle is isolated, a Penrose drain or umbilical tape can be used to protect and maneuver the radial nerve and brachialis muscle bundle. The muscles visible on the distal aspect of the humerus are the anconeus and extensor carpi radialis (ECR). A periosteal elevator is used to move the deltoid and the biceps brachii muscles should that be necessary.

To close, the fascial layer that was incised at the beginning is closed, followed by subcutaneous tissues and skin.

Fracture Management for the Small Animal Practitioner, First Edition. Edited by Anne M. Sylvestre.
© 2019 John Wiley & Sons, Inc. Published 2019 by John Wiley & Sons, Inc.

(a)

(b)

(c)

(d)

(e)

(f)

(g)

(h)

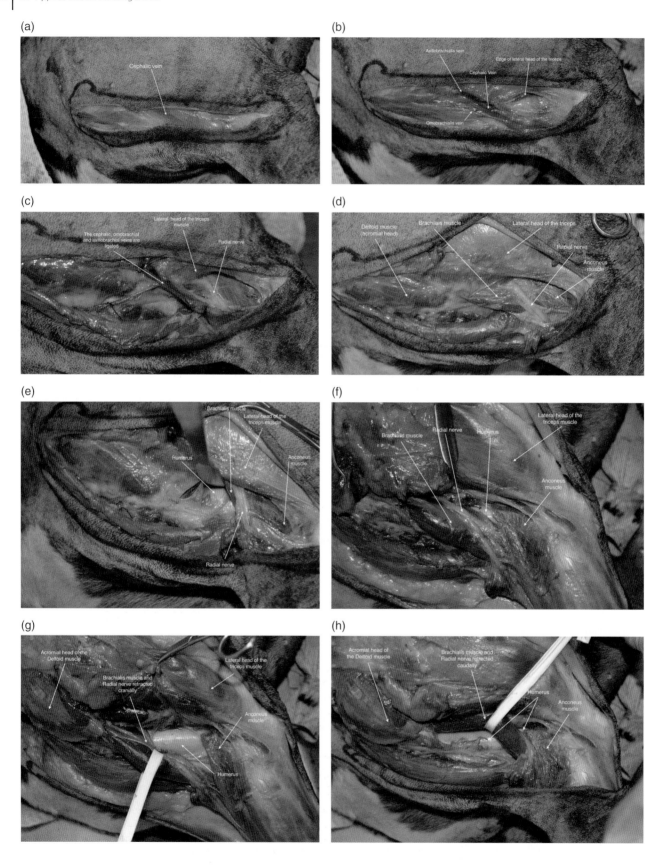

25.2 Approach to the Diaphysis of the Radius

The muscle and tendons of interest in the distal radius are the abductor pollicis longus (APL), ECR, and the extensor digitorum communis (EDC). The ECR divides into two flat tendons over the distal third of the radius. The smaller, more medial tendon inserts on the proximal aspect of the second metacarpal (MC) bone, while the thicker more central tendon inserts on the third MC. One of its functions is to extend the carpus. It is important to preserve the tendons of the ECR in order to maintain carpal extension. The tendon of the APL travels obliquely over the ECR toward the first metacarpal bone where it inserts. It functions to abduct the first digit.

25.2.1 Patient Position (Figure 25.2)

It can be difficult to position the patient for this surgery. Having the patient in sternal recumbency with the head turned away from the fractured limb seems to be the position that allows for the easiest access and view of the fracture site. The patient's head should rest on rolled towels to maintain it elevated, otherwise the weight of the head resting down on the operating table will cause the forelimb to roll inward, making manipulation and visualization more difficult.

Some surgeons prefer to have the patient in dorsal recumbency with the shoulder flexed. The antebrachium can be more readily manipulated in this position but it is not supported, which can make it difficult to work with.

Free draping of the limb is important with the toes wrapped in a sterile drape (Vet Wrap works well for this). The paw wrap needs to be secured in place with a towel clamp as it can easily become inadvertently removed during the surgery.

25.2.2 Surgical Approach (Figure 25.3)

The incision is made over the cranial aspect of the radius, preferably lateral to the cephalic vein, and centered over

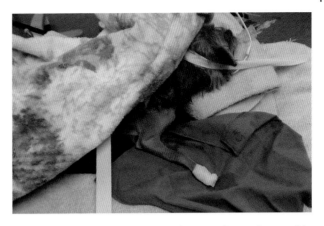

Figure 25.2 The patient is positioned in sternal recumbency with the affected limb extended toward the end of the table. The head is rotated away from the affected limb and rested on a towel to help maintain the patient's body in a propped up position.

the fracture. The medial branch to the cephalic vein can be avoided with this craniolateral approach. The incision typically needs to extend to the proximal level of the carpal joint. A small hypodermic needle can be inserted into the carpal joint to help identify its location. The tendon of the APL muscle can be severed and reflected laterally. A periosteal elevator is used to move the ECR (either medially or laterally) off the cranial surface of the distal and proximal fragments. A sufficient amount of the bone should be exposed to be able to manipulate the fragments and accommodate a plate.

The subcutaneous tissues and skin only need to be closed.

25.3 Approach to the Femoral Diaphysis

The femur is not a superficial bone like the tibia or radius but it is relatively easy to approach from the lateral surface.

25.3.1 Patient Position

The patient is placed in lateral recumbency with the affected limb uppermost. Free draping of the limb is

Figure 25.1 Approach to the lateral diaphysis of the left humerus is demonstrated in this canine cadaver specimen. The patient is positioned in lateral recumbency with the affected limb up. Proximal is on the left side of the pictures. (a) A skin incision is made directly over the lateral aspect of the bone. The cephalic vein can be seen crossing the surgical site in the mid-to-distal third of the bone. (b) The subcutaneous fascial tissues are incised in the same plane as the skin. The cephalic vein and its branches, the omobrachial and axillobrachial veins, are located within the fascial tissue. The fascial plane attaches to the cranial edge of the lateral head of the triceps muscle. (c) The incision in the connective tissue is continued distally and proximally until the veins can be isolated, ligated, and transected. Caution must be exercised as the radial nerve is located distal to the cephalic vein and just deep to the fascial plane. (d) With the vessels transected and the skin retracted caudally, the lateral head of the triceps muscle, the radial nerve, and brachialis muscles are visible. With appropriate dissection, the acromial head of the deltoid and the anconeus muscles are also visible. (e and f) The humerus is located under the brachialis muscle. A periosteal elevator is used to isolate the brachialis muscle from the underlying humerus. In (f) the exposure has been enhanced to aid with identification of the relevant structures. (g and h) A Penrose drain or umbilical tape can be used to protect and maneuver the radial nerve and brachialis muscle bundle.

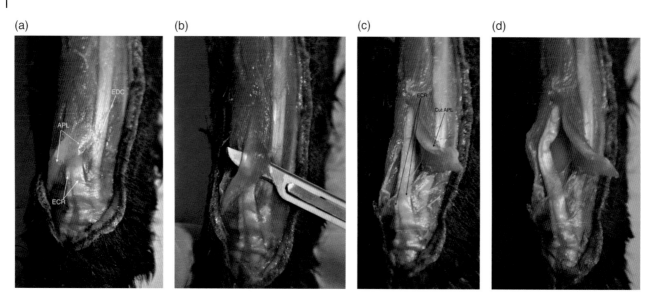

Figure 25.3 Approach to the mid-to-distal diaphysis of the left radius is demonstrated in this canine cadaver specimen. Proximal is at the top of the pictures. A skin incision is made on the cranial surface of the radius, centered over the fracture, and just lateral to the cephalic vein. The subcutaneous connective tissues are incised in the same plane, exposing the abductor pollicis longus (APL), extensor carpi radialis (ECR), and the extensor digitorum communis (EDC) (a). The APL tendon is cut (b) to expose the tendons of the ECR (c). These tendons must be protected. Using a periosteal elevator the ECR is moved medially to expose the cranial surface of the radius (d). The cranial surface of the radius can be easily exposed further proximally by bluntly separating the ECR from the APL and the EDC.

important, with the paw and tarsus wrapped in a sterile drape. A video demonstration of free draping a limb can be viewed at www.focusandflourish.com.

25.3.2 The Surgical Approach

The craniolateral approach to the femur is used (Figure 25.4). The skin is incised just slightly cranial to the femur itself. The tensor fascia lata is then incised just cranial to the biceps femoris muscle. The biceps femoris muscle is retracted caudally and the vastus lateralis cranially. It may be necessary to elevate portions of the adductor muscle from the caudal surface of the femur. As much soft tissue attachment should be maintained on the bone as possible to preserve the blood supply to the fragments. The dissection should be focused at the level of the fracture and then extended proximally and distally until a sufficient amount of bone is exposed to allow for proper positioning of the implants.

Closure begins by re-apposing the tensor fascia lata (TFL) to the edge of the biceps femoris muscle. This is followed by subcutaneous tissues and then skin.

25.4 Approach to the Tibial Diaphysis

The medial approach to the tibial diaphysis is by far the simplest approach as there are no muscles or tendons to be moved. However, the degree of swelling of the

connective tissues overlying bone can be remarkable, making the bone appear deeper than it really is. The saphenous vein does cross the mid-diaphysis and should be preserved.

25.4.1 Patient Position

Place the patient in lateral recumbency with the affected limb down. The contralateral limb is comfortably secured in an abducted position with tape or ties. Free draping of the limb is important, with the paw wrapped in a sterile drape (Figure 25.5). The sterile foot wrap should be secured in place with a towel clamp as it can easily become inadvertently removed during the surgery.

25.4.2 The Surgical Approach

A skin incision is made on the medial aspect of the tibia, with the incision centered over the fracture. The bone is located directly under the skin and swollen subcutaneous tissues. Care is taken to preserve the cranial branch of the medial saphenous vein (Figure 25.6). This is a more difficult bone to "toggle" into place because of the fibula, but it can readily be distracted into reduction and maintained in place with bone holding forceps.

To close, the subcutaneous and skin layers are sutured.

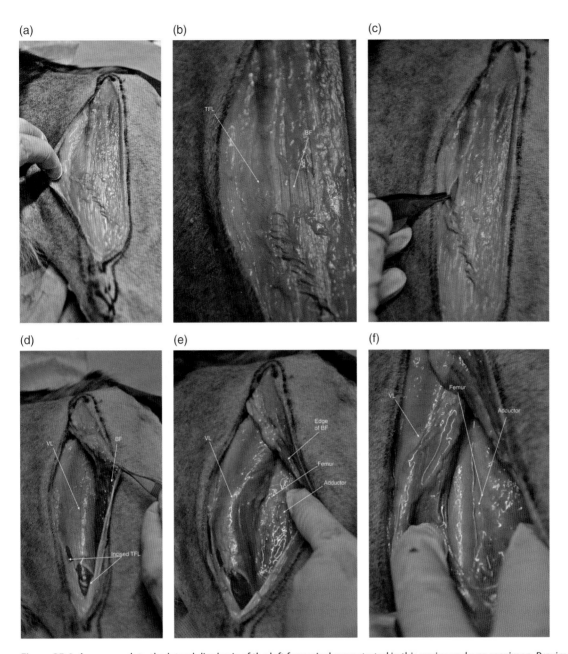

Figure 25.4 An approach to the lateral diaphysis of the left femur is demonstrated in this canine cadaver specimen. Proximal is at the top of the pictures. The patient is positioned in lateral recumbency with the affected limb up. The skin is incised slightly cranial to the femur (a). The subcutaneous connective tissues are incised along the same plane until the biceps femoris muscle (BF) and tensor fascia lata (TFL) can be identified (b). An incision is made in the TFL (c), just cranial to the BF muscle. The incision is then extended proximally and distally using Mayo scissors, exposing the underlying vastus lateralis (VL) muscle (d). The BF is retracted caudally and the VL is retracted cranially, exposing the femur (e) and the adductor muscle. The connective tissues overlying the bone have been cleared making the femur clearly visible (f).

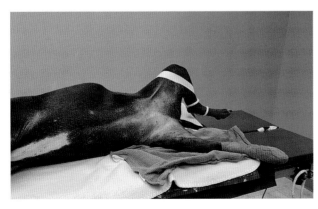

Figure 25.5 The patient is positioned in lateral recumbency with the affected limb down and the upper limb pulled out of the way.

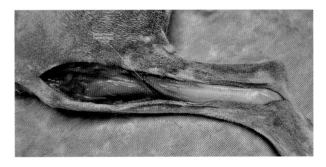

Figure 25.6 An approach to the medial tibia diaphysis of the right tibia is demonstrated in this canine cadaver specimen. Proximal is at the top of the pictures.

Reference

1 Johnson, K.A. (2014). *Piermattei's Atlas of Surgical Approaches to the Bones and Joints of the Dog and Cat*, 5e. Philadelphia, PA: Elsevier.

26

Implants

Harold Wotton

Everost, Inc., Sturbridge, MA, USA

26.1 Maneuvering Orthopedic Implants

Imagine if your patient could tell you exactly how they feel! Imagine if your patient would follow all your post-surgical instructions! Imagine if your patient could use things like crutches or slings. Unfortunately, in veterinary surgery (specifically orthopedic surgery) all we can do is imagine. Your patients need orthopedic implants that have been designed to support immediate loading and cycling of the injured limb.

Over the past 20 years, there have been more orthopedic companies entering the animal health care market than any other type of company. Maneuvering through the increasing number of products provided by these companies and feeling confident that the implants being purchased will perform as expected is becoming very difficult.

Veterinary implant companies are *not* regulated by any outside body to ensure their quality and test methods. Therefore, the burden is on the practice/surgeon to understand what makes a quality implant and where they can be purchased.

There are a few basic things one must understand to make sound decisions on where to purchase orthopedic implants and the good news is there are really only four groups of companies out there.

I) *Human orthopedic companies*: These companies started by providing implants on the human side and entered into the veterinary market. There are only a few of these in the animal health market and they are unable to stray far from the standards set up by governing bodies on the human side. One can always feel comfortable that these are high-quality implants, but they are expensive. Also many of the implants they provide were designed for humans and not for animals.

II) *Veterinary orthopedic implant companies that design and manufacturer their own implants*: This group of companies is small and most often the best option for one's orthopedic needs. They tend to be companies that control their manufacturing process from start to finish. Starting with an engineered drawing, which they own, and finishing with parts manufactured either in their own facility or by a certified manufacturing facility (US Food and Drug Administration (FDA), International Organization for Standardization (ISO), or Conformité Européenne (CE)), which are completely traceable. They provide material certifications and quality documentation upon request, and support any issues there may be with the implants. This is also the group of companies that tends to innovate the most.

III) *Wholesalers of veterinary orthopedic implants*: The number of these companies is the largest among all groups. This type of company simply orders in their implants and sells them most often at the cheapest price with no added value other than price. Their implants are not traceable (lot tracked) and they will not offer any material certifications or quality documents, normally because it is out of their control. Of all the company groups this group comes with the most risk purely due to the unknowns of their material selection, manufacturing methods, and locations, and the lack of quality control.

IV) *Veterinary distributors/wholesalers*: These companies are the companies veterinarians buy most of their non-surgical goods from. The distribution model is to offer products that the customer needs. If a veterinary distributor is offering orthopedic implants, the odds are that they are buying them from one of the types of companies listed above, with the exception of the human orthopedic companies (they do not sell through distribution). Distribution is usually one of the best options for the veterinary clinic because it offers the "one stop shop" benefit and usually comes with free shipping.

The orthopedic implants, for the most part, will be responsible for the outcome of the surgery and healing process. With so many other areas to save on in an orthopedic procedure (white goods, drugs, etc.) the last place to look for the most inexpensive option is the implants. The orthopedic implants are one's signature on the surgery.

26.2 Quality Implants: Essential Information on Quality Implants

A veterinary surgeon's patient is one of the most challenging patients of all. In comparing them to human patients there are several challenging factors for the surgeon, the implant designer, and the owner of the pet.

It starts with the designer. In designing veterinary implants for veterinary surgery, unlike human implant designers, the designer/engineer needs to create a product that can withstand immediate weight bearing, cyclic loading, and still be able to maintain a stable fracture environment. In contrast, on the human side, the patients use braces, crutches, wheelchairs, buggies, and many other tools so not to load the fracture or the implant.

It is important for a veterinary surgeon to truly understand what a quality implant entails. Unfortunately, in the veterinary market there is no regulatory body that oversees implant design or implant production. In the human market the FDA regulates and verifies every aspect of an implant before it can be offered to market. Therefore, the burden of deciding if an implant is truly a quality implant rests with the veterinary surgeon.

In today's market there are large numbers of suppliers of veterinary implants and as a veterinarian this can be very challenging to maneuver. Therefore, a basic knowledge of quality implants would be useful when attempting to make the right choice.

A quality implant requires a comprehensive design process and a quality management system! The comprehensive design process is a very detailed process during which an implant goes from a dream to reality. In summary, there are some essential components of the implant that the end user needs to be comfortable with. *A quality implant needs to be produced from certified implant materials supplied from one of the few FDA-certified mills of implant materials.* Every lot of certified materials is supplied with a certification sheet that should be available to the end user. The implant supplier should be the implant designer to ensure an established design system is in place. The design system

will verify and validate each step of the product design. Part of the design process should be both destructive and non-destructive testing to ensure product performance. During production there needs to be an in-process quality system that will ensure only implants that meet product specifications move onto the next step in the process. The implant supplier needs to have a registered quality system, like ISO. A registered quality system holds the implant provider accountable for all the essential steps of the design and production process. A registered system will need to be audited by a third party to validate the system. Any implant that is placed into the body needs to be marked with both the company logo and the lot number. This is absolutely essential for the traceability of the implant, especially if the implant fails or causes issues with the patient.

Veterinary health implant companies are not required to follow any of these standards and only a few companies in veterinary health do follow such standards. When evaluating an implant provider, one should be sure to ask the appropriate questions to gain a comfort level with the quality of the implant.

Example questions to ask a potential supplier:

1) Do they design their own products?
2) Do they manufacture their products?
3) Are the products manufactured to any FDA, ISO, or American Society for Testing and Materials (ASTM) standards?
4) Are their manufacturers FDA or CE registered?
5) What country are their products manufactured in?
6) Do they perform any testing on their products?
7) Do they use certified medical implant materials?
8) Can they supply the material certifications?
9) Are their products traceable in case of a failure?
10) How do they handle an implant failure?

26.3 Titanium vs Stainless Steel

Which to use and why they cannot be mixed…

The major factor regarding whether mixed metals such as titanium and stainless steel can create clinical problems is related to a corrosion property known as galvanic corrosion. Galvanic corrosion is an accelerated form of corrosion that may occur when two dissimilar metals are coupled in the body. Each metal has a distinct corrosion potential in electrochemically conductive fluids, which are ever-present in the body. These dissimilar metals behave like the positive and negative terminals of a battery and corrosion currents may be generated.

The metal ions released from corrosion reactions can cause inflammatory responses, metal sensitivity reactions, and/or long-term detrimental systematic effects.

In addition, the corrosion process can reduce the mechanical strength of the implants.

The use of mixed metals in the same bone is not a problem as long as the implants are not in direct contact with each other. For example, the use of a stainless steel plate for a distal fracture and titanium plate for a proximal fracture on the same femur is acceptable so long as the implants are not in physical contact with each other.

Implants made from titanium have been successfully used in clinical practice, in the human market since 1965. Medical-grade titanium has a documented history of outstanding biocompatibility. Clinic experience demonstrates that tissue adjacent to titanium implants is well vascularized with a reduced tendency toward capsule formation. Studies (with equine) have shown that titanium causes less inflammation inside the body than traditional stainless steel screws. Titanium also has the added benefit of producing less X-ray visuals than stainless steel, which is crucial when reviewing postoperative films.

Medical-grade titanium is produced using advanced processing methods that significantly increase the strength of the material. Various combinations of strength and ductility are provided to meet the demands of each specific implant application. All medical-grade titanium implants have a special anodized surface finish that increases the thickness of the protective oxide film. The surface finish treatment creates a unique appearance that is a distinguishable feature of many titanium implants.

Improved biocompatibility, proven functional performance, and excellent corrosion resistance are important advantages of medical-grade titanium implants. Additional clinical benefits include the absence of metal allergy reactions, permanent implantation options, and preservation of the biological environment.

Index

Note: Page references in *italics* refer to Figures; those in **bold** refer to Tables.

Fracture Management for the Small Animal Practitioner, First Edition. Edited by Anne M. Sylvestre.
© 2019 John Wiley & Sons, Inc. Published 2019 by John Wiley & Sons, Inc.